PERSPECTIVES
HUMAN
OCCUPATION
Participation in Life

Editor: Timothy L. Julet
Managing Editor: Linda S. Napora
Marketing Manager: Aimee Sirmon
Project Editor: Paula C. Williams
Designer: Risa Clow
Compositor: LWW In-house Compositor
Printer: Maple

Library of Congress Cataloging-in-Publication Data
Perspectives on human occupation : participation in life / [edited by] Paula Kramer, Jim Hinojosa, Charlotte B. Royeen.
    p. ; cm
Includes bibliographical references and index.
ISBN 0-7817-3161-5
    1. Occupational therapy. I. Kramer, Paula. II. Hinojosa, Jim. III. Royeen, Charlotte Brasic.
    [DNLM: 1. Occupational Health. 2. Occupational Therapy. WA 400 P467 2003]
RM735 .P38 2003
615.8′515--dc21

                                                                    2002040593

                                                                            12
                                                                    8 9 10

PERSPECTIVES IN
HUMAN
OCCUPATION
Participation in Life

EDITORS

Paula Kramer, PhD, OTR, FAOTA
Professor and Chair
Department of Occupational Therapy
College of Health Sciences
University of the Sciences in Philadelphia
Philadelphia, Pennsylvania

Jim Hinojosa, PhD, OT, FAOTA
Professor and Chair
Department of Occupational Therapy
The Steinhardt School of Education
New York University
New York, New York

Charlotte Brasic Royeen, PhD, OTR, FAOTA
Associate Dean for Research
School of Pharmacy and Allied Health
Creighton University
Omaha, Nebraska

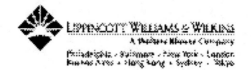

LIPPINCOTT WILLIAMS & WILKINS
A Wolters Kluwer Company
Philadelphia · Baltimore · New York · London
Buenos Aires · Hong Kong · Sydney · Tokyo

*To the founders of the profession —
their commitment to occupation
fostered the development of Occupational Therapy*

and

*To the people in our lives who have enhanced our
thoughts about activities and occupation*

Foreword

The Foreword is "usually written by a person who is prominent in the book's field." The field for this book is clearly the study of occupation and occupational therapy. I am not an occupational therapist, but rather a psychologist who spent 25 years in practice before joining public health. Imagine my surprise at being invited to overview this new product. After reading the chapters of the book, however, I know that in my heart I could have been an OT. The volume is full of well-written and, on the whole, plain language descriptions of the rich historical foundations and philosophical underpinnings of the profession. As a non-occupational therapist, I find many common concepts and yet can clearly see the unique contribution made by the pioneers and current professionals in occupation. The professional perspective provided by this volume should please current writers and doers in occupational theory, practice, and science, as well as students.

This text highlights important aspects of the field. Several chapters point to the multidisciplinary nature of the founders of occupational therapy. The integration of professionals from different backgrounds (medicine, psychology, social work, etc.) struggling and finding common ground from which to help people reach their potential should be a source of pride for the field. This cross-fertilization from the beginning has required the field to be open to new ideas. Although this may have left the emerging field open to second-guessing or wandering from its foundations, this core of conceptual openness is clearly depicted and should be a source of pride.

A second highlight is one rarely found in professional texts. Throughout the chapters there is credit given to academic departments of the authors. What a unique idea—to acknowledge the contributions of one's peers to the advancement of the field. This suggests a level of collegial interaction and collaboration not often observed, much less reported, in university departments. Not coincidental is the revisiting of the importance of trust and relationship as core constructs to the therapeutic interaction. This person/client-centered perspective pervades the volume. Explicitly acknowledging the power of the individual and highlighting trust as central to the therapeutic relationship are affirmed as essential elements of the profession.

A third observation is how relevant the writings from founders continue to be after close to a century has elapsed. The credibility inherent in such longevity of ideas should be a source of strength for the field and vision for students. Probably the most important and revolutionary notion espoused is the powerful impact of the environment. The importance of context as a concept has grounded the profession. Several chapters also allude to the seductions to dissociate individuals from their environment. Reimbursement policies focusing on services to improve the function of the body system with little attention to the environmental factors challenged the underpinnings of the profession for a time. This volume, however, re-energizes the conversation surrounding the core tenets of the field, and looks to the future.

The World Health Assembly approved a new classification to complement the established classification of the etiology of disease in 2001. The new *International Classification of Functioning, Disability, and Health* provides the conceptual framework, a classification system, and a coding scheme that will be the basis for science, program, and policy in the coming generation. Two major tenets of the new system are that the environment and contextual factors play a crucial role in human function generally and in disability specifically. Second, the outcomes for all people are framed as societal participation. These two components of the new *ICF* have been the essence of occupation and occupational therapy since their inception: (a) participation and (b) society. This framework allows occupation and occupational therapy to take a leadership role as the field of health and disability move beyond body function to embrace the assessment of classification of health status. The coding system will allow both positive and negative elements of the environment to be included for research, policy development, and program implementation. Evaluation of activity limitations can now be balanced between domains of the individuals and their environment. New assessment tools and procedures will grow from this model and occupational therapists will be in the forefront. This text provides the foundation from the past and reaches to the future.

DONALD J. LOLLAR, ED.D.
Associate Director, Disability and Health
National Center on Birth Defects and
Developmental Disabilities
Center for Disease Control
Atlanta, Georgia

Preface

"There are three sides to every story: yours . . . mine . . . and the truth. No one is lying."
— Robert Evans, 1994

We read this quote just when we were completing this book and it struck a chord in us. Robert Evans, the famous movie producer of "Chinatown," "The Godfather," and many more films, wrote it in his autobiography, as he remembered the events of his life. The same can be said about the major construct of this book. There are many sides to human occupation and no one sees them quite the same way. This book is all about perspectives, just as the quote above relates to perspectives. Each chapter in this book presents another view of human occupation. They are quite different, some easy to read, some much more complex, but all enlightening and all meant to deepen your understanding of this very complex construct. There is no one truth about human occupation, except that it enriches our lives.

The original idea for this book started with the increased focus on occupation in the 1998 *Standards for an Accredited Educational Program for the Occupational Therapist* (ACOTE, 1998a) and the *Standards for an Accredited Educational Program for the Occupational Therapy Assistant* (ACOTE, 1998b). But it soon became much more, exploring the various theoretical approaches to occupation, looking at how occupation related to the World Health Organization's *International Classification of Functioning, Disability and Health* (WHO, 2001), seeing how this fits with the *Occupational Therapy Practice Framework* (AOTA, January 2002), and, most of all, trying to understand the enormous complexities of this subject.

The book is organized in three sections. All of the chapters have Objectives to focus the reader and Study Questions at the end to test your understanding of the information presented. Section I covers the core concept of occupation. Chapter 1 defines and clarifies the terminology of occupation and how it used today. It focuses occupation as the core concept of the profession of occupational therapy. This chapter highlights the need for occupational therapists to keep the individual's occupations in the forefront of their thoughts throughout the intervention process. Chapter 2 views the profession's use of the term occupation historically. It also delves into ways that this construct has been used in practice, and it presents human occupation in a broader context. The last chapter of this section explores the philosophical basis of occupation and the different ways it has developed in our profession and practice.

The heart of the book is Section II, which presents various perspectives of human occupation. The authors of these chapters are true scholars who have been instrumental in the development of each perspective. Some of the chapters are easier to read and understand than others; however, all are important. You may have to read some chapters several times in order to grasp what the author(s) are trying to impart. You may not agree with all of them, but they will raise questions for you and expand your thinking on the topic. There have been whole books written about some of these perspectives; for others, this chapter may be the most comprehensive information on the perspective. The Objectives at the beginning of the chapters and the Study Questions at the end will help you clarify your understanding of the material.

Section III presents issues of human occupation related to practice. It covers the client-centered approach, the influence of occupation on evaluation and treatment, the ethical issues of human occupation, and a summary focusing on current and future issues.

As editors and educators, our hope is that this book will promote your independent thinking on human occupation. It should challenge you and stretch your thinking. This book is just a start. As a profession, we still have miles to go in both theory development and research about human occupation. And just maybe this will stimulate your thinking to help move both the construct and our profession forward.

PAULA KRAMER
JIM HINOJOSA
CHARLOTTE BRASIC ROYEEN

References

Accreditation Council for Occupational Therapy Education (1998a). *Standards for an Accredited Educational Program for the Occupational Therapist*. Bethesda, MD: American Occupational Therapy Association.

Accreditation Council for Occupational Therapy Education (1998b). *Standards for an Accredited Educational Program for the Occupational Therapy Assistant*. Bethesda, MD: American Occupational Therapy Association.

American Occupational Therapy Association. (2002, January). Occupational therapy practice framework: Domain and Process (Draft XVIII.). Bethesda, MD: author.

Evans, R. (2002). *The kid stays in the picture*. Beverly Hills, CA: New Millenium Press.

World Health Organization. (2001). *ICF: International Classification of Functioning, Disability and Health*. Geneva, Switzerland: World Health Organization.

Acknowledgments

The editors sincerely thank all the contributing authors who graciously shared their ideas about occupation in this comprehensive text. We know that writing these chapters required a great deal of thought, time and effort and so a very special thank you to each contributing authors' spouses, significant others, families, and friends who supported them during this effort. The many people who reviewed chapters of this text are also acknowledged for the time they gave willingly to make certain this was a quality book. Your opinions are very important to us!

Aimee Luebben made important, significant contributions to the completion of this text. She helped us with all the chapter objectives, read through chapters for clarity and had numerous discussions with us that helped us clarify our thoughts and make this a successful book. We are indebted to her for her support and outstanding assistance. And of course, as always, we are all very grateful to our families and significant others who graciously put up with us during this project, and still continue to love and support us.

Certain people and experiences stand out as particularly significant in developing our thoughts and ideas about human occupation.

Paula would like to recognize Stephen Heater and the member of the Accreditation Council for Occupational Therapy Education as moving her ideas about occupation into another realm.

Paula, Jim and Charlotte would like to thank their colleagues at University of the Sciences in Philadelphia, New York University and Creighton University, respectively.

Last, but certainly not least, are our friends at Lippincott Williams & Wilkins. We started this project with Margaret Biblis, who encouraged us to think broadly; Tim Julet challenged us, supported us and always came up with wonderful, interesting ideas; Linda Napora was a constant source of assistance through the ups and downs of the editorial process; and Paula Williams guided the stages of production from manuscript to published book. Thanks to all of you.

Reviewers

Contributors

Sue E. Baptiste, MHSc, OT (Reg)
Associate Professor
Assistant Dean, Occupational Therapy
School of Rehabilitation Sciences
McMaster University
Hamilton, Ontario, Canada

Catana Brown, PhD, OTR, FAOTA
Associate Professor
Department of Occupational Therapy
  Education
University of Kansas Medical Center
Kansas City, Kansas

Janice Posatery Burke, Ph.D.,
OTR/L, FAOTA
Chairman and Associate Professor
Department of Occupational Therapy
College of Health Professions
Thomas Jefferson University
Philadelphia, Pennsylvania

Winnie Dunn, Ph.D., OTR, FAOTA
Professor and Chair
Department of Occupational Therapy
  Education
University of Kansas Medical Center
Kansas City, Kansas

Kirsty Forsyth, Ph.D., OTR, SROT
Lecturer
Department of Occupational Therapy
Queen Margaret University College
Edinburgh, Scotland, United Kingdom
and
Post Doctoral Fellow
Department of Occupational Therapy
College of Applied Health Sciences
University of Illinois at Chicago
Chicago, Illinois
and
Director
UK MOHO Centre for Research and
  Education
University of London
London, England, United Kingdom

Jim Hinojosa, PhD, OT, FAOTA
Professor and Chair
Department of Occupational Therapy
The Steinhardt School of Education
New York University
New York, New York

Roger I. Ideishi, JD, OTR/L
Vice Chair and Assistant Professor
Department of Occupational Therapy
College of Health Sciences
University of the Sciences in Philadelphia
Philadelphia, Pennsylvania

Gary Kielhofner, DrPH, OTR, FAOTA
Wade/Myer Chair, Professor and Head
Department of Occupational Therapy
College of Applied Health Sciences
University of Illinois at Chicago
Chicago, Illinois
and
Foreign Adjunct Professor
Division of Occupational Therapy
Karolinska, Institutet
Stockholm, Sweden
and
Visiting Professor
School of Occupational Therapy
University of London
London, England, United Kingdom

Paula Kramer, PhD, OTR, FAOTA
Professor and Chair
Department of Occupational Therapy
College of Health Sciences
University of the Sciences in Philadelphia
Philadelphia, Pennsylvania

Aimee J. Luebben, Ed.D, OTR, FAOTA
Occupational Therapy Program
University of Southern Indiana
Evansville, Indiana

David L. Nelson, Ph.D., OTR
Professor of Occupational Therapy
Department of Occupational Therapy
School of Allied Health
Medical College of Ohio at Toledo
Toledo, Ohio

Charlotte Brasic Royeen, PhD, OTR,
FAOTA
Associate Dean for Research
School of Pharmacy and Allied Health
Creighton University
Omaha, Nebraska

Janette K. Schkade, Ph.D., OTR, FAOTA
Professor Emeritus
School of Occupational Therapy
Texas Women's University
Denton, Texas

Sally Schultz, Ph.D., OTR
Professor and Interim Dean
School of Occupational Therapy
Texas Women's University
Denton, Texas

Kathleen Barker Schwartz, Ed.D, OTR,
FAOTA
Professor
Department of Occupational Therapy
San Jose State University
San Jose, California

Julie Jepson-Thomas, PhD, OTR/L, FAOTA
Professor and Chair
Department of Occupational Therapy
School of Allied Health
Medical College of Ohio at Toledo
Toledo, Ohio

Ann A. Wilcock, DipCOT, BappScOT, Grad-
DipPublicHealth, PhD
Professor of Occupational Therapy
Deakin University
Victoria, Australia
and
Visiting Professor of Occupational
Therapy
Brunel University
London, England, United Kingdom

Mary Jane Youngstrom, MS, OTR, FAOTA
Clinical Instructor
Department of Occupational Therapy
Education
University of Kansas Medical Center
Kansas City, Kansas

Contents

1

Core Concept of Occupation

Jim Hinojosa, Paula Kramer, Charlotte Brasic Royeen, and Aimee J. Luebben

OBJECTIVES

This chapter will help you to:

- Differentiate between occupation as means and occupation as ends.
- Discuss the evolutionary and recent revolutionary philosophical bases of the term occupation.
- Reflect on your own use of language, perspectives of human occupation, and ideas of occupational therapy.
- Discover the ultimate goal of occupational therapy.
- Consider the future challenges to occupation and occupational therapy.

Every day we engage in many routine tasks. Some are important to us and others are just things that we do. Think for a moment about the things you do each day. Brushing your teeth, washing up, getting dressed; the list is endless. Now think about the things that are very important to you. Kissing a loved one good morning, making dinner, working on a project that you enjoy, tucking a child in at night; again, the list can be long. These are the things that make your life meaningful. Being able to engage in the daily tasks of life, those that are mundane and those that are of utmost importance, is the critical focus of occupational therapy. These daily patterns of our lives — which are meaningful to us — make us who we are. These are our occupations.

Core to the profession of occupational therapy is the concept of occupation. Occupation is composed of the daily tasks and purposeful activities in which we engage coupled with the meaning or personal, subjective value these tasks and activities provide. Our occupations are formed by our cultural background; our interests and aspects of life that are meaningful to us as individuals form our occupations. Occupations have some measure of personal satisfaction. They are self-directed, personally initiated, goal-directed, and organized (Clark et al., 1991; Kramer & Hinojosa, 1995; Krishnagiri, 2000; Yerxa, 1998). Yerxa (1998) states that occupation should be the central idea to a curriculum designed for the future, as occupation is what differentiates us from all other professions.

Traditionally, occupational therapy practitioners have used occupation as a means as well as an end. Occupations are used in our daily interventions with clients (occupation as a means during intervention), yet our goal is to have the client continually engage in the occupations of his or her choice (occupation as an end of intervention). This use of the same terminology in two distinctly different ways is confusing to many individuals. In essence, we are using the term to mean both the process of our interventions and the product or end goal of our interventions.

Occupation as a means is when a specific occupation, determined by the client's choice or interests, is used as a means in therapy to bring about change in a person's performance. The success of occupation as a means is entirely dependent on the meaningfulness or subjective value of the occupation to the individual (Primeau & Ferguson, 1999). The fit between the person and the occupation is most important when occupation is used as a means. Trombly (1995) notes that when occupation is used as a means, it is equivalent to purposeful activity.

Occupation as an end is the goal or the product of intervention. Used in this manner occupation allows the person to participate in meaningful experiences within the context of his or her life. Occupation as end is the performance of activities or tasks that the person deems as important to life, derived from the person's values, experiences and culture (Trombly, 1995).

This book presents various perspectives on occupation that exist in our profession today. It is important to note that there is no one definition or perspective that is recognized by the whole profession. Occupation is an evolving construct that is generally illustrated within the context that it is used.

This chapter defines and clarifies how occupation is used today by occupational therapy practitioners, drawing from official American Occupational Therapy Association (AOTA) documents and current scholarly papers. Beginning with the philosophical basis of the profession, occupation is introduced as a core concept of the profession. Because occupation, and the relative importance of occupation, have changed over time to the profession and for society, this chapter highlights how occupational therapy practitioners need to keep the individual's occupations in the forefront of their thoughts throughout the intervention process. The discussion includes the importance of occupation to the profession, to society, and to education. The importance of occupation will also be related to the *ICF: International Classification of Functioning, Disability and Health* (World Health Organization [WHO], 2001) at the end of this chapter.

PHILOSOPHICAL BASE

Purposeful activity has been identified as a key concept of the profession in the *Philosophical Base of Occupational Therapy* (AOTA, 1979a, Resolution 531-79). In this particular statement occupation was used synonymously with purposeful activity. "Purposeful activity facilitates the adaptive process" (AOTA, 1979a, p. 785), resulting in positive changes in function. Although there has been a scholarly discussion on the relationship between purposeful activities and occupation, this statement continues to be the official philosophical base of the profession. Immediately after, the AOTA adopted, as official association policy per AOTA's Representative Assembly Resolution 532-79 (AOTA, 1979b), occupation as the common core of occupational therapy. Additionally, the Articles of Incorporation of the American Occupational Therapy Association were amended in January 1976, to include the concept of occupation within the third article. Thus, despite recent scholarly discourse on just what constitutes occupation, the concept as the core of the profession has been official policy for more than 25 years.

A profession's philosophical statement outlines the basic belief system of the profession. It is a description of what the profession values and believes to be important. The philosophy of a profession is constantly evolving. A profession's philosophy is dynamic and not static. Yet, key elements within the philosophy of a profession will always remain, like the importance of the individual and his or her right to human dignity. Aspects of our basic philosophy will be the same, regardless of the occupational therapy practitioner's specific interventions, frame of reference, or model of practice.

All professions are built on a philosophical foundation. Philosophy is one of the bases for what is taught in entry-level education. The accreditation process for occupational therapy and occupational therapy assistant education recognizes the importance of the profession's philosophical base. The *Standards for an Accredited Educational Program for the Occupational Therapist* (Accreditation Council for Occupational Therapy [ACOTE®], 1998a) and *Standards for an Accredited Educational Program for the Occupational Therapy Assistant* (ACOTE®, 1998b) (both documents are commonly referred to collectively as the *Standards*), as well as a previous document, *Essentials and Guidelines for an Accredited Educational Program for the Occupational Therapist* (AOTA, 1991a) and *Essentials and Guidelines for an Accredited Educational Program for the Occupational Therapy Assistant* (AOTA, 1991b) (these documents are currently referred to as the *Essentials*), require a statement of the profession's philosophy and an integration of that philosophy with the curriculum design. Further, the *Standards* (ACOTE®, 1998a, 1998b) require programs to articulate their views of humanity and the teaching-learning process. These philosophical statements guide the educational program so that the student will be taught or will learn models of practice, frames of reference, and intervention within this context. It is also critical that students keep this philosophy in mind when approaching and intervening with clients.

Re-emergence of Occupation As a Key Construct

Although the occupational therapy philosophical statement of 1979 uses purposeful activities and occupation synonymously, the term *occupation* has had different meanings to the profession over time. Our founders used the word *occupation* to define the profession. This term was often used in the context of occupying one's time purposefully. Later, the term occupation became synonymous with purposeful activities, and then virtually disappeared from our terminology. From the 1960s through the 1980s, there was some discussion about changing the name of the profession to avoid use of the term occupation and to have a title that better described our interactions (at that time) with clients. Then gradually, the term occupation became more prevalent. Scholars such as Reilly (1962), Kielhofner (1983, 1995, 1997), Yerxa (1967, 1998), Nelson (1988), and Clark (1993) emphasized the importance of occupation to what we do within the profession. Practitioners began to endorse the use of this term. Simultaneously, this emerging emphasis on occupation influenced the educational process. The education process as reflected in the *Essentials* (AOTA, 1991a, 1991b) does not even use the term occupation, whereas the more recent 1998 *Standards* (ACOTE®, 1998a, 1998b) use this term generously and make some distinctions between occupation and purposeful activities.

In the 1990s, the profession recognized the need to clarify its terminology, and the AOTA adopted several official documents on purposeful activities (Hinojosa, Sabari, & Pedretti, 1993), function (Baum & Edwards, 1995), and occupation (Christiansen, Clark, Kielhofner, Rogers, & Nelson, 1995). A statement on the relationship between these three concepts was written, proposing a taxonomy in which occupation was the broadest concept with purposeful activities being an essential aspect of occupation (Hinojosa & Kramer, 1997). The proposed definitions of occupation and purposeful activities were put forth as follows:

> *"Occupations are the ordinary and familiar things that people do every day"* *(Christiansen, et al., 1995, p. 1015). Occupations are the activities people engage in throughout their daily lives to fulfill their time and give life meaning.*

Occupations involve mental abilities and skills, and may or may not have an observable physical dimension. Occupations always have some degree of personal meaning having contextual, temporal, psychological, social, symbolic, cultural, ethnic, and/or spiritual dimensions. Occupations reflect the unique characteristics of the person. A person is defined, to some extent, by the occupations in which he or she engages. A person's preferred occupations may change over time, depending on differing factors or circumstances in his or her life. An understanding of occupations is still evolving, and there is a need for more research on the relationship between occupations and a person's health and well being (Hinojosa & Kramer, 1997, p. 865).

"Purposeful activity refers to goal-directed behaviors or tasks . . . that the individual considers meaningful" (Hinojosa et al., 1993, p. 1081). People continually engage in purposeful activities as a part of their occupations. Purposeful activities have personal meaning combined with a goal-directed quality and are encompassed within occupations. Within this view, goal-directed does not necessarily imply a physical product or an outcome, but does involve active engagement that meets personal goals or needs. Therapeutically, purposeful activities are used to evaluate, facilitate, restore, or maintain an individual's abilities to meet demands in his or her life; in other words, to engage in occupations (Hinojosa & Kramer, 1997, p. 865).

OCCUPATION AS PROCESS AND PRODUCT

Occupation includes a wide variety of life tasks, such as self-care, leisure, work, and contributing to society (Christiansen, 1999; Law, 1998). A person's occupations develop and change over time. One of the key challenges facing occupational therapy is the profession's own use of the term occupation. That is, the term *occupation* as currently used within the field indicates both a process (means) or active doing, and a product (ends) or that which is done (Christiansen & Baum, 1997; Gray, 1998). Using occupation in this dual manner results in an ambiguous term, which can be confusing to practitioners, other professionals, and the general public. To clarify what is meant by occupational therapy in the public eye, a call to use the term *occupation* as a process and the term *activity* as the outcome when communicating with other professionals and the general public has been put forth (Royeen, 2000, 2002).

Developmental Nature of Occupation

Occupations are shaped by our personal interests, desires, and values. We engage in things that we want to do or have to do. Most people engage in the same activities — such as eating, dressing, and bathing — but the things that we want to engage in define who we are, differentiating us from one another. The specific occupations that we want to do are the things that make us unique. Additionally, how one carries out an occupation can also be part of what makes us unique. Descartes' phrase, "I think, therefore I am" can be updated to reflect an occupational perspective, "I feel, therefore I do." A primary motivator in our impetus to do something in particular is based on our emotions, which are the "fires" and desires that get us "to do," or to engage in occupations.

Beginning with childhood, occupations emerge as the individual develops and progresses (Primeau & Ferguson, 1999; Reilly, 1962; Yerxa et al., 1989). Kielhofner (1997) proposes that participation in occupations enhances child development. Initially, infants are predominantly reflexive beings. However, basic behavioral patterns emerge as infants respond to those in their environment. Patterns typically center on establishing homeostasis through eating and sleeping (Royeen, 1995). Each of these fundamental activities becomes a key element of a child's occupation as he or she develops and matures.

In early childhood, primary occupations consist of eating, sleeping, playing, learning, and participating as a family member. In middle childhood, the occupations continue with an increasing focus on studying and learning, with a healthy dose of play and family life included. In later childhood, the beginning of working and leisure occupations emerge, in addition to the existing occupation of studying. During early adolescence, an increasing participation in leisure occupations and work may emerge. In late adolescence, the occupational concerns center around accepting more responsibility and developing occupational patterns for life through the exploration of future roles. Early adulthood signifies specific decisions about occupational roles. Finding partners, establishing lifestyles, working, and parenting are predominant occupations. Middle adulthood may bring the expansion of the parenting occupation, service to the community, commitment to work, and commitment to family. Maturity typically maintains the occupations of working and engaging in self-rewarding leisure activities. Senior status continues some occupations over time, depending on resources and health, and the loss of other occupations. Throughout the life process, very individualistic patterns of occupations emerge (Kramer & Hinojosa, 1995).

The development of individual patterns of occupation does not take place within a vacuum. Individual occupational pattern development is highly influenced by context. People develop within their culture, locality, spiritual affiliation, and socioeconomic background, to name a few influences. This development influences who they are, what they do, and what occupations are meaningful to them.

The Term Human Occupation — Use of Language

The use of the term *human occupation* is not routine or common lay language. To most people, human occupation means the jobs that they do to earn an income or a living. The public view of occupation does not include the wide range of daily activities. Since the term occupation as we mean it is not common language, it may appear to the public that occupational therapy practitioners have overconceptualized the term to give it special meaning. Once we take a term normally used by most people to mean one thing and use it in an entirely different way, do we create situations in which we are not understood by others? If so, this can create circumstances in which we mean one thing and only a very limited group of people can understand what we are saying. For example, when a physician uses language that we do not understand, do we feel included or inferior? We need to be certain that we are effectively communicating what we mean in a way that it can be understood by others. A good example of this is when Florence Clark, describing her seminal well-elderly study, talked about occupational therapy as engaging in *life style redesign* (Clark, 1997; Mandel, Jackson, Zemke, Nelson, & Clark, 1999). Life style redesign was something that most people could understand. It is critical that we use language that people readily understand, and that we simultaneously educate people about the use of language that describes us clearly. In this way, people can begin to appreciate what occupational therapy really means.

Another perspective is that using the term *human occupation* provides occupational therapy with a persona of a highly sophisticated, science-based profession. This is important. All professions have their own language and terminology that make them unique. As occupational therapy practitioners, we need to consider precise meanings of words and intended audiences as we communicate. To communicate effectively with others, we need to explore our terminology in conjunction with the *ICF* (WHO, 2001), a taxonomy that focuses on the individual's ability to engage in activities and participate in society. The essence of the *ICF* is shown Table 1-1.

As a field, we can choose to better align our use of terminology (occupation as process and activity as outcome) with what will likely become the standard across the world for professionals and for third-party payers, or we can continue to employ the word *occupation* in an ambiguous manner, but one in which we as a field might prefer. Note that *ICF* terminology includes the concept of activities. For this reason, occupational therapy is challenged to clarify how and what occupation is in terms of *ICF* terminology. For example, what do we as occupational therapists mean by *activity*? Is it the same as what is intended by *ICF* use of *activity*? Since the *ICF* has been accepted on a global level, we are challenged to clarify to ourselves and to others how our use of terms is similar and how it is different. Only by providing such clarification can occupational therapy position itself effectively in the public mind.

The way language is used reflects on your personal perspective as an occupational therapy practitioner. In writing this chapter, we struggled with our own comfort with the language. Although we all are committed to the profession's refinement of the construct of human occupation, we each have our own perspective on the use and value of the terminology. An enjoyable part of editing this book has been the opportunity to reflect on our own development, views, and beliefs about occupation and occupational therapy. The following are personal reflections by the authors on some ideas of the profession and perspectives on occupation. In Narrative 1.1, Jim describes his view on the importance of purposeful activities and his journey to acceptance that human occupation is one core construct for the profession. In Narrative 1.2, Paula describes her views, based on a life experience with occupational therapy. In Narrative 1.3., Charlotte describes the importance of occupation throughout her life. Aimee describes how her nontraditional background has affected the way she "listens" to our profession's terminology in Narrative 1.4.

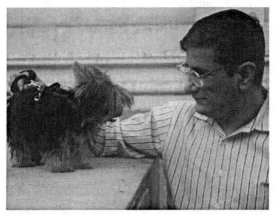

Jim playing with his dog Gizmo.

NARRATIVE 1.1. *Jim*

A Journey of Acceptance of the Term Occupation

When I graduated from the Occupational Therapy Program at Colorado State University in the 1970s, I had no understanding of why the profession was called occupational therapy. I accepted the explanation that the title came from a historical perspective. I really did not question this historical rationale and did not have an invested opinion in debate at the time of whether the profession should change its title to something else. I accepted that as therapists we were concerned with the activities that people engaged in to occupy their lives and give it meaning. As a student, I learned that therapists used activities to

Table 1-1   ESSENCE OF THE ICF: INTERNATIONAL CLASSIFICATION OF FUNCTIONING, DISABILITY, AND HEALTH

Parts	I: Functioning and Disability		II: Contextual Factors	
Components	Activities and Participation	Body Functions and Structures	Environmental Factors	Personal Factors
Domains	Life areas • Tasks • Actions	• Body functions • Body structures	External influences on functioning and disability	Internal influences on functioning and disability
Constructs	• Capacity (executing tasks in a standard environment) • Performance (executing tasks in the current environment)	• Change in body function (physiology) • Change in body structure (anatomic)	Facilitating or hindering impact of features of the physical, social, and attitudinal world	Impact of attributes of the person
Positive aspects	*Functioning*		Facilitators	Not applicable
	• Activities • Participation	• Functional integrity • Structural integrity		
Negative aspects	*Disability*		Barriers	Not applicable
	• Activity limitations • Participation restrictions	• Impairments		

Adapted with permission from World Health Organization. (2001). *ICF: International classification of functioning, disability and health* (p. 11). Geneva, Switzerland: Author.

engage people in meaningful, purposeful activities. I learned that engagement in activities directed the attention to the tasks and that skills would address a person's physical, psychosocial, developmental, or cognitive deficits. As a student I learned a wide range of activities, from self-care to recreation to specific arts and crafts. I particularly enjoyed the learning of various activities and fondly remember cooking class, woodworking lab, weaving lab, and square dance calling. Occupational therapy students were encouraged to broaden their perspectives to include a wide range of activities that we might need to know when dealing with clients in a variety of settings. We learned by doing. I studied anatomy, neuroanatomy, kinesiology, and chemistry, but I loved the arts and crafts classes.

My upbringing and personal background may have influenced this love for crafts. Raised in Colorado, my father was a highly skilled carpenter and my mother always did needle work. My father built our home and my mother decorated it. Family activities included fishing, hiking, and taking family trips. As an occupational therapist, I use purposeful activities as a primary tool and feel that I need to justify them. I am uncomfortable with a current trend in the profession to label everything that we do as occupation. I personally cannot believe that brushing my teeth or being able effectively to use toilet paper in the bathroom is an occupation. I do believe that they are important purposeful activities. I have come to realize that the combination of these two activities is fundamental to be able to complete personal hygiene occupations. Throughout this text, you will read various scholars' perspectives on human occupation and in the end, you must come to your own perspective. I truly believe that one strength of occupational therapy is the diversity of opinions and views. I believe that our discussion of our individual ideas will lead to a greater understanding.

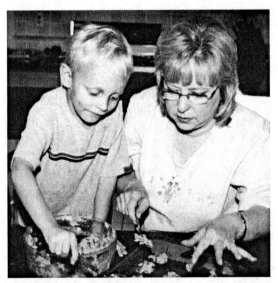

Paula baking cookies with her son Andrew.

NARRATIVE 1.2. *Paula*

A Life Experience of Activities to Occupation

My views of occupational therapy came from a very personal experience. As a pre-adolescent, I had a spinal fusion to correct scoliosis. Back in the 1960s, the procedure required 3 months of hospitalization, lying flat in bed the whole time, and then 8 more months at home in the same position. Quite a bit different than the way such things are handled today. My doctor referred me to occupational therapy to keep me busy, as I recall. I received occupational therapy 5 times per week for 1 hour a day. The therapist spent quite a bit of time asking me about what I liked to do. We spoke about my love of needlework, specifically knitting, crocheting, and needle point, as well as cooking and going shopping with my friends. She showed me how to knit and crochet in bed, how to operate a sewing machine and make clothes, which I had never done before, and even arranged for me to cook lunch for some of my favorite personnel in the hospital. She helped arrange pizza parties with my friends and other social gatherings. Over time the relationship between the therapist and client became quite intense. We shared a lot and gradually I learned that, despite my body brace and surgery and not being able to even sit up, I was still the same person I had always been and I was still capable of doing many things. When I was able to verbalize this to her, she was elated. "You've got it, that's the purpose of all the things we've been doing," she said. This was a great revelation. I understood occupational therapy to mean occupying one's time purposefully and that this purposeful use of time brought skills and personal understanding. I knew that I wanted this to always be a part of my life, and my first occupational therapist remains dear to me to this day.

Occupational therapy education strengthened this belief for me. We never used the word occupation, but the importance of "activities and doing" was always stressed. I learned how much foundational knowledge, in science and psychology, was necessary to truly understand the process of "doing." I found the sciences difficult, the psychology exciting, the personal exploration threatening but growth-inducing, and the crafts fun. However, it all fit with the focus on doing that I had grown up with (i.e., what you did defined who you were, and if you could engage in activities that you enjoyed, you were healthier and whole). My mother was always doing needlework or knitting and was very involved in many volunteer organizations, always telling us that giving our time to things we believed in was important. My father was always organizing playful outings, skating, sledding, planning trips. For me, the current focus on occupation is a way of clarifying who we are to the outside world. Occupation is the larger heading, the umbrella of what we do. Occupations are the broad patterns of our lives. They are categories of meaning in our lives, while purposeful activities are the specific tasks in which we engage that bring our lives meaning and pleasure. I think as occupational therapists, we need to embrace this core concept of occupation to bring clarity and understanding of our profession to the outside world, but not to the exclusion of others. Purposeful activities taught me who I was when I was younger, occupying my time in a meaningful way. Together these activities comprised occupations that shaped me, even though I did not know it.

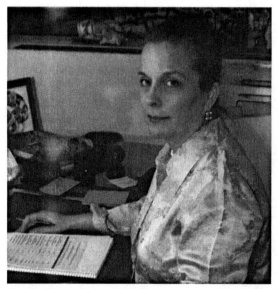

Charlotte working.

Narrative 1.3.*Charlotte*

To Do with Meaning Is To Live

My belief in the power of occupation has always been a guiding force in my life. Early in life, I can clearly recall using purposive activities such as games and songs to make my home more friendly during after school hours when I was the first person home. I can recall building forts behind the television, as well as singing songs to the furniture, in order quell anxiety of being home alone. I also recall my father teaching me how to roller skate, not through words or books, but through the "doing" of it.

Further, I can remember the exhilaration of high school when engagement in multiple occupations ranging from student to actor to artist gave rise to a wonderful sense of well-being. My high school summers were spent as an occupational therapy aide in what at that time was New Jersey Neuropsychiatric Unit in Skillman, New Jersey, wherein I was able to participate in the power of occupation in the rehabilitation of those with chronic mental disease, alcoholism, and drug abuse. The essential link of occupation as a human bond was reinforced from that experience.

These early experiences inevitably led me to the field of occupational therapy, where my entry-level studies focused on traditional crafts, the wonder of neuroscience, a holistic approach to practice, and the application of purposeful activities or occupations for promotion of better living. I recall very deliberately choosing what was considered a "traditional, conservative" school. It appears that, perhaps, it was so traditional that the foundations in occupation and purposeful activities, as originally defined by the profession's founders, were most consistent with my education. Perhaps it was so traditional that it was timeless in the roots of occupational therapy (e.g., occupation).

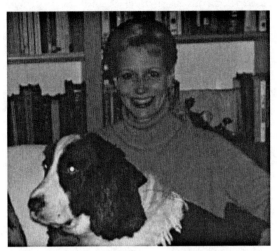

Aimee enjoying quality time with her dog Wellington.

NARRATIVE 1.4. *Aimee*

Occupation, Activity, and Practice: Whispering Words

Words whisper to me. A teacher of classical languages, I have listened to whispering words for more than three decades. Because words speak quietly to me, my reflections on our profession and occupation reflect my educational background. My story is somewhat different. Unlike Paula, Jim, and Charlotte (although they are my contemporaries), I did not discover the phrase *occupational therapy* until I was almost 30, a time in my life when I needed to heal some personal wounds. Knowing that I

heal best by learning new things and realizing the job market for Latin teachers in the mid 1970s was abysmal, I decided to change professions. I wanted to hold on to my first love, Latin, so I identified two broad professional areas: law or medicine. Paging through various job guides, I narrowed my choices to two professional roles: attorney or occupational therapist, the latter a career choice I just happened to stumble across.

I applied to several occupational therapy curricula, choosing one of the earliest educational programs. In school the history of our profession was my favorite part, understandingly because in those days before I became a futuristically thinking occupational therapist, my orientation was to the past (my first degree also included geology). Although my educational program at that time was fairly heavily invested in what I now call "component-land," I bucked the system even then by practicing at the occupation-level because of my passion for what our profession's rich history taught me and the fact that the words *occupation, activity,* and *practice* were telling me how to provide occupational therapy services.

In 1992, when I moved to the University of Southern Indiana to design an occupational therapy curriculum, an educational program designed to be occupation-focused from the beginning, I found a history professor willing to tutor me in classical Greek. From that time, I have listened to words in two languages that are considered dead by many people but are very much alive to me. From an etymological standpoint (I always have to remind a friend that *etymology*-without the letter *n*-is the study of words, not bugs), pairings of the words *occupation, activity,* and *practice* have similar meanings. For example, "doing" is one of many meanings for *ago*, the derivation of activity, and πρασσω (transliterated as *prasso*), the derivation of practice (this same Greek word also gave rise to the words *pragmatic* and *praxis*.) Although classical languages can be translated in many different ways, "keeping busy" or "being engaged" is a shared meaning of *occupo* (*ob*, meaning "over" + *capio*, meaning "experience," "take," "seize"), the derivation of occupation and that same Greek derivation of practice. I have to confess I am also thrilled that the nouns — *occupatio, actio,* and πραξη — are feminine, even though I know these nouns were originally derived from verbs.

I have to say I smile whenever I become aware of the latest salvo in the great terminology debate — occupation versus activity — especially since the dueling camps both emphasize the "doing" aspect of the words. Of these hotly debated words, *activity* is derived from *actus*, the fourth principal part of *agere*, which means "to do" (and also "to perform"). In Latin, the fourth principle part is the masculine subject form of the perfect passive participle. This type of participle is often the ending of a process or the product of a process completed. I also smile when I read the word *engage* used in conjunction with the word *occupation* because of the redundancy of the two words. For example, since *occupatio* can mean "engagement," the phrase *engage in an occupation* becomes for me: *engage in an engagement*.

Interestingly, the Greek and Latin words that can mean "doing" have had sexual connotations at some time in history. In ancient Greece, the word for *practice* (πραξεις, transliterated as *praxis*) was a euphemism for sexual intercourse, and in the 16th and 17th centuries, *occupy* virtually disappeared from use because of the word's sexual meaning. Evidence of this latter change in meaning comes from Shakespeare whose character, Doll Tearsheet, a prostitute at the Boar's Head Tavern, said (primarily to Falstaff), "These villains will make the word as odious as the word *occupy*, which was an excellent good word before it was ill sorted" *2 Henry IV* (Act 2, Scene 4, ll. 138-140). Within this same vein, I also find fascinating the fact that today the word *doing* has a sexual connotation.

Although I listen to words, I tend to use *occupation* and *activity* interchangeably. I do not worry about adding the adjective *purposeful* to activity because those whispering words have linked *purposeful* and *activity* in my brain. Over the years I have changed the way I talk about our profession, moving from using *activity* with a smattering of *occupation* to equal parts of both words and then to a heavy emphasis on *occupation*. When I talk to future occupational therapists who are learning about our profession's uniqueness — occupation — I return to my classical language roots to teach about the PAP, an acronym for present active participle, which is a verb that has ongoing action in the current timeframe and that is not passive. I tell students that when they practice they should listen for people's words that end in -*ing*. By hearing these whispering PAPs, the students are most likely to identify people's occupations. In the next few years, my utilization of the two words is likely to become more balanced again because of the preeminent role *activity* plays in the *ICF* (WHO, 2001). In addition, my teaching students about occupation by focusing on the participle form mirrors the heavy emphasis of the word *participation* in this same global taxonomy. I firmly believe that to remain a viable and even thriving profession, we may need to shout, not whisper, both words: *occupation* to members of our profession and *activity* to people outside occupational therapy.

Learning Activity

Think about your own life and the role activities and occupation play in it. Reflect on a typical day in your life and list those activities. Try to categorize these activities into occupations, based on their meaningfulness and value to you. Think about which were easy to categorize and which were more difficult to categorize. Take some time and reflect on the role of occupations in your life and the relationship of this to your choice of occupational therapy as a profession.

THE INDIVIDUAL'S OCCUPATION AND OCCUPATIONAL THERAPY

To design and develop an intervention that will be meaningful to an individual, the occupational therapy practitioner must spend time talking and/or interacting with the client and learning about who he or she is. We cannot expect to design an intervention that is meaningful to the client if we do not understand that individual. The occupational therapist does not decide what is important, the client identifies what is important to him or her. If the client loves to build models and needs to work on fine motor coordination, then an intervention plan that involves building models or something along those lines would have a greater chance of engaging the client. People tend to respond well to the activities they like to do. If we use something pleasurable for treatment, the intervention may engage clients but also distract them from the difficult task of building or rebuilding skills. Occupational therapy can be a difficult and painful process, but if there is an aspect of enjoyment, the individual is more likely to engage. Think of a diet. Diets are difficult; they are restrictive and take some of the wonderful pleasures out of life. Nevertheless, once you agree that the diet will be helpful (a degree of motivation), you are more likely to at least start the diet. The initial stages can be difficult, but once you begin to see results, you are more likely to continue.

As a client in occupational therapy, Sam was reluctant to get involved in the intervention process. He had peripheral nerve involvement, causing limited sensation in his hands. He had been an engineer and built many complex models. His hobby was building things, from simple to the complex. His disability limited his ability to create the projects he wanted. However, more simple projects seemed beneath him, a constant reminder that he could no longer do the things that he used to do. In this scenario the occupational therapy practitioner has two challenges: to work creatively with Sam on developing new and satisfying occupations that build on his engineering background (e.g., using computer graphics), and to assist him in accepting the limitations his disability has placed on his occupations.

Occupations enrich our lives. By being able to do something that is meaningful, we enhance our daily existence. But this is a very individualized experience. Roller blading may bring excitement to an uneventful day to one person, while being able to sit and talk to a loved one may be pleasurable to another person. We often use the phrase *quality of life* to encompass this concept. Inherently, we have an idea of what that means, how individuals live, the joy they take in specific activities, their ability to engage in life. However, quality of life can mean different things to different people. For some, quality of life is being involved in outdoor sports, for others this phrase means reading to one's children, and to still others, quality of life may mean simply being alive and able to interact in some meaningful way with others. It is critical that the individual be able to define what are his or her significant occupations.

Kielhofner (1997) synthesized the salient features of many scholarly definitions of occupation as follows:
- Comprises work, play/leisure, and daily living activities.
- Arises as a response to and fulfills a specific motive or need.
- Involves doing or performance that calls upon specific capacities.
- Entails completion of a specific form.
- Interrelates with the sociocultural context.
- Provides meaning.
- Interweaves with the developmental process (p. 55).

More recently, Crabtree (1998) has alluded to the cultural and familial relationship of occupation as meaning: "Occupation is intentional human performance organized in number and kind to meet the demands of self maintenance and identity in the family and community" (p. 208). Further, Yerxa (1998) has provided a definition that reflects a conceptualization of occupation consistent with recent work in chaos theory and complexity: "Occupational may be organized into a view of the human as a multileveled, open system acting upon and responding to the environment over a developmental trajectory, from birth to death" (p. 366).

Participation in Meaningful Occupations — The Ultimate Goal

As our profession returns to its roots in embracing occupation, we must be cognizant of the road we have traveled. A variety of areas have become part of our practice over time.

Many models of practice, theories, and frames of reference have emerged. We have moved from a profession that was defined by crafts to one that embraces many different types of interventions. In our movement to embrace occupation, it is critical that we continue to acknowledge all other aspects of our profession. The various frames of reference used in practice with our clients — whether designed for those with psychosocial dysfunction, physical dysfunction, or pediatric disabilities — are significant contributions to our applied body of knowledge. Frames of reference provide important information for intervention and need ongoing development and refinement. The overall concern of occupational therapy is to ensure that an individual can function in society so that he or she can participate in purposeful activities and occupations. It is the unique composition and combinations of purposeful activities that comprise human occupations. In the wide range of therapeutic interventions, the occupational therapy practitioner uses a variety of frames of reference and strategies to assist the client to achieve his or her desired goals. To view our practice only within the context of occupation would be a mistake. Yet, at the same time, all practice should include engagement in meaningful occupation as an ultimate goal. The readers of this text are encouraged to read the work of others who have focused primarily on models of practice and frames of reference (Bruce & Borg, 1993; Kielhofner, 1997, 2002; Kramer & Hinojosa, 1999; Mosey, 1986; Trombly & Radomski, 2002) and purposeful activities (Cynkin, 1979; Cynkin & Robinson, 1990; Fidler, 1996; Fidler & Fidler, 1978; Fidler & Velde, 1999; Hinojosa & Blount, 2000; Mosey, 1986).

The focus of this book is to provide information on the basic tenets of occupation. You will acquire a firm foundation on the emerging perspectives of occupation. This book will give you an understanding of where the profession is today and introduce you to various scholars contributing to the profession's view of occupation. These scholars' unique perspectives will provide you with a foundation for the development of your future practice.

FUTURE CHALLENGES TO OCCUPATIONAL THERAPY

The previous sections of this chapter focused on the past and present in terms of philosophy and underpinnings of occupation and occupational therapy. This section provides a summary view of current and future events that may influence occupational therapy.

Two key changes are influencing how we use the word *occupation* and how we think about practice. The first change is the latest revision of the occupational therapy profession's uniform terminology taxonomy. The second change, as mentioned earlier in this chapter, is the most recent version of the global taxonomy, the *ICF*. Each taxonomy is discussed briefly here.

The first version of our profession's uniform terminology taxonomy document (AOTA, 1979c) was developed in response to federal regulations that required uniform reporting systems for all hospital departments. Although these federal regulations were never implemented, the next version, *Uniform Terminology, 2nd Edition* (AOTA, 1989), was reorganized to (a) emphasize the occupational performance areas and components addressed in direct service delivery and (b) delete the indirect aspect of service delivery and the Product Output Reporting System (which were integral aspects of the original document). *Uniform Terminology, 3rd Edition* (AOTA, 1994), which was expanded to incorporate context as an element of occupational performance, provided a generic outline of the occupational therapy domain of concern and created common terminology for individuals inside and outside the profession. The purpose of the uniform terminology docu-

Table 1-2   COMPARISON OF THREE TAXONOMIES: ICF, UTIII, AND THE FRAMEWORK

	Part I: Functioning and Disability		Part II: Contextual Factors	
ICF	Activities and Participation	Body Functions and Structure	Personal Factors	Environmental Factors
UTIII	*Performance Areas:* Activities of Daily Living; Work and Productive Activities; Play or Leisure Activities; *	*Performance Components:* Sensorimotor; Cognitive; Psychosocial	*	*Performance Contexts:* *; Environment; Temporal Aspects
Framework	**Areas of Occupation:** ADL; IADL; Work; Education; Social Participation; Play; Leisure	**Performance Skills:** Process Skills; Communication/Interaction Skills; Motor Skills	**Client Factors:** Body Functions; Body Structures — **Performance Patterns:** Routines; Habits; Roles	**Activity Demands:** Objects† — **Context:** Physical; Cultural; Social; Spiritual; Temporal; Virtual

*Aspects not addressed in UTIII.

†The aspect, Activity Demands, includes Objects Used and Their Properties, Space Demands, Social Demands, Sequencing and Timing, Required Actions, Required Body Functions, Required and Body Structures.

ICF, *International Classification of Functioning, Disability, and Health* (WHO, 2001); UTIII, *Uniform Terminology for Occupational Therapy, 3rd Edition* (AOTA, 1994); Framework, *Occupational Therapy Practice Framework: Domain and Process* (AOTA, 2002).

ment has changed with each iteration; the most recent revision includes a transformation in name and scope. The *Occupational Therapy Practice Framework: Domain and Process* (adopted by the AOTA Representative Assembly 2002 and called the *Framework*) is the "next evolution in a series of documents that have been developed over the past several decades to provide consistency in the profession's focus and language" (AOTA, 2002,

p. 70). The *Framework* is intended "(a) to describe the domain that centers and grounds the profession's focus and action and (b) to outline the process of occupational therapy evaluation and intervention that is dynamic and linked to the profession's focus on and use of occupation" (p. 1). This new document updates, revises, and incorporates *Uniform Terminology, 3rd Edition's* primary elements (performance areas, components, and contexts), adding and expanding older definitions that now reflect current practice, providing relevant practice examples, and making linkages to *ICF* terminology.

The *ICF* (WHO, 2001) is a conceptual taxonomy with a goal that is similar to that of the occupational therapy profession's uniform terminology taxonomy, but for a much larger audience. Replacing the medical model of disease in WHO's previous international classifications with a social model of health, the *ICF* provides consistent language across varying countries and cultures to use when describing how individuals with disabilities participate in society. To understand how *Uniform Terminology, 3rd Edition* (AOTA, 1994) and the *Framework* (AOTA, 2002) fit with the *ICF*, a summary is presented in Table 1-2.

Note that in Table 1-2, *ICF* terminology includes the concept of activities. For this reason, occupational therapy is challenged to clarify how and what occupation is in terms of *ICF* terminology. Only by providing such clarification can occupational therapy position itself effectively in the public mind.

SUMMARY

This chapter reviews how occupation is used in our profession today. Occupation is a core concept of occupational therapy. Occupation is composed of daily tasks and purposeful activities, intertwining with the meaning or personal, subjective value these tasks and activities provide to individuals. Occupations are shaped by individuals, formed by our cultural background, our interests, and aspects of life that are meaningful. Our occupations are formed in childhood and change during our life span. Occupational therapy practitioners are unique in their use of occupations, using occupation as a means as well as an end. This dual use of the construct *occupation* has led to some confusion about its meaning. As the profession clarifies its understanding of occupation, the terminology will become clearer and better understood by practitioners and by society as a whole.

STUDY QUESTIONS AND LEARNING ACTIVITIES

1-1. What are your daily patterns of occupation? List them.

1-2. What daily occupations do you most value? Or, which daily occupations give you the most personal satisfaction? Select the top five, or the five that are most important to you, and place a star by them as listed from question 1-1.

1-3. Hypothesize as to why the five occupations identified in question 1-2 are meaningful to you.

1-4. Speculate what an educational curriculum based on occupation would look like. Speculate what fieldwork experiences based on occupation would look like.

1-5. Contrast occupation as a means with occupation as an end.

1-6. Hypothesize why occupation has no single definition embraced by the entire profession of occupational therapy.

1-7. Trace the profession of occupational therapy's use of the term occupation over time.

1-8. Explain why or how the term occupation is used in an ambiguous manner.

1-9. What is the relationship between emotions and occupation?

1-10. Provide an example of an individual's pattern of occupation.

1-11. What is effective communication about occupational therapy?

1-12. What is the *ICF*, why is it important, and how does it affect communication about occupational therapy?

1-13. Generate your own personal definition of the term occupation. Reflect on your definition. How is it the same or how is it different from the definitions used in this chapter?

1-14. Generate your own story about how you came to value occupation.

1-15. Define occupation for someone outside the profession.

References

Accreditation Council for Occupational Therapy Education. (1998a). *Standards for an accredited educational program for the occupational therapist.* Bethesda, MD: American Occupational Therapy Association.

Accreditation Council for Occupational Therapy Education. (1998b). *Standards for an accredited educational program for the occupational therapy assistant.* Bethesda, MD: American Occupational Therapy Association.

American Occupational Therapy Association. (1979a). Philosophical base of occupational therapy, resolution #531-79. *American Journal of Occupational Therapy, 33,* 785.

American Occupational Therapy Association. (1979b). Occupation as the common core of occupational therapy, resolution #532-79. *American Journal of Occupational Therapy, 33,* 785.

American Occupational Therapy Association. (1979c). *Occupation therapy output reporting system and uniform terminology system for reporting occupational therapy services.* Bethesda, MD: Author.

American Occupational Therapy Association. (1989). *Uniform terminology for occupational therapy services (2nd ed.). American Journal of Occupation, 43,* 1047–1054.

American Occupational Therapy Association. (1991a). Essentials and guidelines for an accredited educational program for the occupational therapist. *American Journal of Occupational Therapy, 45,* 1077–1084.

American Occupational Therapy Association. (1991b). Essentials and guidelines for an accredited educational program for the occupational therapy assistants. *American Journal of Occupational Therapy, 45,* 1085–1092.

American Occupational Therapy Association. (1994). Uniform terminology for occupational therapy (3rd ed.). *American Journal of Occupational Therapy, 48,* 1047–1054.

American Occupational Therapy Association. (2002, February). Occupational therapy practice framework: Domain and process (draft XVIII). Bethesda, MD: Author.

Baum, C., & Edwards, D. (1995). Occupational performance: Occupational therapy's definition of function. *American Journal of Occupational Therapy Association, 49,* 1019–1020.

Bruce, M. A., & Borg, B. (1993). *Psychosocial occupational therapy: Frames of reference for intervention* (2nd ed.). Thorofare, NJ: Slack.

Christiansen, C. H. (1999). Defining lives: Occupation as identity: An essay on competence, coherence, and the creation of meaning. *American Journal of Occupational Therapy, 53,* 547–548.

Christiansen, C., & Baum, C. (1997). *Occupational therapy: Enabling function and well-being.* Thorofare, NJ: Slack.

Christiansen, C., Clark, F., Kielhofner, G., Rogers, J., & Nelson, D. (1995). Position paper: Occupation. *American Journal of Occupational Therapy 49,* 1015-1018.

Clark, F. (1993). Occupation embedded in a real life: Interweaving occupational science and occupational therapy. *American Journal of Occupational Therapy, 47,* 1067–1078.

Clark, F. (Interviewee). (1997, October 22). *CNN News.* Atlanta, GA: Cable Network News.

Clark, F., Parham, D., Carlson, M. E., Frank, G., Jackson, J., Pierce, D., Wolfe, R. J., & Zemke, R. (1991). Occupational science: Academic innovation in the service of occupational therapy's future. *American Journal of Occupational Therapy, 45,* 300–310.

Crabtree, J. L. (1998). The end of occupational therapy. *American Journal of Occupational Therapy, 52,* 205–214.

Cynkin, S. (1979). *Occupational therapy: Toward health through activities.* Boston: Little, Brown and Company.

Cynkin, S., & Robinson, A. (1990). *Occupational therapy and activities health: Toward health through activities.* Boston: Little, Brown and Company.

Fidler, G. S. (1996). Lifestyle performance: From profile to conceptual model. *American Journal of Occupational Therapy, 50,* 139–147.

Fidler, G. S., & Fidler, J. W. (1978). Doing and becoming: Purposeful action and self-actualization. *American Journal of Occupational Therapy, 32,* 305–310.

Fidler G. S., & Velde, B. (1999). Activity: Reality and symbol. Thorofare, NJ: Slack.

Gray, J. M. (1998). Putting occupation into practice: Occupation as ends: Occupation as means. *American Journal of Occupational Therapy, 52*, 354–364.

Hinojosa, J., & Blount, M. L. (2000). *The texture of life: Purposeful activities in occupational therapy.* Bethesda, MD: American Occupational Therapy Association.

Hinojosa, J., & Kramer, P. (1997). Statement: Fundamental concepts of occupational therapy: Occupation, purposeful activity, and function. *American Journal of Occupational Therapy, 51*, 864–866.

Hinojosa, J., Sabari, J., & Pedretti, L. (1993). Position paper: Purposeful activity. *American Journal of Occupational Therapy, 47*, 1081–1082.

Kielhofner, G. (1983). *Health through occupation: Theory and practice in occupational therapy.* Philadelphia, PA: F.A. Davis.

Kielhofner, G. (Ed.). (1995). *A model of human occupation: Theory and application* (2nd ed.). Baltimore, MD: Williams & Wilkins.

Kielhofner, G. (1997). *Conceptual foundations of occupational therapy* (2nd ed.). Philadelphia, PA: F.A. Davis.

Kielhofner, G. (Ed.). (2002). *A model of human occupation.* (3rd ed.). Philadelphia, PA: Lippincott Williams & Wilkins.

Kramer, P., & Hinojosa, J. (1995). Epiphany of human occupation. In C. B. Royeen (Ed.), *AOTA self study series: Human Occupation.* Bethesda, MD: American Occupational Therapy Association.

Kramer, P., & Hinojosa, J. (1999). *Frames of reference for pediatric occupational therapy* (2nd ed.). Philadelphia, PA: Lippincott Williams & Wilkins.

Krishnagiri, S. S. (2000). Occupations and their dimensions. In J. Hinojosa, & M. L. Blount (Eds.), *The texture of life: Purposeful activities in occupational therapy* (pp. 35–50). Bethesda, MD: American Occupational Therapy Association.

Law, M. (Ed.). (1998). *Client-centered occupational therapy.* Thorofare, NJ: Slack.

Mandel, D. R., Jackson, J. M., Zemke, R., Nelson, L., & Clark, F. A. (1999). *Lifestyle redesign: Implementing the well elderly program.* Bethesda, MD: American Occupational Therapy Association.

Mosey, A. C. (1986). *Psychosocial components of occupational therapy.* New York: Raven Press.

Nelson, D. L. (1988) Occupation: Form and performance. *American Journal of Occupational Therapy, 42*, 633–641.

Primeau, L., & Ferguson, J. (1999). Occupational frame of reference. In P. Kramer & J. Hinojosa (Eds.), *Frames of reference for pediatric occupational therapy* (2nd ed., pp. 469–516). Philadelphia, PA: Lippincott, Williams & Wilkins.

Reilly, M. (1962). Occupational therapy can be one of the great ideas of 20th century medicine. *American Journal of Occupational Therapy, 16*, 1–9.

Royeen, C. B. (1995). The human life cycle: Paradigmatic shifts in occupation. In C. B. Royeen (Ed.), *The practice of the future: Putting occupation back into therapy.* Bethesda, MD: American Occupational Therapy Association.

Royeen, C. B. (2000). Occupation reconstructed. Paper presentation at the Education Special Interest Section Workshop, American Occupational Therapy Association Annual Conference, March 29.

Royeen, C. B. (2002). Occupation reconsidered. *Occupational Therapy International, 9*, 112–121.

Trombly, C. A. (1995). Occupation: Purposefulness, and meaningfulness as therapeutic mechanisms. The 1995 Eleanor Clarke Slagle lecture. *American Journal of Occupational Therapy, 49*, 960–972.

Trombly, C. A. & Radomski, M.V. (2002). *Occupational therapy for physical dysfunction* (5th ed.). Philadelphia, PA: Lippincott Williams & Wilkins.

World Health Organization (2001). *ICF: International classification of functioning, disability and health.* Geneva, Switzerland: Author.

Yerxa, E. J. (1967). Authentic occupational therapy. *American Journal of Occupational Therapy, 21*, 1–9.

Yerxa, E. J. (1998). Occupation: The keystone of a curriculum for a self-defined profession. *American Journal of Occupational Therapy, 52*, 365–372.

Yerxa, E. J., Clark, F., Frank, G., Jackson, J., Parham, D., Pierce, D., Stein, C., & Zemke R. (1989). An introduction to occupational science: A foundation for occupational therapy in the 21st century. *Occupational Therapy in Health Care, 6*, 1–17.

2

History of Occupation

Kathleen Barker Schwartz

INTRODUCTION

To understand the evolution of the term occupation we must go back to the founding years when the profession was first established. The founders came from a variety of professional backgrounds. Their varying perspectives created a rich, complex vision of occupation, one that probably would not have happened had they been from the same disci-

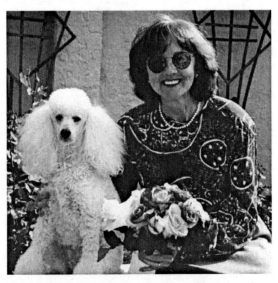

Kathleen with her miniature poodle, Jake, in her rose garden.

pline. This complexity and richness is something we value highly in the profession today. However, it also presented a challenge to the founders and to practitioners today: How do you define occupation to the public and professional colleagues in one short phrase that will be understandable? Thus, language was as much of an issue to the founders as their beliefs and values. This chapter examines the founders' conceptions of occupation, the philosophy of occupation as they articulated it, and the issues they faced in choosing a name for the profession. The evolution of the term occupation is traced to the present day, and an overview of the relative importance of occupation as it has changed over time within the profession is provided.

ORIGINS OF OCCUPATION

Meaning of Occupation to the Founders

On March 15, 1917, five professionals who shared a common belief in the benefits of occupation met together to found the National Society for the Promotion of Occupational Therapy (NSPOT) (later to become the American Occupational Therapy Association) (Fig. 2-1). They were William Rush Dunton, George Edward Barton, Eleanor Clarke Slagle, Susan Cox Johnson, Isabell G. Newton, and Thomas Bessell Kidner. Susan Tracy was invited but was unable to attend. Dunton was a psychiatrist, Barton and Kidner were architects, Slagle came from a social service background, Johnson was a teacher of arts and crafts, and Tracy was a nurse. This variety of professional backgrounds helped to shape each of their perspectives on occupation and its use in treatment.

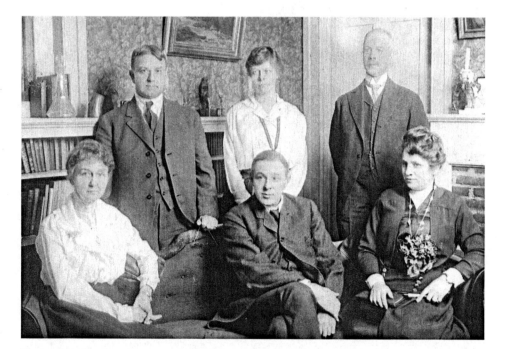

Figure 2-1. Founders of the National Society for the Promotion of Occupational Therapy Association (1917). Front row (L-R): Susan C. Johnson, George E. Barton, Eleanor Clarke Slagle. Back row: William R. Dunton, Jr., Isabel G. Newton, Thomas B. Kidner. (Reprinted with permission from the Archives of the American Occupational Therapy Association, Inc.)

William Rush Dunton began as an assistant physician at Sheppard Asylum (later renamed Sheppard Pratt Hospital), where he was introduced to therapeutic occupations by Edward Brush, MD, then superintendent. When in 1902 a separate building for occupation classes was created, Dunton took much of the responsibility for enlarging the patient activities to include leatherwork, weaving, art, metalwork, bookbinding, electrical repair work, and printing (Fields, 1911). Dunton's conception of occupation can be found in a published outline of lectures (AOTA, 1925) of which he was the primary author. In the document, occupational therapy was defined as a "method for training the sick or injured by means of instruction and employment in productive occupation" (p. 280). It specified that authentic occupational therapy must be of interest to the patient, "useful, not aimless, progressive, individualistic, and carried on by encouragement, not criticism" (pp. 278-279). Treatment guidelines specified that the choice of occupation should be based on the patient's "estimated interests and capability," that occupations should be graded to gradually increase "strength and capability," and group work should be encouraged to stimulate "social adaptation." It stipulated that treatment should be prescribed and under medical supervision, and that the "only reliable measure of the treatment is the effect on the patient" (p. 280). Dunton was a leading advocate for the profession through his prolific writing and numerous professional publications. He was also instrumental in establishing and editing the profession's official journal. Dunton was president in the association's early years, and throughout his career worked closely with Slagle to establish the viability of the profession.

In later years Eleanor Clarke Slagle was characterized as a "pioneer by nature, with a searching mind and a keen interest in social problems and their psychological aspects" (Robeson, 1937). Initially attracted to occupation by her association with Julia Lathrop and Jane Addams of Hull House, Slagle saw its potential to restore the seriously mentally disabled to self-sufficiency and participation once again in society. She conceptualized the idea of "habit training" while director of occupational therapy at Phipps Clinic, under the supervision of Dr. Adolph Meyer. Slagle applied habit training to the most profoundly involved patients, those Meyer characterized as suffering from severely "disorganized habits" (Wilson, 1929). In habit training, Slagle designed a program for small groups of patients who followed a strict schedule that included self-care and personal hygiene, walks and other physical activities, occupation classes, and meals. "To visualize the picture more clearly, let us consider a group of sixteen untidy, destructive, assaultive, abusive and rapidly deteriorating young women . . . . These patients were placed on a twenty-four hour program drawn up by the director of occupational therapy and accepted by the medical superintendent . . . At the end of considerably less than a year's intensive work fifteen of the group are entirely retrained in decent habits of living and are now being trained in carefully graded tasks . . ." (Slagle, 1924). Slagle's work reflected her definition of occupation as "purposeful activity of mind or body . . . [which] may be therapeutic, educational, vocational or economic" (Slagle, 1918) (Fig. 2-2). Slagle went on to hold leadership positions ranging from president to secretary-treasurer of the American Occupational Therapy Association for the next 25 years and is legendary for her administrative and political skill.

George Barton was an architect whose interest in occupation came about as a result of his own efforts to cure himself from tuberculosis and paralysis. With no motion possible in his left hand and arm, he used his own body as a clinic to work out the problem of rehabilitation himself (Newton, 1917). Barton bought a small house and barn in Clifton Springs which he named Consolation House and in 1914 opened a school, workshop, and a vocational bureau for convalescents (Barton, 1914). Consolation House was Barton's answer to the inhumanity and unhealthful conditions he personally experienced in the san-

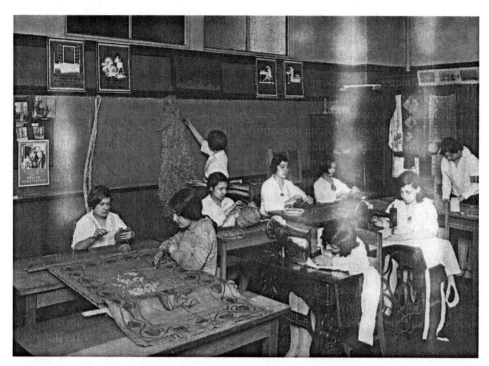

Figure 2-2. Productive occupation for women based on the patient's interest in vocational training. (Reprinted with permission from the Archives of the American Occupational Therapy Association, Inc.)

itariums and medical institutions of that time. In contrast, he created a humane, comfortable place where he felt people could get well and become self-supporting through engagement in occupations. In his view occupation strengthened the body, clarified the mind, and offered "a new life upon recovery" (Barton, 1920, p. 307). He believed an important component of this recovery should include the ability to make a living. In his conception, the occupational therapist would work under the prescription of the doctor, who would specify the desired physical and mental results. Barton's contribution to occupation was important but brief. He died in 1923.

As a former teacher of arts and crafts, Susan Johnson brought a background in education, a value of handicrafts, and a belief that occupations could improve the physical and mental condition of patients. She was asked to join the founding group as a result of her work in therapeutic occupations for New York State. Before this, she has been an arts and crafts teacher in Berkeley, California, and had also taught crafts while residing in the Philippines. In her view the purpose of therapeutic occupation was to, "divert the mind from destructive tendencies, substitute normal interests and constructive activity, and crystallize them into right mental habits" (Johnson, 1920, p. 69). In addition to aiding in the cure of mental illness, Johnson also saw the physical benefits of occupation in restoring "functional" power to stiffened joints, contracted muscles, and injured nerves. She emphasized occupation's role in training in adaptation and the importance of using a wide range of occupations, depending on the condition of the individual. Johnson noted that handcrafts had a special therapeutic value: "The regaining of self-confidence, satisfaction in accomplishment, the direction of thought into wholesome and normal channels, and graded physical exercise producing a healthful tired feeling without overstrain which in turn brings its demand for relaxation, rest, and sleep, are all factors within the therapeutic value of handcrafts" (p. 70). She warned, however, that handcrafts must be "rightly directed as a step in graded training," or there was the risk of having the patient become demoralized from "routine occupations which provide exercise for muscles only and call forth little or no mental activity or self-expression" (p. 70). In 1923 Johnson left the occupational therapy department she helped to establish at Montefiore Hospital. Until her death in 1932 she directed the Convalescent Workshop in New York City.

Thomas Kidner's contribution to occupation was the idea of the "pre-industrial shop" which had as its purpose to "assist the patient in his re-adjustment to normal living by affording opportunity for the development of habits of industry that have been impaired by disease or accident" (Kidner, 1925, p. 188). As Vocational Secretary to the Canadian Military Hospitals and a former architect, Kidner was particularly interested in how the shops would be designed to enable the convalescent soldier to return to a vocation by which he could support himself (Fig. 2-3). His vision of occupational therapy included four components: "First, the habit training; next, the group work on the wards; then, the Occupational Therapy center; all these activities being purely therapeutic. Then . . . the pre-industrial shop. From this shop, the patient passes on to community life; either in the institution or the outside world" (pp. 187-188). He acknowledged that his conception was difficult to implement because "the work of the shop is of a dual nature. In part, it is therapeutic, but on the other hand it must partake largely in its methods of the nature of a trade or industrial school and, even more, of a commercial workshop or factory" (p. 188). The solution, he proposed, was either to "superimpose upon the training of an occupational therapist some training methods of commercial shops" or to select trade workers who would be amenable to "some training in the aims, principles and methods of occu-

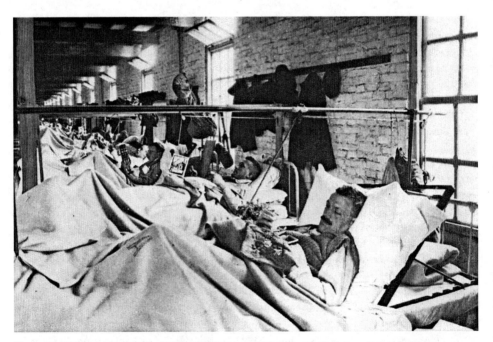

Figure 2-3. Men in an army hospital engaged in meaningful occupation to restore physical functioning. (Reprinted with permission from the Archives of the American Occupational Therapy Association, Inc.)

pational therapy" (p. 189). Kidner served as president of the association from 1923 to 1928.

Dunton credits Susan Tracy with giving a strong stimulus to occupational therapy through her book *Studies in Invalid Occupation* (1910). He also characterizes her as the first to give "systematic training in occupation" (Dunton, 1921, p. 15). Invalid occupation was indeed one of the first comprehensive discussions of the use of therapeutic occupation. In it she described methods of teaching, qualifications, and necessary equipment; she also included case study examples of patients who had benefited from therapeutic occupations. As director of the nurses' training program at the Adams Nervine Asylum in Boston, Massachusetts, Tracy led the effort to build and equip a house devoted to occupation treatment at the asylum. "Much importance was placed on the occupation room, wherein opportunity was provided for various forms of interesting and useful work. Weaving rugs and finer fabrics, basket work, bookbinding and clay modeling were employed at the start." In her view a patient's engagement in occupation "became the source of new purposes, of changed avenues of thought and of stimulated ambitions" (p. 7) (Fig. 2-4). She specified that a therapeutic occupation should always "possess a certain dignity. Do not encourage the employment of time on unworthy materials and purposeless productions" (p. 15). Throughout her career Tracy continued her advocacy for the therapeutic value of occupation and for the nursing profession to be the teachers of occupation.

Choosing the Name Occupation

Because the term occupation represented the embodiment of the founders' values and beliefs, we must examine the issues surrounding the choice of the term. The founders recognized it was not a simple matter of semantics, but a critical factor in the successful estab-

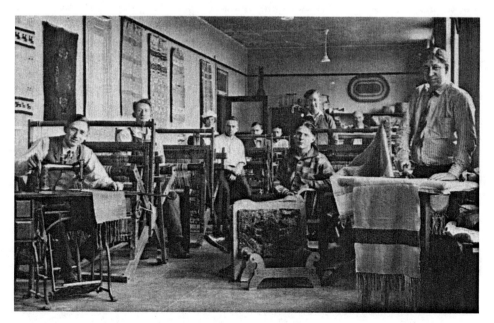

Figure 2-4. Using valuable occupation to promote health. (Reprinted with permission from the Archives of the American Occupational Therapy Association, Inc.)

lishment of the profession as legitimate. In choosing the term occupation, the founders faced several obstacles. One was that many terms were used interchangeably to mean occupation. Dunton illustrated this at the founding meeting of the National Society for the Promotion of Occupational Therapy, when he presented a paper that chronicled the pioneering efforts of those who advocated the use of occupation in the 1800s to treat mental illness (Dunton, 1917a). He noted that before 1910 in the United States the terms labor, employment, amusements, and moral treatment were all used to refer to treatment using occupation with the mentally ill. It was only after 1910 that the term occupation began to be used in the literature (Dunton, 1921). There were some examples of the term occupation used in the 1800s in Europe. Dunton cited an article on lunatic asylums of England, which described how Bethlehem Hospital developed a program in which patients were provided with "materials for occupation" (Dunton, 1917a, p. 381). He also cited an article describing Pinel's work: "Since Pinel has demonstrated the happy effects of occupation in asylums, all physicians concur in the opinion that it is one of the most important employments in the treatment of the insane . . ." (p. 381).

Not only were many terms used to mean occupation in the professional literature, there were several meanings to the term in the lay language (Oxford English Dictionary, 1989). One meaning was, "The being occupied or employed with, or engaged in something" (p. 682). Although this meaning did accurately reflect what the founders intended, there was a fear that occupation might be too common a word and therefore readily dismissed by the scientific community. Dunton's statement illustrates the founders' concern: "Various names are given, such as occupation, diversion, diversional occupation, occupational diversion, occupation and amusement, employment, work cure, occupational therapy, and ergotherapy. The last is probably the best, and certainly the most scientific term, but as yet it has not come into general use, and the more simple term occupation will probably be used for some time" (Dunton, 1917b, p. 5). As a physician, Dunton understood the importance of being seen as scientifically valid, thus his support for ergotherapy, a term that he believed would be more impressive to the scientific community.

Conversely, the term occupation did satisfy the founders' desire for a word broad enough to encompass all its possible aspects. The 1921 definition satisfied all the founders: "Occupational Therapy may be defined as any activity, mental or physical, definitely prescribed and guided for the distinct purpose of contributing to and hastening recovery from disease or injury" (Dunton, 1950, p. 4). The definition makes it clear that occupation could be used to treat any mental and physical condition, and that a variety of occupations should be used to suit each individual. This breadth of definition was an asset when there were few established health professions. However, turf problems would later develop when more came into existence, and each tried to carve out a particular area of practice. Then occupational therapy was criticized for being too broad and not sufficiently focused (Ambrosi & Schwartz, 1995).

The second meaning of the word occupation is, "A particular action in which one is engaged habitually; an employment, business, or calling" (Oxford English Dictionary, 1989, p. 682). Thus we can see the root of a problem that the profession faces today: It is commonly thought that occupational therapists are concerned with getting people jobs. This was confusing even in the early years because the founders' view of occupation did encompass prevocational treatment, but not vocational. It is doubtful that many people in the early 1900s understood the distinction either.

Then there was the question of who actually coined the term occupational therapy. There are two views: One that Dunton originated the term; the other that Barton did. The case was made for Dunton by Bing (1987), when he argued that the first instance of Dunton's use of the term occupation therapy was in lecture notes written in 1911 for a course for nurses. According to Bing, Dunton wrote, "Occupation therapy serves many purposes, such as keeping the mind occupied, awakening new interests, directing the patients from delusions and hallucinations . . ." (p. 193). In 1921 Dunton published *Occupational Therapy: A Manual for Nurses*. Breines (1987) made the case for Barton, when she argued that in 1914 Barton gave an address before the Massachusetts State Board of Insanity in which he used the words occupational therapy. His address was reprinted in the *Trained Nurse and Hospital Review* (Barton, 1915). Rather than viewing this as a contest between Barton and Dunton, perhaps it is best to see it as an evolution in which many people played a role. "Its beginning was so gradual, and yet so general, it is impossible to give any one person credit as discoverer, or dignify any form of occupation as having been first used to restore a diseased mind . . . possibly the credit belongs to a number of patients . . . [and] the physician, if he was intelligent enough to note the cause of improvement" (Dunton, 1921, p. 11).

Philosophy and Science of Occupation

The fact that occupational therapy has its origins in a philosophy and a science is of paramount importance in understanding the history of occupation. The philosophy came first, and this makes it unique among the other medical professions. For early practitioners this meant that they had to understand thoroughly the belief system underlying the use of occupation in the absence of many scientific guidelines for practice. For today's practitioners it means that using scientific techniques and modalities is not sufficient; one must also understand the beliefs and values — the philosophy — that underlie the practice of occupation.

The roots of occupational therapy can be traced to the philosophical movement known as moral treatment (Dunton, 1917a). Philippe Pinel, the father of moral treatment, was a physician, scholar, and philosopher. He proposed a "revolution morale," which replaced the view that the mentally ill were instruments of the devil and should be locked away from society, with a humane approach based on a belief in the individual's ability to reason and a compassion for the nature of the affliction. Pinel (1809) proposed a carefully planned treatment approach based on the use of "occupational activities of different kinds according to individual taste; physical exercise, beautiful scenery, and from time to time soft and melodious music" (p. 260). His work, along with that of William Tuke in England, stimulated the moral treatment initiatives in the United States implemented at Friends, Bloomingdale, and McLean Hospitals.

Adolph Meyer (1922), a professor of psychiatry at Johns Hopkins University and a mentor of Dunton's and Slagle's, took the ideas fundamental to moral treatment and built on them to create a 20th century "philosophy of occupational therapy." In this paper read at the Fifth Meeting of the National Society for the Promotion of Occupational Therapy, Meyer argued that occupational therapy represented an important, new "human philosophy" in which there is a "valuation of time and work" and a focus on "reality and actuality rather than of mere thinking." Mental problems were seen as "problems of living, and not merely diseases of a structural and toxic nature . . . or of a final lasting constitutional disorder" (p. 4). In this conception, occupational therapy addressed the "habit-deterioration of the mentally ill through systematic engagement of interest, and concern about the actual use of time and work" (p. 4). He gave an example of the use of therapeutic occupations at the Phipps Clinic: "Groups of patients with raffia and basket work, or with various kinds of handiwork and weaving and bookbinding and metal and leather work, took the place of the bored wall flowers and of mischief-makers. A pleasure in achievement, a real pleasure in the use and activity of one's hands and muscles and a happy appreciation of time began to be used as incentives in the management of our patients, instead of abstract exhortations to cheer up and to behave according to abstract or repressive rules" (p. 3). He argued that occupational therapy should consist in giving "opportunities rather than prescriptions. There must be opportunities to work, opportunities to do and to plan and create, and to learn to use material" (p. 7).

Although recognizing its basis in philosophy, the founders also advocated the development of a science of occupation. As a physician, Dunton recognized the importance of being able to establish scientifically the effectiveness of occupation if the profession was going to succeed. He led an effort to analyze occupations scientifically through the Committee on Installations and Advice (Dunton, 1928). He advocated for funding to perform research. "An increase in the number of sustaining members will make it possible for the society to extend its research . . . To the present it has not been possible to make any grants for research, and all that has been done has been by the self sacrifice of individuals . . The foundation of a research fund to be administered by the Board of Management, is especially desirable . . ." (NSPOT, c1923, p. 3). In addition to funding problems, occupational therapy also faced a methodological problem. A profession based on a philosophy of humanism and social concern, and a necessarily broad definition of practice, did not lend itself to the reductionistic paradigm of the physical sciences. In 1934 Dunton addressed the issue at a meeting of psychiatrists: "[We] are unable to present the results of research because psychologists have not yet given us the formulae for judging the emotional effect of pounding a copper disk into a nut dish . . . In other words, we lack a quick and snappy means of measuring the emotions" (p. 325). He urged occupational therapists to use other methods of research, such as systematic observation, and to develop new methods that would avoid reducing the occupational therapy process to "fractions, tangents, and cosines" (p. 325).

In summary, the founders' conceptions of occupation were guided by a humanistic philosophy that recognized the full complexity of the individual and the therapeutic process that would enable patients to adapt to the problems of living. They acknowledged the importance of developing a science of occupation and worried that the term occupation might sound too simple and therefore not adequately represent the complex processes underlying it. Although they had a variety of views on the use of occupation, the founders shared a common understanding of the value of occupation. They shared the belief that engagement in occupations should have meaning and purpose and bring joy to the individual. They defined the use of occupation broadly, to include habit training, handcrafts, graded physical exercise, and the pre-industrial shop. They established community settings, such as Consolation House, to provide an optimal environment for individuals to engage in occupations that would "arouse interest, courage, and confidence; exercise mind and body; overcome disability, and re-establish capacity for industrial and social usefulness" (AOTA, 1925). Thus, the founders offered a vision that foreshadowed the many aspects of occupation that would be emphasized by future generations of practitioners.

Occupational therapy in the 1930s consisted primarily of "bedside and ward occupations" conducted in mental health facilities, tuberculosis sanitoriums, orthopedic units of general hospitals, convalescent homes, and crippled children's hospitals (Figs. 2-5 and 2-6) as well as prevocational treatment in curative workshops (Kidner, 1930). By the mid-1940s, however, there was a shift away from a generalist approach and toward one of specialization within occupational therapy in mental health, physical rehabilitation, or pediatric practice. With this shift, there was a decreased reliance on general occupations and an increased use of techniques and modalities specific to the area of specialization. World War II resulted in the rapid growth in the profession, particularly in the area of physical rehabilitation.

RE-EMERGENCE OF OCCUPATION

A Quiet Revolution

The protests began quietly in the 1960s, with a few of the profession's leaders speaking out; it swelled in the 1970s to a chorus of voices urging therapists to return to their roots in occupation. The Slagle Lectures presented by Mary Reilly (1962) and Elizabeth Yerxa (1967) illustrated the nature of the concern. Reilly (1962) challenged the profession to return to the founders' vision and to develop a body of knowledge based on a thorough understanding of the nature of occupation. She criticized the movement away from occupation, citing both the delimiting effects of psychoanalytic theory on psychosocial occupational therapy practice and the heavy emphasis on muscle efficiency and enabling devices in physical dysfunction practice. She left open the question of whether the profession could fulfill the founders' "truly great and magnificent" vision: that individuals "through the use of [their] hands as they are energized by mind and will, can influence the state of [their] own health" (p. 62). Yerxa (1967) proposed a vision of what she called "authentic occupational therapy," in which therapists would collaborate with patients in choosing occupations that had purpose and meaning. She urged therapists to think for themselves and described the high price therapists paid by relying on the doctor's prescription in "the reduction of our potential to help clients because we often stagnated at the level of applying technical skills" (p. 2).

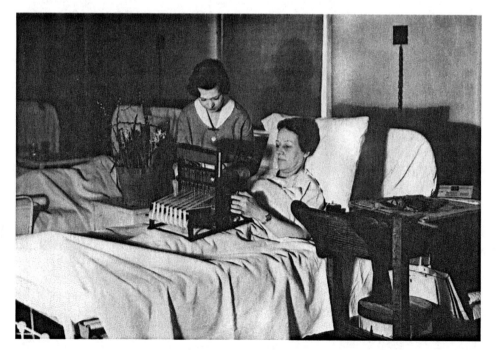

Figure 2-5. Bedside occupational therapy in a women's ward circa the early 1930s. (Reprinted with permission from the Archives of the American Occupational Therapy Association, Inc.)

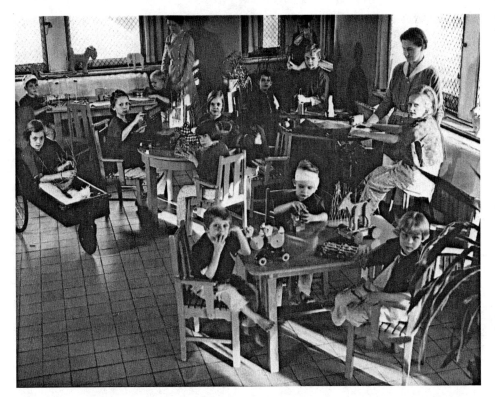

Figure 2.6. Occupational therapy in a children's ward in Indianapolis in the mid-1930s. (Reprinted with permission from the Archives of the American Occupational Therapy Association, Inc.)

Leaders who presented a further analysis of the problem joined these voices in the 1970s. Shannon (1977) saw the "derailment of occupational therapy" and its replacement with a "technique philosophy." He perceived two philosophies at odds with each other. One viewed the individual as a "mechanistic creature susceptible to manipulation and control via the application of techniques." The other, based on the early philosophy of moral treatment, held a holistic and humanistic view of the individual. Kielhofner and Burke (1977) described the situation as a conflict between two paradigms: One based on the paradigm of occupation and moral treatment, the other based on reductionism, a mode of thinking characteristic of the medical model. In Fidler's (1981) view, therapists had replaced occupation with modalities that eliminated the "self as the doer-agent and place[d] the causative agent outside the self." She warned that "when occupational therapists are comfortable labeling a significant part of their practice as unproductive activity, the fundamental principles of occupational therapy are denied" (p. 567). Bockoven, a psychiatrist, urged occupational therapists to build on the legacy of moral treatment. "Does it sound too visionary," he asked, "to suggest that there be a consolation house within walking distance of every urban dweller?" (1971, p. 224). He went on to describe his view of the essence of occupational therapy, one that represented the philosophy of moral treatment and Meyer's philosophy of occupational therapy: "It is the occupational therapist's inborn respect for the realities of life, for the real tasks of living, and for the time it takes the individual to develop his modes of coping with his tasks, that leads me to urge haste on the profession . . . to assert its leadership in fashioning the design of human services programs . . ." (p. 225).

The Challenge to Occupation-Centered Practice

What happened in the intervening years to move the profession away from its founding premise? There were several causes. One was rooted in the rehabilitation movement, which began with World War II and grew to encompass the civilian population by the 1970s. Because therapists working in this environment were required to possess specialized medical knowledge and technological skills, this prompted the creation of a specialty within occupational therapy dedicated to treating individuals with physical dysfunction. Therapists sought to attain credibility within the medical model by working under a doctor's prescription and using what was viewed as the latest scientific techniques and modalities. A second important event was the funding of Medicare and Medicaid in 1965. This legislation increased demand for medical services for the chronically ill and elderly and also signaled the importance of the third-party payer. When federal money began to run out in 1980, only those services that were deemed "medically necessary" were reimbursed. Other third-party payers followed Medicare's lead, holding the same narrow view of what constituted legitimate service. This resulted in even more pressure for occupational therapists to do only what fit within a medical paradigm of treatment. This situation recalls the concerns over language and perception first voiced by the founders: that occupation can seem deceptively simple and not scientific and therefore not of value from a medical perspective. Dunton voiced this fear when he advocated that we call ourselves ergotherapists because it seemed more scientific. Associated with this was the ongoing issue of the difficulty the profession had in reducing the complexity of occupation into one simple definition for the public or colleagues.

The pressure to conform to a paradigm that did not really fit resulted in a lack of confidence among occupational therapists. This was remarked on by colleagues outside the profession such as Kutner, a psychiatrist, who was characterized by Woodside (1971) as expressing concern about what he saw as feelings of "professional inferiority among occupational therapists . . .that we think we can't really influence developing programs and patient improvement" (p. 230). Woodside's remarks were directed at a serious concern that had developed within the profession, the question as to the viability of mental health practice. "The hypothesis is that the next ten years may witness the death of at least one area of our profession, our work with the mentally ill . . . Psychiatric occupational therapy could cease to exist because other professions are rapidly absorbing our body of knowledge, they appear to the public to be offering the same services that we offer, and they are selling their programs to other professionals and the public more effectively than we are" (p. 229). The solution, according to Bockoven (1971), was to return to the profession's roots in moral treatment. This meant establishing itself outside the constraints of medical institutions. "It would be most unfortunate for all society but especially for the mentally ill if occupational therapy were to limit itself by continuing to be satisfied with running dinky little sideshows in large medical institutions" (p. 224). "Don't drop dead," he exhorted, "take over instead!" (p. 225).

The lack of a science unique to occupation, or theories of practice, or research that proved the efficacy of practice, deeply hampered therapists' efforts to establish credibility in all areas of practice. The richness and complexity of occupation is not evident if one cannot articulate the underlying rationale and its basis in a recognizable science. Only as this issue has begun to be addressed in the past two decades have therapists appeared to regain the confidence to retain and reintroduce occupation as the centerpiece of therapy. Efforts of the profession's academic leaders have been focused on creating a science of occupation (Clark et al., 1991), defining theories to guide practice (Kielhofner, 1997), producing research that demonstrates the effectiveness of occupational therapy (Case-Smith, 2000), and defining the best approaches to treatment by examining evidence-based practice (Tickle-Degnen, 2000). The profession's struggle with language — one that this chapter demonstrates goes back to the founding years — is being addressed by Hinojosa and Kramer (1997) and others. What is purposeful activity? What is meaningful activity? What is occupation? After all, if we cannot decide among ourselves the meaning of terms, how can we expect others to understand? Lastly, it is important to acknowledge the difficulty the profession faces in going against the dominant paradigm. Occupation does not fit neatly into one specific paradigm; therefore, it will always be an uphill battle. Nevertheless, as this chapter shows, our heritage as fighters goes back to the founders. It is helpful to keep in mind Meyer's (1922) words regarding those who practice occupation therapy: It takes "rare gifts and talents and rare personalities to be real pathfinders in this work . . . it is all a problem of being true to one's nature and opportunities and of teaching others to do the same with themselves" (p. 7). After all, occupation is not only the best idea of the 20th century, but also the 21st.

Acknowledgment

The author extends her warmest thanks to Mary Binderman, Director of Information Resources at the Wilma F. West Library, for her assistance. She is a true friend to the historical scholar. The author also thanks Bob Bing, PhD, OTR, FAOTA, for his willingness to help clarify some of the more obscure points of our history.

STUDY QUESTIONS

2-1. Discuss key contributions to occupational therapy made by each of the following individuals:
   a. William Rush Dunton
   b. George Edward Barton
   c. Eleanor Clarke Slagle
   d. Susan Cox Johnson
   e. Thomas Bessell Kidner

2-2. What were synonyms for the word occupation in the early 1900s? What words might be synonyms for the word today?

2-3. The founders' use of the term occupation implied its use as a process. Explain.

2-4. When and how was the term occupational therapy first used?

2-5. When and how did a research emphasis in the profession first occur?

2-6. Explain and discuss the complexity of occupational therapy as it initially emerged. Specifically address the problem this created when contrasted to the prevailing scientific approach.

2-7. Discuss reductionism. Discuss moral treatment.

2-8. Explain and discuss the statement, "Occupation can seem deceptively simple and not scientific and therefore not of value from a medical perspective."

2-9. Imagine that you are going to open a moral treatment center where you live. What would such a center look like?

2-10. Discuss whether occupation is referred to as a process or product in this chapter. Provide evidence for your statements.

2-11. Explain why and how occupational therapy goes against today's current dominant scientific paradigm.

References

Ambrosi, E., & Schwartz, K. B. (1995). The profession's image: 1917–1925. Occupational therapy as presented in the media. *American Journal of Occupational Therapy, 49*, 715–719.

American Occupational Therapy Association. (1925). An outline of lectures on occupational therapy to medical students and physicians. *Occupational Therapy and Rehabilitation, 4* (4), 277–292.

Barton, G. E. (1914). A view of invalid occupation. *Trained Nurse and Hospital Review, 52*, 327–330.

Barton, G. E. (1915). *Occupational therapy*. Reprints from the Trained Nurse and Hospital Review, 15–22. Wilma L. West Library Archives.

Barton, G. E. (1920). What occupational therapy may mean to nursing. *Trained Nurse and Hospital Review, 64*, 304–310.

Bing, R. K. (1987). Who originated the term occupational therapy? The author's response. *American Journal of Occupational Therapy, 41*, 192–194.

Bockoven, J. S. (1971). Legacy of moral treatment: 1800's to 1910. *American Journal of Occupational Therapy, 25*, 223–225.

Breines, E. (1987). Who originated the term occupational therapy? Letters to the editor. *American Journal of Occupational Therapy, 41*, 192–194.

Case-Smith, J. (2000). Effects of occupational therapy services on fine motor and functional performance in preschool children. *American Journal of Occupational Therapy, 54*, 372–380.

Clark, F., Parham, L. D., Carlson, M., Frank, G., Jackson, J., Pierce., Wolfe, R., & Zemke, R. (1991). Occupational science: Academic innovation in the service of occupational therapy's future. *American Journal of Occupational Therapy, 49*, 1015–1018.

Dunton, W. R. (1917a). History of occupational therapy. *The Modern Hospital, 8* (6), 380–382.

Dunton, W. R. (1917b). The growing necessity for occupational therapy. An Address delivered before the class of Nursing and Health, Teachers College, Columbia University. Wilma L. West Archives.

Dunton, W. R. (1921). *Occupation therapy: A manual for nurses*. Philadelphia, PA: W.B. Saunders.

Dunton, W. R. (1928). *Prescribing occupational therapy*. Springfield, IL: Charles C. Thomas.

Dunton, W. R. (1934). The need for and value of research in occupational therapy. *Occupational Therapy and Rehabilitation, 13*, 325–328.

Dunton, W. R. (1950). A lecture on occupational therapy. Wilma L. West Library Archives.

Fidler, G. S. (1981). From crafts to competence. *American Journal of Occupational Therapy, 35*, 567–573.

Fields, G. E. (1911). The effect of occupation upon the individual. *The American Journal of Insanity, 68*, 103–109.

Hinojosa, J., & Kramer, P. (1997). Statement: Fundamental concepts of occupational therapy: Occupa-

tion, purposeful activity and function. *American Journal of Occupational Therapy, 51*, 864–866.

Johnson, S. C. (1920). Instruction in handcrafts and design for hospital patients. *The Modern Hospital, 15* (1), 69–72.

Kidner, T. B. (1925). The hospital pre-industrial shop. *Occupational Therapy and Rehabilitation, 4* (3), 187–194.

Kielhofner, G. (1997). *Conceptual foundations of occupational therapy* (2nd ed.). Philadelphia, PA: F.A. Davis.

Kielhofner, G., & Burke, J. P. (1977). Occupational therapy after 60 years: An account of changing identity and knowledge. *American Journal of Occupational Therapy, 31*, 674–689.

Meyer, A. (1922). The philosophy of occupation therapy. *Archives of Occupational Therapy, 1* (1), 1–10.

National Society for the Promotion of Occupational Therapy. (c 1923). Circular of information. Sheppard Hospital Press. Wilma L. West Library Archives.

Newton, I. G. (1917). Consolation house. Wilma L. West Library Archives.

Oxford English dictionary (2nd ed.). (1989). 10, 681–683.

Pinel, P. (1809). *Traite medico-philosophique sur l'alienation mentale* (2nd ed.). Paris: J.A. Brosson.

Reilly, M. (1962). Eleanor Clarke Slagle lecture: Occupational therapy can be one of the great ideas of 20th century medicine. *American Journal of Occupational Therapy, 16*, 1–9.

Robeson, H. A. (1937). Eleanor Clarke Slagle. *American Journal of Occupational Therapy*, September, 3–5.

Shannon, P. D. (1977). The derailment of occupational therapy. *American Journal of Occupational Therapy, 31*, 229–234.

Slagle, E. C. (1918). Lecture. Wilma L. West Library Archives.

Slagle, E. C. (1924). A year's development of occupational therapy in New York state hospitals. *The Modern Hospital, 22* (1), 98–104.

Tickle-Degnen, L. (2000). Monitoring and documenting evidence during assessment and intervention. *American Journal of Occupational Therapy, 54*, 434–436.

Tracy, S. E. (1910). Studies in invalid occupation: A manual for nurses and attendants. Boston: Whitcomb & Barrows.

Wilson, S. C. (1929). Habit training for mental cases. *Occupational Therapy and Rehabilitation, 8*, 189–197.

Woodside, H. H. (1971). The development of occupational therapy, 1910–1929. *American Journal of Occupational Therapy, 225*, 226–230.

Yerxa, E. J. (1967). Eleanor Clarke Slagle lecture: Authentic occupational therapy. *American Journal of Occupational Therapy, 21*, 1–9.

3

Philosophical Basis of Human Occupation

Janice Posatery Burke

OBJECTIVES

This chapter will help you to:
- Describe the philosophical basis of occupation.
- List the purposes of philosophical principles.
- Differentiate between conceptual models and frames of reference.
- Discover the key concepts and ideas of early occupational therapy practitioners.
- Discuss the key concepts and ideas of contemporary conceptual and practice models.

INTRODUCTION

Occupational therapy was born from the need to provide treatment for individuals who had severe mental problems. These individuals were unable to participate in everyday activities, were isolated in insane asylums and considered beyond help, had no structure and organization to their day, and had little hope for returning to a "normal" life. As physicians and other care-oriented people began to closely examine the needs of these populations, they generated and defined their ideas about the kind of perspective or mind set that might

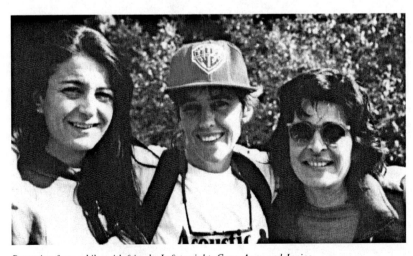

Returning from a hike with friends. Left to right: Cara, Amy, and Janice.

prove helpful. In doing so, a philosophical explanation to support treatment was developed along with the concomitant principles and practices that would guide that treatment as well as outline the knowledge and skills that would be needed by those who provided it to patients.

This chapter offers an in-depth look at the underlying philosophy and principles that are the foundation of occupational therapy. These were the ideas that first carved out what occupational therapy would be, including the kinds of problems therapists would attend to and the strategies they would use to understand and reason about what to do with people who required their care. Along with this historical view of occupational therapy, the chapter also examines contemporary views of occupation, occupational therapy, and occupational science to uncover evidence of the influence of early foundations on current practice and scholarship in the field.

The early philosophy and principles of occupational therapy laid out the problems that were identified as "occupational" deficits. Additionally, the language that would be used to label and describe those deficits, the knowledge that would be used to support the description of those deficits, and the approaches that would be used to address them were also articulated.

Occupational therapy founders, early scholars, educators, and practitioners were clearly focused on the critical role of occupation as a restorative agent for individual patients who were displaced from their roles and their worlds due to chronic health issues. Among the first to be given occupational interventions were patients with neuropsychiatric diseases and disabilities. In time, individuals with physical disabilities and diseases were also included in occupational therapy. Occupational problems for this second group of patients began to emerge along with medical advances that enabled physicians to save more lives. With improved medical care came the need for treatment that would remediate or ameliorate residual limitations. For example, this included soldiers who returned from wars with injuries that required rehabilitation and people who had industrial accidents and injuries that resulted in the need to relearn skills and habits for independence in everyday living.

Why Is It Important To Consider Philosophical Underpinnings?

Phi-los-o-phy, n., the study or science of the truths or principles underlying all knowledge and being (or reality), a system of principles for guidance in practical affairs (American College Dictionary, 1964).

Philosophical principles provide a platform for organizing both thinking and action for an academic discipline or profession. They provide a system for ordering key ideas and the supporting evidence that will guide their further definition. The articulation of philosophical principles allows a group of individuals to feel confident that they share a common focus of concern. Further, philosophical principles establish the parameters of inquiry, guide the development of a language to explain the phenomena of interest, outline related areas of regard, and explain the methods that will be used to guide thought and reason.

Within occupational therapy it is common to find the organization of ideas about occupation explained in conceptual models (Table 3-1) or frames of reference. In each case, authors order their ideas into categories with clear definitions of concepts and descriptions about how the ideas relate to one another. Conceptual models allow

Table 3-1 **CURRENT CONCEPTUAL AND PRACTICE MODELS**

Type	Organizational Strategy	Key Concepts and Ideas
Model of Human Occupation Purpose: Establish a paradigm/conceptual framework for organizing and using interdisciplinary knowledge in occupational therapy practice (first published in 1980, see Kielhofner & Burke)		
Interdisciplinary from social sciences	Open system theory	• Occupational behavior is a result of internal and external factors, including the environment, that support and constrain behavior • Open systems theory is used to explain dynamic nature of human system in interaction with the environment • Input, throughput, output, and feedback are used to illustrate the system • Internal systems are hierarchically organized as subsystems: volition, habituation, and production • Change over time is depicted as a trajectory • Additional concepts include personal causation, interests, values, goals, habits, roles, and biopsychosocial skills
Occupational Science Purpose: To explicate the scientific, systematic study of the human as an occupational being (first published in 1991, see Clark et al.)		
Interdisciplinary	Open systems theory	• Doing as it influences health, self-respect, and sense of dignity • Occupation as unique human enterprise influenced by complexity of factors • Work, rest, leisure, and play; culturally and personally meaningful activity • Activity carries a symbolic vehicle • Occupation components: form, function, meaning, sociocultural, and historical contexts • Open systems model of subsystems: physical, biological, information processing, sociocultural, symbolic-evaluative, and transcendental

Person-Environment-Occupation Model
Purpose: To explicate the theoretical and clinical applications of person-environment interactions (first published in 1996, see Law et al.)

Multidisciplinary

- Transactional relationship between person, environment, and occupation produces occupational performance
- Occupations and roles in work and play
- Contextual influences, temporal factors, physical and psychological characteristics shape meaning and affect behavior
- Personal, social, and physical environments
- Person-environment congruence or fit. *Person*: unique, assumes roles, unique set of attributes and experiences. *Environment*: unique context for each person and included cultural, socioeconomic, institutions, physical, and social considerations
- Activity, task and occupations, temporal aspects, occupational performance

Ecology of Human Performance
Purpose: A framework providing guidelines for including context in occupational therapy research and practice (first published in 1994, see Dunn, Brown, & McGuigan)

Occupational therapy and social sciences

- Physical environment and social, cultural, and temporal factors comprise context that influences behavior and performance and key factors in assessment and intervention planning
- Interrelationships (interactional) of organisms and their environments
- Consider what the environment means for the person. Nonlinear, dynamic perspective: systems as multiply determined, complex and self-organizing.
- Components of behavior and performance: person includes experiences, skills, and abilities (sensorimotor, cognitive, psychosocial)
- Tasks: objective sets of behaviors needed to reach goal
- Environmental cues: support performance
- Context: supports performance and shapes meaning
- Life roles as constellations of tasks

(continues)

Table 3-1 **CURRENT CONCEPTUAL AND PRACTICE MODELS** *(Continued)*

Type	Organizational Strategy	Key Concepts and IdeasLife-Style Performance Model
Life-Style Performance Model Purpose: Outline personal and interpersonal aspects of daily activities and activity patterns to reflect person harmony/ disharmony or balance and to guide intervention. Create a broad, holistic practice model to guide intervention (first published in 1982, see Fidler)		
Social sciences and psychiatry as a resource for conceptualizing human behavior		• Each individual develops "patterns of doing" based on internal and external factors across four domains (self-maintenance, personal gratification, welfare of others, and interpersonal relationships) • Derive sense of satisfaction and quality of life from doing; an individual's strengths and limitations impact activity patterns (disrupt) • Model is configured to identify: relationship of activity patterns to individual needs, identity, social contributor • Holistic framework, sense of competence, adaptation, active participation, purposeful activity/occupation
Occupation Form and Performance Purpose: Establish definitions, eliminate ambiguity for occupational therapy including: occupational form, occupational performance, adaptation, meaning, and purpose in occupation. Provide a framework for applying concepts in treatment and stimulate scholarly inquiry (first published in 1988, see Nelson)		
Occupational therapy	Organizational framework	• Occupational form: pre-existing structure that elicits human performance (physical stimuli, environmental surround, human context, sociocultural reality) • Occupational performance: human actions in response to form (motor and cognitive behaviors) • Occupation: relationship between occupational form and performance • Meaning, developmental structure, purposefulness, adaptation, and levels of occupat ion needed for analysis are also considered

researchers to pursue lines of inquiry about occupation. For example, a conceptual model will define occupation and the behaviors that can be observed as occupational. In so doing, the conceptual model defines how occupational behaviors may vary when they are influenced by health, disease, and disability. Further, a conceptual model provides detailed explanations of the components or parts of occupational behaviors. These are described in detail and are linked to one another through a system of defined relationships. These organized systems of ideas allow scholars to study specific features of occupations and related behaviors and to support both research and practice efforts designed to further develop and elaborate a shared interpretation of occupation.

Frames of reference also provide a set of definitions and descriptions to guide thinking. Unlike conceptual models, a frame of reference is put in place to establish and facilitate a specific perspective on treatment and support the assessment and treatment efforts of practicing therapists. Frames of reference do not typically contain the more rigorous definition of and clarification of concepts and concept relationships that are needed for research. Rather, concept definition is provided to guide overall program development and treatment perspectives. For example, therapists who use a specific frame of reference in their practice are able to share and document an interpretation of patient problems, approaches to evaluation, program planning, and patient performance and outcomes.

Commitment to Occupation

A close look at the philosophy that forms the foundation of occupational therapy reveals an ever-present commitment to the relationship of occupation and health. The foundational concept of occupation clearly plays a part in the description of the mission of the field and the target of intervention. Patient problems were characterized as "problems of living" in early documents that carved out the need for and eventual practice of occupational therapy. Idleness, lack of activity, lost interest and motivation, loss or lack of skills and habits, and separation from the demands and rhythms of everyday life were identified as a complex of problems affecting recovery and health and the successful enactment of occupations.

To address these concerns, a therapy was called for that would use a coordinated approach with consideration for the biological, psychological, and social needs of a person. The approach would require an assessment of the individual with a deliberately planned intervention that included opportunities to engage in a variety of activities over the course of a day, those that were oriented to work, play, recreation, and rest (Figs. 3-1 and 3-2). The actual prescription for occupational therapy was carefully designed based on assessment findings. For example, patients who were anxious and overly sensitive to noise and disruption were exposed to activities that had rhythm and predictability, such as weaving. Patients who were underaroused were given more stimulating activities including outdoor work, woodworking, and metalwork. There were activities for invigorating the body, such as calisthenics and gar-

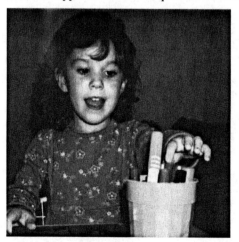

Figure 3-1. Engaging in meaningful occupation.

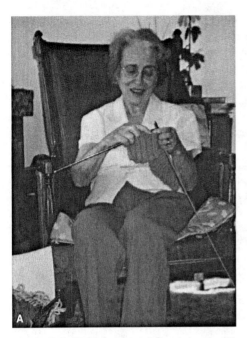
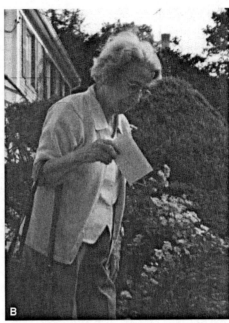

Figure 3-2. (A,B) Doing as it influence health, self-respect, and sense of dignity.

dening, as well as those that would stimulate social interaction including games, picnics, group singing, and dancing.

The basic philosophical tenets of occupational therapy continue to have an enduring presence in today's world of human health and illness. Occupation and related concepts — such as interests and individual preferences, the importance of the environment in stimulating and supporting activity, and the fit of the activity to the person — continue to be applicable to people who have problems related to disability, disease, or other chronic debilitating conditions. As a field devoted to the study of occupation, occupational therapists and occupational scientists have remained committed to the founding principles. These principles are embedded in recognition of the potency of occupation as a catalyst for health.

Adolf Meyer, an early spokesperson for the field, is credited as among those who articulated the philosophical base of occupational therapy (Table 3-2). As early as 1892-1893, he advocated for "proper use of time in some gratifying activity" as a "fundamental issue in the treatment of any neuropsychiatric patient" (Meyer, 1922/1977, p. 639). Meyer focused on problems of adaptation and called for the use of occupation as an intervention. Meyer believed that occupation would be more effective than the traditional "set of medicine and diet" that was the typical treatment of the day.

Soon after Meyer introduced systemized activity as a treatment, he made the following observations: "Groups of patients with raffia and basket work, or with various kinds of handwork and weaving and bookbinding and metal and leather work, took the place of the bored wallflowers and of mischief-makers. A pleasure in achievement, a real pleasure in the use of activity of one's hands and muscles and a happy appreciation of time began to be used as incentives in the management of our patients, instead of abstract exhortations to cheer up and to behave according to abstract or repressive rules" (Meyer, 1922/1977, p. 640).

Table 3-2 **EARLY PHILOSOPHICAL PRINCIPLES**

Use of time
Pleasure in achievement
Engagement of interest
Daily rhythm of rest and activity to maintain balance
Habit training

This first documentation of the value to be found in activity that involves time and work led Meyer to label mental problems as "problems of living." His total commitment to the potency of occupation as a modality to address mental disorders was clear in his call for "systematic engagement of interest, and concern about the actual use of TIME and work an obligation and necessity" (Meyer, 1922/1977, p. 640). With these early discoveries regarding the effects of occupation, others joined the discussion of how certain activities could be used to harness the attention and motivation of patients.

Occupations were also valued for the variation in amount and kind of activity they elicited. Some occupations were important because they were considered work, required the person to be attentive and directed, and evoked a feeling of accomplishment. Others were considered recreation; this would include hobbies that allowed for feelings of pleasure in doing and the opportunity for self-expression. Similarly, activities that were characterized as rest and self-maintenance were also valued, because they filled out the normal round of daily activities that were important for a person to master if he or she was to live an independent life.

The importance of habits and habit training was recognized by early occupational therapists including Eleanor Clarke Slagle and Thomas Kidner (Kidner, 1925, 1930; Slagle, 1922). They focused on habit training as a method for developing needed skills in patients. Habits were considered the basic structures that were needed to support everyday routines of living. In a sense, the automatic nature of habits provided the fuel for everyday actions in everyday environments.

Occupational therapy emerged in the United States as a focused effort for intervention with patients who had "mental disorders" during the early 1900s, when attitudes and actions toward individuals with mental diseases were changing. In the introduction of the *Occupational Therapy Source Book* (1948), the role of occupational therapy in the recovery of a patient was reflected on by Dr. Burlingame, Psychiatrist in Chief of the Institute of Living in Hartford, Connecticut. He viewed occupational therapists as able to prepare patients to "take their places as constructive members of society" (Burlingame, 1948, p. iii). He wrote, "Certainly if inactivity, mental or physical, exerts a desocializing influence because it is foreign to 'normal' living, it follows that anything foreign to normal living contains the same insidious factor. Thus, we know that our patients must not only be kept busy, but that they must be kept busy in a constructive manner, in some way that will prepare them better to take their places as constructive members of society" (Burlingame, 1948, p. iii).

Contemporary Iterations of Philosophical Principles in Occupational Therapy

Occupational therapists and occupational scientists continue to be committed to a thorough understanding of the relationship of occupation to both physical and mental health in their current scholarship and research. Contemporary scholars are exploring these principles through research efforts that explore and describe occupation in specific groups of individuals as well as facilitate the development of conceptual and practice models (Table 3-3 provides some contemporary examples).

A Holistic View of the Person

A significant, core principle that underscores all conceptual and practice models in occupational therapy is holism. This principle emphasizes the importance of considering the person as a whole, with a range of internal influences on behavior. Such a perspective underscores the complexity of human behavior and rejects a mechanistic view of the person. A holistic, multidimensional view includes full consideration of physical, social, cognitive, psychological, and spiritual factors as shaping behavior. It is the combination of these factors that presents a unique profile of a person. In addition to an understanding of each person as a combination of influences, occupational therapists also view an individual as unique in the occupational roles that he or she selects to enact in everyday life, thus adding another dimension to the profile of a person.

The use of organizational concepts, such as systems thinking and systems theory, have been helpful in hypothesizing about the ways multidimensional human systems — in conjunction with an external environment — work and how such information can be explained and organized.

Table 3-3   PRINCIPLES AND COMPONENTS OF CONTEMPORARY OCCUPATIONAL THERAPY AND OCCUPATIONAL SCIENCE

Principles	Components
Holistic view of the person	The importance of considering the physical, social, cognitive, psychological, and spiritual dimensions of each person
Occupational behavior	A focus on the behavior that occurs based on the kinds of internal and external factors influencing a person; also referred to as occupational performance and occupational role performance
Influence of culture on occupation	An understanding of the role of culture in informing and shaping an individual's perception of occupationally relevant roles and behaviors; an understanding of the importance of culturally specific rituals, symbols, and meanings
Dynamic relationship between the person and environment	The importance of environment in supporting occupation and the feelings of competence and well-being that result from success in occupation
Emphasis on the uniqueness of the individual	A commitment to the uniqueness of each individual; the use of interest, motivation, and novelty as instigators of occupation
Significance of occupation to health and well-being	This includes consideration of a number of behaviors including competence, achievement, motivation, doing, and active engagement in meaningful and purposeful activity that occur in conjunction with occupation

Occupational Behavior

Occupational behaviors are manifested in regularly occurring activities that take place throughout the day, week, month, and year. They are composed of the skilled actions and habits that are part of one's work, play, leisure and recreation, self-care, and life management roles. For individuals to enact their chosen occupational roles, they must have the requisite set(s) of skills and habits (patterns of behaviors) that support everyday occupational behaviors (Fig. 3-3). For example, to enact the role of a fifth grade student, one must have skills in areas such as handling common classroom objects (paper, pencil, books, backpack) as well as effectively moving in the environment, listening, attending, and other cognitive skills to support learning, social and behavior skills, and communication skills. Similarly, those skills must be sufficiently developed to form patterns of behavior or habits that will support everyday enactment of the behaviors. Habits become automatic, to some extent, when they are used regularly.

Influence of Culture on Occupation

Similar to the appreciation of each individual as unique, occupational therapists subscribe to an understanding of the important and powerful role of culture. Culture provides scaffolding for informing and shaping an individual's perception of the different roles and behaviors that are important in the social group. Culture influences an individual's recognition and selection of valued occupational roles and behaviors (and the importance of specific rituals and symbols that accompany those roles and behaviors) (Fig. 3-4).

Dynamic Relationship Between the Person and the Environment

Occupational therapists continue to recognize the role of human and nonhuman environments in supporting or suppressing occupational behavior. Ideas such as the "just right challenge," grading activities, adapting the environment, context, environmental press, and ther-

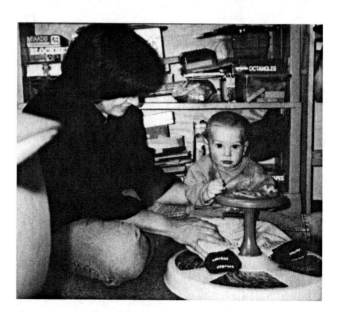

Figure 3-3. Carefully balancing environmental demands.

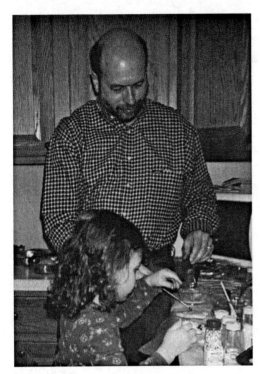

Figure 3-4. Cultural influences on roles and behaviors

apeutic use of self are examples of the attention that occupational scientists and therapists give to the environment when occupational performance is being developed. In addition to assessing an individual's strengths and weaknesses, therapists will often assess the human and nonhuman environments. Along with direct intervention for person-oriented skills, changes in the environment are also very much the purview of occupational therapy.

Emphasis on the Uniqueness of the Individual

Occupational therapy practice and conceptual models continue to emphasize a commitment to the uniqueness of each individual and the importance of assessing and intervening based on individually designed plans. The idea of patent plans or pathways for treating a condition are rejected based on their failure to consider individuals and what will be specifically meaningful to them. Careful consideration of a person's patterns of interests, motivation, values, and goals provides a platform for launching a specific plan of action. By taking the time to develop a profile of the individual, the therapist is able to select and use objects and activities that will create a sense of novelty and thus instigate behaviors associated with occupation. The complexity of reasoning and judgments that must be made by a therapist during this aspect of care has gained increasing attention in the literature associated with clinical reasoning and clinical mastery (Burke & DePoy, 1991; Mattingly & Fleming, 1994).

Significance of Occupation to Health and Well-being

Perhaps one of the most compelling, yet least understood, principles of occupational science and occupational therapy concerns the way occupation triggers feelings of health and well-being. Outcomes of occupation-oriented activities, those that have embedded meaning for an individual person, have been noted to produce feelings of competence, a sense of being effective, a sense of achievement, and the adaptive response. Of note is the difficulty that occupational scientists and occupational therapists have had in carefully measuring this effect. This difficulty has been speculated to be in part due to the widespread effect of occupation-oriented intervention on the person and their occupational performance (Burke, 1996; Wood, 1996). Emerging evidence of the relationship between active engagement in personally meaningful and purposeful activity promises to demonstrate methods that can be used to understand such effects (Clark et al., 1997; Zimmerer-Branum & Nelson, 1995).

SUMMARY

The philosophical principles that provided the impetus for the development of the field of occupational therapy have proven timeless in their utility for understanding how humans find meaning in their everyday lives through active engagement in activity. Because of this initial commitment to the power of activity, generations of practitioners, scholars, and researchers have elaborated on the human and nonhuman factors that affect occupational performance. For many, the notions and ideas that are embedded in occupational science and occupational therapy are "common sense." Yes, indeed they are. For those of us who regularly experience the pleasure of doing, the feelings of pride and enjoyment, the suspension of time, and the release from the more basic pressures of place and person, these ideas are second nature. However, that knowledge, that common sense understanding, comes with the successful experience of occupation that is not so common in populations throughout the world. For many, the complications of physical and psychological stressors, environmental demands and constraints, and limited opportunities for development of skills and habits have made the acquisition and use of this common sense knowledge out of reach. It is because of these human failures and struggles that occupational scientists and therapists have come to understand the complexity that is embedded in the common sense principles of occupation.

STUDY QUESTIONS

3-1. What is a philosophy? Why is a philosophical basis critical for a profession?

3-2. Of what purpose is a conceptual model? Of what purpose is a frame of reference? How are they similar? How are they different?

3-3. Does this chapter discuss occupation as a process or as a product? Explain.

3-4. Discuss holism in relation to occupational therapy and occupational science.

3-5. What role do habits play in occupational behavior?

3-6. What role does culture play in occupational behavior?

3-7. Speculate about the role of occupation in health and well-being. How could you begin to support or provide evidence to back up your speculations?

3-8. Occupational therapy has been referred to as a profession of common sense. Explain and justify this statement.

References

American College Dictionary. (1964). New York: Random House.

Burke, J. P. (1996). Moving occupation into treatment: Clinical interpretation of "legitimizing occupational therapy's knowledge". *American Journal of Occupational Therapy, 50,* 635–638.

Burke, J. P., & DePoy, E. (1991). An emerging view of mastery, excellence, and leadership in occupational therapy practice. *American Journal of Occupational Therapy, 45,* 1027–1032.

Burlingame, C. C. (1948). Foreword. In S. Licht (Ed.), *Occupational therapy source book.* Baltimore, MD: Williams & Wilkins.

Clark, F. A., Azen, S. P., Zemke, R., Jackson, J., Carlson, M., Mandel, D., Hay, J., Josephson, K., Cherry, B., Hessel, C., Palmer, J., & Lipson, L., (1997). Occupational therapy for independent-living older adults: A randomized controlled trial. *Journal of the American Medical Association, 278,* 1321–1326.

Clark, F. A., Parham, D., Carlson, M., Frank, G., Jackson, J., Pierce, D., Wolfe, R., & Zemke, R. (1991). Occupational science: Academic innovation in the service of occupational therapy's future. *American Journal of Occupational Therapy, 45,* 300–310.

Dunn, W., Brown, C., & McGuigan, A. (1994). The ecology of human performance: A framework for considering the effect of context. *American Journal of Occupational Therapy, 48,* 595–607.

Fidler, G. S. (1982). The life style performance profile: An organizing frame. In B. Hemphill (Ed.), *The evaluation process in occupational therapy.* Thorofare, NJ: Slack.

Kidner, T. B. (1925). The hospital pre-industrial shop. *Occupational Therapy and Rehabilitation, 4,* 187–188.

Kidner, T. B. (1930). *Occupational therapy: The science of prescribed work for invalids.* New York: W. Kohlhammer/Stuttgart.

Kielhofner, G., & Burke, J. P. (1980). A model of human occupation: Part I. Conceptual framework and content. *American Journal of Occupational Therapy, 34,* 572–581.

Law, M., Cooper, B., Strong, S., Stewart, D., Rigby, P., & Letts, L. (1996). The person-environment-occupation model: A transactive approach to occupational performance. *Canadian Journal of Occupational Therapy, 63,* 9–23.

Mattingly, C., & Fleming, M. (1994). *Clinical reasoning: Forms of inquiry in a therapeutic practice.* Philadelphia, PA: F.A. Davis.

Meyer, A. (1922/1977) The philosophy of occupational therapy. *American Journal of Occupational Therapy, 31,* 639–642.

Nelson, D. (1988) Occupation: Form and performance. *American Journal of Occupational Therapy, 42,* 633–641.

Slagle, E. C. (1922). Training aides for mental patients. *Archives of Occupational Therapy, 1,* 11–17.

Wood, W. (1996). Legitimizing occupational therapy's knowledge. *American Journal of Occupational Therapy, 50,* 626–634.

Zimmerer-Branum, S., & Nelson, D. (1995). Occupationally embedded exercise versus rote exercise: A choice between occupational forms by elderly nursing home residents. *American Journal of Occupational Therapy, 49,* 397–634.

4

Model of Human Occupation

Kirsty Forsyth and Gary Kielhofner

OBJECTIVES

This chapter will help you to:

- Discuss the three Model of Human Occupation constructs: person, environment, and occupational performance.
- Differentiate among the three components of the person construct: volition, habituation, and performance capacity.
- Characterize these volition aspects: causation, values, and interests.
- Distinguish habits from roles as aspects of habituation.
- Discriminate between the physical and social aspects of the environment construct.
- Explain participation, occupational forms, and skills as aspects of the occupational performance construct.
- Apply the Model of Human Occupation to practice situations.
- Describe various Model of Human Occupation resources for practice.

⌐ABOUT THE AUTHORS

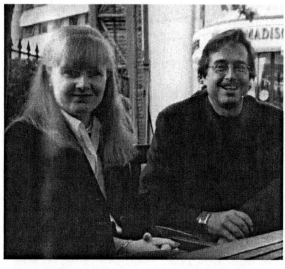

Kirsty and Gary enjoying a break at a cafe in the United Kingdom.

Gary was introduced to occupational therapy while running a recreational program out of an occupational therapy department. At the time, he was a conscientious objector who had an interest in pursuing a political science degree with a focus on peace studies. His background in philosophy and theology as well as his interest in psychology led him to become intrigued with what was going on during occupational therapy. This led to his pursuit of professional education in occupational therapy. However, his initial experiences in occupational therapy education were disillusioning to the point that he contemplated pursuing another career. Fortuitously, he met Dr. Mary Reilly at an AOTA conference and decided to drop out of the occupational therapy program in which he was enrolled and begin his studies again with Dr. Reilly.

He credits Dr. Reilly with providing him with commitment and value for occupational therapy: "There was something about the way that Reilly thought and the way that she processed ideas that I really got! And that I liked!" Gary's devotion to practice has been with him since these early experiences. When talking about his early experiences at the University of Southern California, he describes the importance of being able to relate what he was learning to practice. Based on these experiences, in 1980 he published — with Janice Burke and Cindy Igi Heard — a series of articles about a model of human occupation that could be used to address the gap between occupational behavior and practice. This focus on the relationship of theory to practice characterizes his professional career.

Gary describes himself as a visual thinker who is creative not only in intellectual work but also in management. He sees the big picture and has the ability to articulate it. His ideal is to develop knowledge in concert with practice. He believes that the profession needs to focus on occupation and to create a strong empirically supported practice that uses meaningful occupations to help people with disabilities. Consistent with this belief, he has continually worked closely with clinicians to develop sound clinical assessments and articulate theoretically based protocols for intervention. His advice for students is as follows:

> Everybody participates in the foundations of the field. The story about the client that I saw last week is just as contextually valuable as the published set of theoretical concepts. So I try to give students a perspective that from the very beginning that they are going to learn theory. And the reason they are learning theory is as language — and as a lens through which they are going to see their practice. Students need to learn about theories for them to become alive. Theories have got to be in their heads, in their hearts, theory has got to be driving how students see clients, what they understand about clients, what they do with clients, . . . if theory is not an active thinking tool then that is a real problem. I really believe it is really important for the students to become active consumers of theory. So that they can hold theories accountable. It is sort of like a mechanic, if you give him a broken wrench, or a wrench that doesn't work, he's going to say, "This damn thing doesn't work. I can't use this!" And I think that clinicians ought to say the same thing (personal interview, 2001).

Commitment to theory and practice continues to be the focus of Gary's work and refinement of the Model of Human Occupation. With his colleagues, he is systematically applying theory in practice. Some questions being explored are the following. What is the actual mechanism for change? How does it change? Why does it change? What do you do? What does the client do? When something does not change, why does it not change? While trying to understand the underlying process, he and his colleagues are currently engaged in ongoing research on these issues, producing protocols for intervention, starting to test these interventions empirically, and publishing the results.

As he looks to the future, Gary is thinking about who will continue his work. One key person is Kirsty Forsyth. Kirsty received her occupational therapy degree at Queen Margaret's College in Scotland. She then attended the University of Illinois, where she earned a post-professional master's degree and expanded her knowledge about the Model of Human Occupation. When she completed her degree, Gary encouraged her to continue working toward a doctorate. Instead of continuing right away, she went back to Scotland to apply what she had learned. A few months later, she contacted Gary and enrolled in a doctoral program to learn longitudinal research and sophisticated statistical designs. After completing her doctorate, Kirsty then continued in a part-time post-doctoral program in addition to teaching at Queen Margaret's College.

INTRODUCTION

During the 1960s and 1970s, Dr. Mary Reilly led the development of the occupational behavior tradition that aimed to recapture the field's focus on occupation as the media and method of the field (Reilly, 1962; Reilly, 1969). The occupational behavior tradition was pivotal in returning occupational therapy's paradigm to a focus on occupation (Kielhofner, 1997). Much of current occupation-focused theory and practice of the field today stem from this perspective.

The Model of Human Occupation grew out of this occupational behavior tradition. Originally, three of Reilly's students (Kielhofner, Burke, and Heard), who were concerned with how the concepts of occupational behavior could be more directly applied in practice, set out to articulate a conceptual model of practice. Consistent with the occupational behavior tradition, one goal of the conceptual model of practice was to provide a deeper understanding of the nature of occupation in human life and its role in health and illness. However, the main emphasis of the model was to synthesize many of the themes of occupational behavior into a framework suitable to guide practice. In contrast to the occupational behavior tradition, which aimed to capture a wide range of themes to characterize occupational therapy's fundamental nature and mission, the model sought to be a tool of everyday practitioners. During the time the conceptual model of practice was first developed and prepared for publication, its three original authors were working as practitioners. To this day, one of the central features of this conceptual model of practice is the extent to which practitioners shape how its theory is articulated and applied.

The basic outline of the conceptual model of practice was originally expressed in an unpublished Master's thesis (Kielhofner, 1975). The conceptual model of practice was first published 5 years later, after refining the concepts and experimenting with them in practice (Kielhofner, 1980a, 1980b; Kielhofner & Burke, 1980; Kielhofner, Burke, & Heard, 1980). In 1985 the book, *A Model of Human Occupation: Theory and Application*, introduced an expanded theory and a wide range of clinical applications (Kielhofner, 1985). A revision of the conceptual model of practice was completed in 1995 with the publication of the second edition of this book. The third edition was published in 2002. *A Model of Human Occupation: Theory and Application* is the authoritative and most current understanding of this theory and its application. It is the primary reference on the conceptual model of practice. This text is a necessary resource for therapists who wish to apply the Model of Human Occupation to their work.

Other published literature on the Model of Human Occupation provides additional, rich sources of theoretical discourse, discussions of programmatic applications, cases examples, and research findings. The literature on this model is extensive and worldwide. More than 235 articles and chapters discussing theoretical, applied, or research aspects of the model have been published in the English language. The Model of Human Occupation Clearinghouse, maintained at the University of Illinois at Chicago, distributes a wide range of materials, including assessment manuals, case videotapes, and other monographs detailing application of the model. Information on the Clearinghouse can also found on the website. A current bibliography of literature on the model can be found at http:/www.uic.edu/hsc/acad/cahp/OT/MOHOC.

This chapter provides an overview of the Model of Human Occupation theoretical constructs, resources, and case materials. Additional literature on the model can be found in the bibliography and at the website mentioned previously.

MODEL OF HUMAN OCCUPATION: THEORETICAL CONSTRUCTS

A conceptual model of practice proposes theory to address certain phenomena with which the model is concerned (Kielhofner, 1997). The Model of Human Occupation provides theory aimed at explaining aspects of healthy occupation and problems that arise in association with illness and disability. Its concepts address the:

- Motivation for occupation
- Routine patterning of occupational behavior
- Nature of skilled performance
- Influence of environment on occupation

As a conceptual model of practice, the Model of Human Occupation should be constantly tested empirically and revised to reflect both research findings and theoretical developments in related interdisciplinary concepts on which the model is based. The theoretical arguments underpinning this model are currently undergoing major revisions. Therefore, the presentation of the Model of Human Occupation below is based on existing published literature but also points to new developments. The following sections address the main conceptual ideas in the Model of Human Occupation: (1) how occupation is organized, (2) components of the person, (3) environment, and (4) occupational performance.

How Occupation Is Organized

The Model of Human Occupation asserts that what a person does in work, play, and self-care is a function of motivational factors, life patterns, performance capacity, and environmental influences. Because the Model of Human Occupation includes such a wide range of concerns in its theoretical constructs, it must relate these diverse constructs together. The model has consistently drawn on contemporary systems theory to consider how the many factors that contribute to occupation are organized together. The model's systems view of the human being has traditionally emphasized two main points.

The first point is that behavior is dynamic and context-dependent. That is, a person's inner characteristics interact with the environment to create a network of conditions that influence how one is motivated, what one does, and how one performs.

The second point is that occupation is essential to self-organization. That is, by doing things people shape who they are. For example, in doing things, people engage in occupations and thus maintain or alter their capacities and generate ongoing experiences that affirm or reshape their motivation. Therefore, how each of us is put together is a reflection of what we have done in the past. People become, to an extent, what they do.

Consistent with this principle, the model views therapy as a process in which people are helped to do things in order to shape their abilities, self-concepts, and identities. Occupational therapy engages people in occupational behavior, which helps to maintain, restore, or reorganize their occupational lives.

Components of the Person

To explain how occupational behavior is chosen, patterned, and performed, the Model of Human Occupation depicts the human as composed of three elements: volition, habituation, and performance capacity. Volition refers to the process by which persons are motivated toward and choose what they do. Habituation refers to a process whereby doing is organized into patterns and routines. Performance capacity refers both to the underlying objective mental and physical abilities as well as the lived experience that shapes performance. Each of these three components of the person will be discussed in more detail.

Volition

Choices for Action

Decisions about what to do shape the content of our unfolding hours, days, and weeks. Although some aspects of each day will be part of a routine (and thus governed by habituation), there are throughout each day opportunities to decide what to do next, when to terminate an activity, and when to go on to another. These kinds of everyday decisions are referred to as activity choices. Examples of activity choices are when we chose one activity over another, such as deciding to go out for dinner with a friend versus eating at home while watching television, or going for a walk versus reading the newspaper. Other activity choices occur spontaneously when opportunity emerges, such as the child who wakes to a new snowfall and heads out to play.

Individuals also make larger choices concerning occupations that will become an extended or permanent part of their lives. This kind of decision is called an occupational choice. Occupational choices involve commitments to enter into a course of action or to sustain regular performance over time. Examples of occupational choices are decisions to enter an occupational role such as becoming a student or a parent, or taking a job. Another example of an occupational choice is joining a health club to exercise regularly, taking up a new hobby, or undertaking a project like painting one's house or apartment. Together, activity choices and occupational choices influence, to a large extent, what kinds of things we do in our daily lives. These choices are a function of volition.

Drive for Action

Volition begins with the drive for action that all humans inherit as a function of their complex nervous systems. Evolution has programmed humans to have a strong desire to do things. However, what each individual ultimately is motivated to do depends on highly personal characteristics. These will now be described.

Volitional Thoughts and Feelings

At the core of volition are thoughts and feelings about doing things, such as enjoying, valuing, and feeling competent. These thoughts and feelings are shaped by previous experience, interpretation of that experience, and anticipation of the future (Fig. 4-1). For example, our feeling of attraction to doing some leisure occupation, such as hiking in the woods, might be based on the experience of satisfaction or pleasure in doing it as well as the subsequent recognition that we liked it because it provided contact with nature, exercise, and quiet time for reflection. Given that experience and interpretation, we are more likely to look for (anticipate) opportunities to do the same or similar occupations in the future and to choose to do so when there is opportunity. As this example points out, volitional thoughts and feelings and the choices they influence are part of an ongoing process. The process of anticipating, choosing, experiencing, and interpreting occupational behavior represents an ongoing cycle that can sustain or alter our motivation. Thus, for example, the child who is good at and enjoys sports will choose to participate in sports, generally enjoy them, and do well, thus reinforcing the interest. Some middle-aged persons, who have engaged in sports all their lives, will begin to experience decreased physical capacity and pain that may lead them to reconsider their enjoyment and capacity and thus make new choices in the future. Persons with illness or trauma that alters their capacities significantly may have dramatically altered experiences and have to radically rethink what they can and want to do.

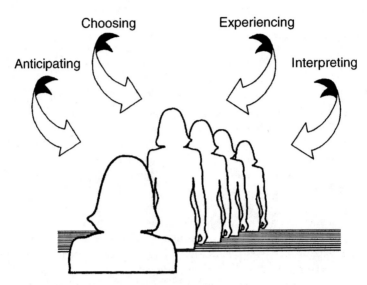

Figure 4-1. Volitional Process: Reflecting on Self in Action over Time. Reprinted with permission from Kielhofner, G. (1995). *A model of human occupation: Theory and application* (2nd ed.). Baltimore, MD: Williams & Wilkins.

Content of Volitional Thoughts and Feelings

The thoughts and feelings we have about doing things ultimately turn on the issues of our own mastery, enjoyment, and valuation of what we have done. Consequently, volitional thoughts and feelings pertain to:

- How effective one is in acting on the world
- What one holds as important
- What one finds enjoyable and satisfying

These three areas are referred to as personal causation, values, and interests, respectively. Each is discussed below.

Personal Causation. We all observe ourselves through the common sense lenses of our cultures, building up a store of knowledge about what kind of capacities we have in relationship to what our context demands and expects of us. As we do things, we generate thoughts along with feelings of confidence or insecurity about our physical, mental, or social abilities. We reflect on how effective we are in using our capacities to achieve our desired outcomes. Consequently, we also develop thoughts and feelings about how effective we are in using our capacities and how compliant or resistant life is to our efforts. These are all components of personal causation.

Personal causation is reflected in our awareness of present and potential abilities and our sense of how able we are to bring about what we want. As previously mentioned, personal causation is always situated in one's particular context. Our own culture and social environment tell us what capacities we should have and why they matter. A performer on stage, a taxi driver in a large city, a grade school teacher, and a farmer in the countryside will each be concerned about very different kinds abilities. Whether they emphasize and care about personal expressiveness, physical strength, social skills, or mental skills will depend on what others in their everyday work care about and what they need to be able to do to complete their work.

Similarly, the course of development results in changing concerns about capacity. For a small child, achieving milestones like walking are occasions when a new sense of power is realized and there is significant social recognition of competence. Soon these milestones become taken for granted and new challenges that result in success or failure shape personal causation. For example, performance in sports, school achievement, and skill in interacting with peers become paramount issues of personal causation in later childhood. In adult life productive employment is often a dominant concern, and our performance in a work situation has a large impact on our feelings of competence and efficacy. In old age, personal causation can become dominated with feelings of loss of capacity and control. Consequently, personal causation is never static, but rather a dynamic unfolding set of thoughts and feelings about our capacities and our efficacy in achieving what we want. As we proceed through life, new experiences can alter our views of our capabilities and how they matter.

Our unique personal causation influences how we anticipate, choose, experience, and interpret what we do. We feel confident or insecure about our physical, intellectual, or interpersonal abilities. Consequently, we tend to choose to do things that provide opportunities to use those capacities and to avoid tasks that are likely to overtax our capacities. When we know ourselves to be capable and skilled, we are disposed to act and generate further evidence of our ability. When we know ourselves to be incapable, we feel compelled in the opposite direction. Consequently, the thoughts and feelings that make up personal causation are powerful motivational influences.

Values. Choices for occupations are also influenced by our values. Values are composed of beliefs and commitments that define what is good, right, and important. They influence our view of what is worth doing and what is the proper way to act. Values are felt as obligations, and we cannot behave contrary to values without feeling guilty or inadequate (Bruner, 1990). Conversely, we experience a sense of belonging and correctness when following values.

Our values derive from our context. From childhood on, we interact with a cultural milieu that embodies values within a coherent worldview. Values are expressed in the common sense of that world and the kind of life that persons in that cultural world lead (Bruner, 1990). These values define what is good, right, and important, serving as principles to guide human conduct (Grossack & Gardner, 1970; Kalish & Collier, 1981; Klavins, 1972; Lee, 1971; Smith, 1969). For example, an elderly person's values may be organized around a traditional small town viewpoint with its own definitions of right and wrong connected to a religion-based view of what is important. A very different set of convictions may underlie an adolescent living in the inner city who learns on the street a code of gang solidarity, territoriality, survival by aggression, and other non-mainstream views of life. Whereas these perspectives are clearly distinct, each represents a value-laden way of viewing self and world.

Thus, values specify for an individual what is worth doing, how one ought to perform, and what goals or aspirations deserve one's commitment. Values belong to a common sense, cultural view of life and are usually associated with strong emotions (e.g., feelings of security, worthiness, belonging, or accomplishment). Persons perceive value when they see a course of action as how one ought to act (Lee, 1971).

Values determine one's view of the worth of different occupations. Therefore, values influence the sense of self-worth that one derives from succeeding at occupations. For example, in a family in which academic achievement is valued, a child who does well in school is more likely to evaluate himself positively.

Interests. Interests begin with natural dispositions (e.g., the tendency to enjoy physical or intellectual activity). They further develop through the acquisition of tastes. Consequently, interests are generated from the experience of pleasure and satisfaction in engaging in occupations (Matsutsuyu, 1969). Therefore, the development of interests depends on available opportunities to engage in occupations.

Being interested in an occupation means that one feels an attraction based on anticipation of a positive experience. This attraction may come from positive feelings associated with the exercise of capacity, intellectual or physical challenge, fellowship with others, aesthetic stimulation, or other factors. We are more likely to enjoy what we can perform with some level of proficiency when skill is involved in the performance. Csikszentmihalyi (1990) describes flow, a form of ultimate enjoyment in activities that occurs when a person's capacities are optimally challenged.

Other pleasures associated with the performance of occupations may emanate from sensory pleasures that arise during performance (we may enjoy how tools feel in our hands, how our cooking smells, the visual pleasure of country scenery on a hike or bicycle ride, and even the vestibular pleasure associated with such activities as snow skiing). Interest may emerge from aesthetic arousal or intellectual intrigue such as that we may gain from painting or reading a book. Since many occupations produce outcomes or products, satisfaction may emanate from what we have accomplished or produced. One may find a craft particularly satisfying because of the pleasing or useful product that results. Enjoyment may come from the sense of association and fellowship experienced in occupations performed with others. Attraction to any particular occupation most likely represents a confluence of several of these factors.

As they develop, people form a propensity to enjoy particular ways of performing or particular activities over others. This preference is often manifested as a pattern of related interests such as athletic interest or cultural interests, including theater and art. On the other hand, persons may have very diverse and seemingly unrelated preferences. Preferring certain occupations over others influences what we chose to do.

Summary. We have seen that volition is a pattern of thoughts and feelings concerning the occupations in which we engage. These volitional thoughts and feelings are imbedded in a cycle of anticipation, choice, experience while doing, and subsequent interpretation. Our volition predisposes us to attend to the world and anticipate possibilities for action in particular ways. That is, our attraction to occupations, beliefs about capacity, and convictions about performance first and foremost influence what we notice and search out in the world. They also influence what we are likely to feel or think about prospects for involvement in the occupational opportunities we encounter. We tend to be unaware of that in which we have no volitional investment and, conversely, more versed in what corresponds to our competence, interests, and commitments. This means that what is "out there" in the world for people is very much a function of how their volition is organized. In the same way, our choices for what occupations to engage in and who we want to become are a function of our volition.

Volition influences how we experience occupational forms. Over the course of time we engage in a variety of occupations, which we find more or less enjoyable or valuable and in which we feel more or less able. Volition also influences how we interpret our actions and experience. Our values may have an important influence on the meanings we assign to what we do. For example, the high school senior who is committed to going to college will interpret a "C" grade differently from the one who envisions himself working as a carpenter in 3 months. In similar fashion, personal causation can influence how one interprets performance. An individual who does not believe he can influence his grade outcomes is more likely to assign the outcome of a good grade to luck and a bad grade to teacher bias. Experience is thus filtered through a process of sense-making that emanates from our particular volitional organization. Volition is more than an aggregate of feelings and thoughts about competence, values, and interests. It is an interrelated worldview in which themes of personal causation, value, and interest function as common sense comprehensions of self and the world.

Volition, Disability, and Therapy

The role of volition in the lives of persons with disabilities may vary widely depending on the nature of a person's impairment and lifestyle. Volition may lead to activities and occupational choices that are the sources of dysfunction. Acquired impairments may threaten and alter previously positive volition and can lead to a downward spiral into helplessness and demoralization. An example is the young father who worked in a physically demanding job and then sustained an on-the-job injury that resulted in chronic disabling back pain. He was no longer able to do the work he had enjoyed. He could no longer function as the primary bread winner of the family. His former hobby of body-building was disrupted, and his self-image as someone who was physically strong and athletic eroded. His relationship with his son, which had been based on their doing sports activities together, began to deteriorate. As a result of the convergence of these factors he became increasingly withdrawn, depressed, and focused on his pain.

As the example illustrates, the impact of impairments on personal causation, interests, and values can lead to a breakdown of morale and motivation in the individual. The future can seem bleak with goals obliterated, pleasure in activity diminished, and meaning and purpose in life eroded. When persons perceive that they have little or no possibility of influencing the course of their lives, they will not make adaptive choices.

Volition is also central to any process of adjusting to or overcoming the challenges of a disability. For example, to adjust to significant impairments, people must come to terms with their remaining abilities and limitations. They must find new ways to achieve satisfaction and enjoyment in life. They must recreate, to an extent, the common sense world of values in which they previously existed.

For those whose disability brings loss and suffering, volition can offer a means of finding a place in life. For example, the novelist Price (1994) describes how his ability to cope with quadriplegia and chronic pain from a spinal tumor is tied to his passion for writing. The centrality of volition in therapy and in adaptation to disability is evident if we consider that the capacity for engaging in occupations means little if a person does not choose to use that capacity. Nor will people seek to develop new capacities or make adjustments for limitations unless they can see these efforts as providing one occasion to undertake a life with value and satisfaction.

Habituation

The habituation subsystem organizes occupational behavior into the recurrent patterns of behavior that make up much of our daily routines. These patterns integrate us into the rhythms and customs of our physical, social, and temporal worlds. Moreover, they allow us to efficiently and automatically do what we regularly do.

Habituation connects us to and makes us functional within our habits (i.e., through familiar social scene, physical context, and weekly schedule). Habituation also depends on and uses the regularity in our environments to guide how we behave. Thus, the rhythms of day and night and of the week, the patterned comings and goings of others, and the stability of the physical environment are all the foundation on which habituation is built.

Habituated behavior is not mechanically produced according to internal instructions. Rather, habituation relies on an appreciation or an ability to appraise the action-significance of our environment and what goes on within it. For example, we unthinkingly recognize the appearance of an acquaintance as occasion for a greeting, the buzzing of our alarm clock as time to rise, or the approaching landmark as the place to make a left turn on the way to work. Such appreciations enable us, without deliberation or attention, to do what has become habituated in the right way, place, and time.

Habituated patterns of doing are established by repeated action. By virtue of developing a way of doing something likely to be repeated again and again, habituation evokes the very actions that sustain it. Hence, altering what has become habituated is very difficult.

Habituated patterns of action are governed by habits and roles. Together, they weave the patterns with which we typically traverse our days, weeks, and seasons; our homes, neighborhoods, and cities; and our families, work organizations, and communities. In each of these temporal, physical, and social contexts we engage in a wide range of occupations. Habits and roles give regularity, character, and order to what we do and how we do it.

Habits

Habits involve learned ways of doing occupations that unfold automatically (Fig. 4-2). Through repeated experience, a person acquires a way of understanding and behaving in familiar environments. Although habits do regulate behavior according to some kind of broad pattern or template, habitual behavior requires improvisation to accommodate the inevitable novel elements of each new behavioral situation. Dewey (1922) recognized that habits operate in cooperation with context: "Habits are ways of using and incorporating the environment in which the latter has its say as surely as the former" (p. 15). This means that a habit regulates behavior not by strict instructions for behavior, but by providing a

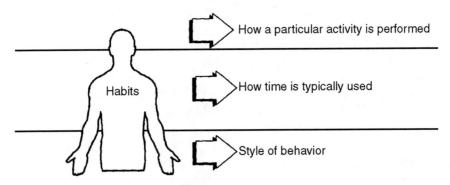

Habits

How a particular activity is performed

How time is typically used

Style of behavior

Figure 4-2. Influence of Habits on Occupation. Reprinted with permission from Kielhofner, G. (1995). *A model of human occupation: Theory and application* (2nd ed.). Baltimore, MD: Williams & Wilkins.

manner of dealing with environmental contingencies. Habits give us our bearings, locating us in unfolding events and allowing us to steer our behavior to the next occurrences that we tacitly anticipate.

Roles

People see themselves as students, workers, parents, etc. and recognize that they should behave in certain ways to enact these roles. Much of what we do is done as a spouse, parent, worker, student, and so on. The presence of these and other roles help assure that what we do has both regularity and relevance to appropriate social systems (Fig. 4-3).

The expectations that others hold for a role and the nature of the social system in which each role is located serve as guides for learning how to behave within that role. Thus, through interaction with others, one internalizes an identity, an outlook, and a way of behaving that belongs to the role. Once internalized, this role serves as a kind of framework for looking out on the world and for acting. Thus, when one is engaging in an occupation within a given role, it may be reflected in how the person dresses, the demeanor of the person, the content of the person's actions, and so on. We need only reflect on how we behave within our worker role versus our role as a parent, spouse, or friend to see how the role we are in shapes our behavior.

Roles not only shape what we do and how we look out onto the world. They also profoundly influence our sense of who we are. We see ourselves as students, workers, parents, friends, and other roles because we recognize ourselves as occupying a certain status or position and also because we experience our selves behaving through these roles. Seeing ourselves reflected in the attitudes and behaviors of others toward us also shapes the identity we derive from our roles (Sarbin & Scheibe, 1983). We all tend to see each other in terms of the roles we hold. Seeing a boss, teacher, or colleague outside the ordinary context in which these roles are played out can seem oddly strange at first, because we are accustomed to seeing these other people in terms of their roles.

Summary. Habituation regulates the patterned, familiar, and routine features of what we do. It involves an appreciative process though which we more or less automatically recognize features and situations in the environment and construct a routine that collaborates with those aspects of the environment. Habituation always involves transaction between the habit and/or roles we have internalized and the unfolding events and external context.

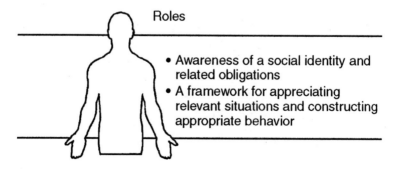

Figure 4-3. Roles. Reprinted with permission from Kielhofner, G. (1995). *A model of human occupation: Theory and application* (2nd ed.). Baltimore, MD: Williams & Wilkins.

When a habit or role is invalidated or terminated, a degree of disorientation and disorganization can follow. For example, if we change jobs, then the familiar route to work, the pattern of relationships with others, the times when we get up in the morning and when we return home from work, and a host of other daily details may change. Until we have waded through the new circumstances enough times to establish new roles and habits, we will need to put forth extra effort and attention. What was formerly familiar and comfortable becomes, at least temporarily, awkward and uneasy.

The extra effort and attention that is required during times of change in our habituation points to the important role of habituation in allowing our everyday action to unfold. Because much of what we do is habituation, we do not need to attend to it and we are free to consciously engage in other thoughts or actions while the habituated behavior unfolds in the background. For example, while driving to work, we can plan aspects of the day, listen to the radio, or carry on a conversation. Such layering of activity allows us to complete more than one thing at a time. This layering of action characterizes much of our daily routine. Habituation also allows us to think in action, rather than having to plan all our behavior ahead of time. We instinctively know how to deal with a whole range of circumstances that arise within our compliment of roles. Thus, in the course of a day we might ask a favor of a friend, give feedback to a co-worker, comfort our children, and support our spouse. These role-related things we do are subtly guided by our awareness of our roles. Habits similarly steer us through myriad daily circumstances that we can manage without having to reflectively attend to them. In the end, habituation plants us comfortably and efficiently in our ordinary habitat.

Habituation, Disability, and Therapy

When habituation is affected by a disability, people can lose a great deal of what has given life familiarity, consistency, and relative ease. Impairments can invalidate established habits and require a person to develop new habits for much of everyday life. New habits may be needed to accommodate or manage the disability. Habits can also be eroded by long periods of enforced inactivity or destabilized by fluctuations or progressive deterioration of one's impairments. When additional time is needed for routine tasks, the rest of the routine must change. Consequently, the onset of a disability may necessitate changing much of the manner of accomplishing the daily things that were at once taken for granted and familiar.

Persons with disabilities may lack opportunities to learn or enter occupational roles while also finding themselves assigned to marginal roles (Hahn, 1985, 1993). Limitations of capacity can disrupt or terminate role performance or major modifications in how one enacts the role. Role strain may occur when a person cannot meet the multiple obligations or aspirations represented in several roles. One of the major tasks of living with disability is to construct for oneself a habituated pattern that allows one to live effectively and comfortably in accord with personal desires and needs. Reconstructing life following onset of a disability means moving from the known to the unknown. One must re-encounter the world within one's altered condition in order to reconstruct a pattern of living represented in new or altered roles and habits. Habits and roles are the source of security, familiarity, and identity for individuals. The whole fabric of the familiar world and the known self is dependent on the recurrent patterns of behavior and experiences sustained by habits and roles.

Therapy must respect the fact that habits and roles are naturally resistant to change. Therefore, sustained practice is necessary to change habituation. Each of us can readily recall how resistant even minor habits of action are to change. Because habituation organizes action to be effective within a specific environment, new habits and roles are best learned in the environments in which they will be performed. Moreover, changing habits and roles often requires changes in the environment.

Performance Capacity

The capacity for performance is affected by the status of one's musculoskeletal, neurologic, cardiopulmonary, and other bodily systems that are used when doing things. Performance also calls on mental or cognitive abilities such as memory and planning. A number of occupational therapy conceptual models seek to explain capacities that make occupational performance possible. These models provide detailed concepts for understanding some aspect of performance capacity. For example, the biomechanical model seeks to explain human movement as the function of a complex organization of muscles, connective tissue, and bones (Trombly & Radomski, 2002). The sensory integration model (Ayres, 1972, 1979, 1986; Bundy, Lane, & Murray, 2002) explains how the brain organizes sensory information for executing an adaptive motor response.

Because a variety of occupational therapy models already address performance capacity as represented in physical and mental performance components, the Model of Human Occupation does not address this aspect of performance capacity. Consequently, occupational therapists using the Model of Human Occupation will also need to use other conceptual models for understanding and addressing performance capacity.

A new theory within the Model of Human Occupation (Kielhofner, Baz, Hutson, & Tham, 2002) offers a different but complimentary way of addressing performance capacity. Other occupational therapy models address the problem of performance capacity from an objective point of view focusing on the physical and mental capacities as phenomena, which can be observed, measured, and modified. The Model of Human Occupation's new view of performance focuses on subjective experience and its role in how people perform. This approach builds on phenomenological concepts from philosophy (Husserl, 1962; Merleau-Ponty, 1962). This concept brings the concepts of mind and body together, demonstrating how they are dual aspects of the same thing. It also offers a way of going beyond current concepts of body and mind to understand how the body is mindful and the mind embodied. These concepts emphasize how the body has an intelligence of its own, especially as pertaining to everyday performance. They also point out how the foundations of abstract mental process are found in bodily experience.

The concept of the lived body also includes the idea that experience is not simply an artefact or consequence of doing. Rather, experience is central to how we perform. The fundamental argument is that to learn any performance, we must discover how it feels (i.e., locate the experience). Performance is guided, then, by how it feels to engage in occupation.

The concept of the lived body offers not only a different way to understand the capacity for performance, but also different ways to appreciate disability.

Performance Capacity, Disability, and Therapy

Disability involves objectively describable impairments of body and/or mind. The concept of the lived body calls attention to the fact that disability is also a particular way of being. This way of being constitutes the reality of the person with a disability — a reality that must be lived.

The unique experiences of having a particular disability are realities, which must be managed and used in dealing with the disability. For example, Murphy (1987) and Sachs

(1993) described their experience of disability as including alienation from one's own body. This alienation involves experiencing the body or some part of the body as not belonging to the self. Persons who experience such alienation must find a way of coming to terms with it. Understanding the subjective experience of disability reveals aspects of a person's functional capacity not accounted for in existing objective approaches. How people perform emanates from how they subjectively encounter themselves and their worlds.

It is through this same realm of experience that effective strategies of change are discovered. Because this is a new approach, applying it to the understanding of disability and adaptation to disability is just emerging. Kielhofner, Baz, Hutson, and Tham (2002) include three studies that illustrate how disability and change can be illuminated by concepts of the lived body. Inasmuch as this approach is a radical departure from traditional ways of looking at performance capacity, it promises to offer fresh ideas and innovative strategies for addressing impairments of performance capacity.

Interdependence of Volition, Habituation, and Performance Capacity

The things we do reflect a complex interplay of our motives, habits and roles, and performance capacity. Volition, habitation, and the lived body always operate in concert with each other, making simultaneous contributions to our doing. We cannot fully understand occupation without reference to all these contributing factors.

Every moment is potentially infused with influences from and interactions of volition, habituation, performance capacity, and the environment. Volition, habituation, and performance capacity always resonate together, creating conditions out of which our thoughts, feelings, and behavior emerge. Examples of such resonation are the anxiety from a lack of belief in skill interfering with performance, old habits interfering with new volitional choices, and the pull of values that keep us going despite pain. In these and endless other circumstances, values, interests, personal causation, role, habits, and performance capacity are always tethered together into a dynamic whole. What we do, think, and feel comes out of that dynamic whole.

Environment

It has just been emphasized how volition, habituation, and performance capacity are organized into a coherent whole. Just as these three components of the person are interrelated and interdependent, persons and their environments are also inseparable. As the discussions above illustrated, the environment always figures intimately in our motives, our habituated action, and our performance.

Each environment potentially offers opportunities, resources, demands, and constraints. Whether and how these environmental potentials affect persons depends on their values, interests, personal causation, roles, habits, and performance capacities. Because each individual is unique with regard to these aspects of self, any environment will have somewhat different effects on each individual within it. The features of an environment and its actual impact on specific persons within that environment are not identical. Nonetheless, characteristics of the environment are important as they have some impact on persons within them. The following sections discuss characteristics of the physical and social environment and the effects on occupation.

The physical environment consists of the natural and human-made spaces and the objects within them (Fig. 4-4). Spaces can be the result of nature (e.g., a forest or a lake) or

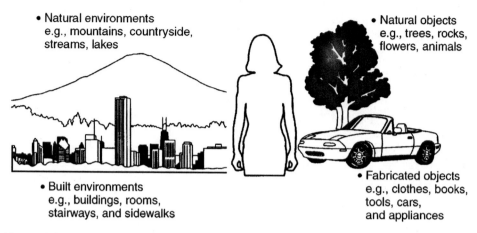

- Natural environments
  e.g., mountains, countryside,
  streams, lakes

- Natural objects
  e.g., trees, rocks,
  flowers, animals

- Built environments
  e.g., buildings, rooms,
  stairways, and sidewalks

- Fabricated objects
  e.g., clothes, books,
  tools, cars,
  and appliances

Figure 4-4. Physical Environment. Reprinted with permission from Kielhofner, G. (1995). *A model of human occupation: Theory and application* (2nd ed.). Baltimore, MD: Williams & Wilkins.

the result of human fabrication (e.g., a house, classroom, or theater). Similarly, objects may be those that occur naturally (e.g., trees and rocks) or those that have been made (e.g. books, cars, and computers). What we do within spaces and with objects depends, of course, on the characteristics of these elements of the physical world and how they affect us.

The social environment consists of groups of persons and the occupational forms that persons belonging to those groups perform (Fig. 4-5). Groups provide and assign roles to their members, and they constitute social space in which those roles are acted out according to group ambience, norms, and climate. Thus, groups allow and prescribe the kinds of things their members can do.

Occupational forms are rule-bound sequences of action that are oriented to a purpose, sustained in collective knowledge, culturally recognizable, and named. Simply said, occupational forms are the things that are available to do in any social context.

Any setting within which we perform is made up spaces, objects, occupational forms, and/or social groups. Typical settings in which we engage in occupational forms are the home, neighborhood, school, or workplace. It is the collective influence of the spatial arrangement, object, available occupational forms, and social groups that influence us. For example, a person whose neighborhood is a small town in the countryside will have quite

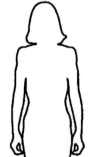

- Social groups
  e.g., families, church groups,
  coworkers

- Occupational forms
  e.g., biking, dressing,
  mowing the lawn, fishing

Figure 4-5. Social Environment. Reprinted with permission from Kielhofner, G. (1995). *A model of human occupation: Theory and application* (2nd ed.). Baltimore, MD: Williams & Wilkins.

different opportunities and resources, demands, and constraints than someone whose neighborhood is the area surrounding public housing in an inner city.

Environment, Disability, and Therapy

The environment can be both a barrier and an enabler for persons who are disabled. Just a few of the kinds of effects the environment can have on disabled persons are noted here. Natural spaces can provide a variety of problems for the person with a disability. For example, snow dampens the sounds used by blind persons to help them navigate and also makes terrain inaccessible to the someone who uses a wheelchair. Much of the built environment limits opportunities and poses constraints on those with disabilities because it is designed for persons without impairments. On the other hand, careful design of spaces can facilitate daily functioning of disabled persons. Similarly, while most fabricated objects in the environment are created for use by able-bodied, sighted, hearing, and cognitively intact individuals, there are also a large number of objects designed to compensate for impairments. Persons with disabilities often must live with many such objects that can carry deep symbolic messages. For example, using a wheelchair can change one's social identity and interactions with others.

Social attitudes often betray discomfort about the person with a disability. Persons with physical and mental impairments often go against cultural values, making others uncomfortable and evoking reactions that range from disgust to pity to derision. Disability may remove people from or alter the positions they can assume in groups. For example, persons with disabilities frequently have access to fewer non-kindred relationships, depending significantly on the family for emotional, financial, and other forms of support. The combination of being severed from ordinary social groups and being placed in specialized groups in which the typical opportunities for roles and activities are severely restricted can constrain the person with a disability.

The occupational forms available to the person with a disability may be limited or altered. Performance limitations can make doing some forms impossible. Persons with disabilities often must give up or relinquish to others occupational forms that have become impossible to do.

In short, the environment can have a multitude of positive or negative effects on the person with a disability, which can make all the difference in that person's life. While the environment is a pervasive factor influencing disability, it is also the therapist's only tool for supporting positive change in the disabled person's life. A therapist may purposefully alter the physical setting to remove constraints on function or to facilitate function. Examples of this are a ramp that replaces inaccessible steps. Therapists can remove objects that are barriers or provide objects such as assistive technology that facilitate functioning. The therapist may provide, monitor, or seek to change social groups such as families, co-workers, and colleagues. Finally, the therapist may provide a client with new occupational forms or help the client to select or modify occupational forms.

Occupational Performance

Personal causation, values, and interests motivate what we chose to do. Habits and roles shape our routine patterns of doing. Performance capacities and subjective experience make possible the details of what we do. The physical and social environment provides opportunities, resources, demands, and constraints on our doing. We can also examine the doing itself and what consequence it has over time. First, doing can be examined at three different levels: (1) participation, (2) performance of an occupational form, and (3) skill.

Occupational Participation

Occupational participation refers to engagement in work, play, or activities of daily living that are part of one's sociocultural context and that are desired and/or necessary for one's well-being . Examples of occupational participation are working in a full- or part-time job, engaging routinely in a hobby, maintaining one's home, attending school, and participating in a club or other organization.

Occupational Forms

Occupational participation involves doing a variety of occupational forms. For example, a professor's work may include lecturing, writing, administering and scoring exams, creating courses, and counseling students. When we complete an occupational form, we perform. For example, when persons do such tasks as walking the dog, baking a chicken, vacuuming a rug, or balancing the check book they are performing those occupational forms.

Skills

Within occupational performance we carry out discrete purposeful actions. For example, making coffee is a culturally recognizable occupational form in many Western cultures. To do so, one engages in such purposeful actions as gathering together the coffee, coffee maker, and a cup; handling these materials and objects; and sequencing the steps necessary to brew and pour the coffee. These actions that make up occupational performance are referred to as skills. Skills are goal-directed actions that a person uses while performing (Fisher, 1998; Fisher & Kielhofner, 1995; Forsyth, Salamy, Simon, & Kielhofner, 1997).

In contrast to performance capacity that refers to underlying ability, skill refers to the discrete functional actions. There are three types of skills: motor skills, process skills, and communication and interaction skills (Fig. 4-6). Detailed taxonomies of the skills that make up each of the three types of skills have been developed as part of creating assessments of skill (see below for further information on these assessments). Fisher and colleagues have developed the taxonomies of motor and process skills which make up an Assessment of Motor and Process Skills (Bernspang & Fisher, 1995; Doble, 1991; Fisher, 1993, 1998). Forsyth and her colleagues have developed a taxonomy of

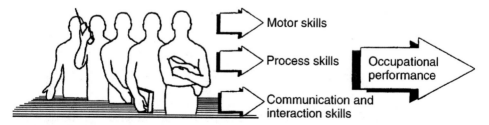

Figure 4-6.   Social Environment. Reprinted with permission from Kielhofner, G. (1995). *A model of human occupation: Theory and application* (2nd ed.). Baltimore, MD: Williams & Wilkins.

communication/interaction skills that make up the Assessment of Communication/Interaction Skills (Forsyth, Lai & Kielhofner, 1999; Forsyth, Salamy, Simon, & Kielhofner, 1997).

Skill is embedded within performance, and the latter within participation. Thus, whenever persons are participating in their occupational role, they complete a number of occupational forms and use a wide range of skills.

RESOURCES FOR PRACTICE

As noted in the beginning of this chapter, the Model of Human Occupation was initiated with the specific goal of developing resources to guide and enhance practice. Today those resources are quite extensive and fall in the following categories: (1) a range of assessments that operationalize concepts from the model; (2) a large number of published case examples as well as videotapes that illustrate application of the model in assessment, treatment planning, and intervention; and (3) published articles and manuals that describe the implementation of programs based on the model.

For the therapist working in almost any area of practice, there will be a variety of these resources. In addition, inquiries may be made directly to a Model of Human Occupation e-mail address (MOHOC@uic.edu), or practitioners may join a Listserv that allows them to dialogue internationally with other practitioners as well as scholars who are working on testing and developing the model and its resources. The following section provides an overview of the resources for practice and how to access them.

Assessment Tools

Over the past 20 years, practitioners have collaborated in the development of a wide range of assessment tools. Most of these tools grew out of needs in specific settings, and their developments were initiated by practitioners. The tools are summarized on Table 4-1. Table 4-1 also identifies where the reader can obtain the tests.

By looking over Table 4-2, the reader will see that some constructs have been extensively covered, whereas others are still in early stages of development. For example, there are a range of tools available for gathering data on volition, designed for a variety of patient needs. Some constructs, such as the environment, are less extensively covered, and work continues in these areas.

Assessment of Communication and Interaction Skills

The *Assessment of Communication and Interaction Skills* (ACIS) is a formal observational tool designed to measure an individual's performance in an occupational form and/or within a social group of which the person is a part. The instrument aims to assist occupational therapists in determining a client's ability in discourse and social exchange in the course of daily occupations. The ACIS has been developed for use in a wide range of settings. Observations are carried out in contexts that are meaningful and relevant to the client's lives. The occupational therapist then completes a 20-item rating form. Data can be combined with observations from other settings to give a more complete picture of the client's skills in communication and interaction.

Administration of the ACIS consist of two steps: (1) observation of the client's social skill during an occupational form and/or within a social group of which the person is a part and (2) rating and entering comments on the score sheet. The ACIS consists of 20 skill items divided into 3 communication and interaction domains: physicality, information exchange, and relations. These items were devised following extensive literature review. The items are arranged into domains by commonality among items.

To administer the ACIS, the occupational therapist observes the client's social skill during an occupational form and/or within a social group of which the person is a part. The total administration time varies from 20-60 minutes. Observation time ranges from 15-45 minutes. Rating time ranges from 5-20 minutes depending on experience using the ACIS; it may be possible to observe more than one person during an observation session. The rating is completed following conclusion of the session. Skills are scored on a four-point scale (4 = competent, 3 = questionable, 2 = ineffective, 1 = deficit) following the scoring criteria for each item provided in a manual. Comments that describe behaviors for a given rating may be entered on the form.

Assessment of Motor and Process Skills

The *Assessment of Motor and Process Skills* (AMPS) represents a fundamental and substantive re-conceptualization in the development of occupational therapy functional assessments. The AMPS is a structured, observational evaluation. The AMPS is used to evaluate the quality or effectiveness of the actions of performance (motor and process skills) as they unfold over time when a person performs daily life tasks. The daily life tasks included in the AMPS are both personal and domestic activities of daily living. The tasks included in the AMPS manual vary in difficulty from simple to complex, with the easiest tasks being less difficult than many self-care tasks, including dressing and toileting.

Since the occupational therapist using the AMPS rates specific motor and process skills according to how each skill contributes to successful task performance, the results provide the occupational therapist with therapeutically useful details about (1) why a person is having difficulty completing a task and (2) how complex a task the person has the ability to perform. Through computer scoring of the client's test results, ability measures for ADL motor skills and ADL process skills can be generated which take into account the challenge of the tasks the client performed and the severity of the ratings of the therapist who observed and scored the performance.

The AMPS is intended to be administered and scored within a 30- to 60-minute period. In most cases, the client completes two or three tasks that take 10-20 minutes each to perform. The administration of the AMPS involves six steps: (1) interviewing the client, with the interview culminating in the client choosing two or three AMPS tasks that he or she will perform; (2) establishing collaboratively the constraints of the tasks to be performed (setting the task contract); (3) setting up the environment; (4) reviewing the contract; (5) administering the assessment; and (6) scoring and interpreting the results. For each task performed, the client is rated on 16 motor skill items and 20 process skill items. The items are rated by a trained occupational therapist who uses a four-point rating scale from 4 (competent) to 1 (deficit).

Assessment of Occupational Functioning

The *Assessment of Occupational Functioning* (AOF) is a semi-structured interview designed to identify strengths and limitations in areas of occupational functioning derived

Text continues on page 70

Table 4–1 **OUTLINE OF THE INSTRUMENTS**

Instrument Name	Format	Purpose
Assessment of Communication and Interaction Skills (ACIS)	Observation Assessment	Gathers information about the communication skills that a person displays while engaged in occupation
Assessment of Motor and Process Skills (AMPS)	Observation Assessment	Gathers information about the motor and process skills that a person displays while engaging in occupation
Assessment of Occupational Functioning (AOF)	Semi-structured self-report	Gathers information on a broad range of qualitative information that may influence occupational performance Includes volition, habituation, and occupational performance skills
Interest Checklist	Self-report Paper-and-pencil form	Gathers information on 68 activities or areas of interest Includes information on strength of interest as well as present and future engagement in activity of interest
NIH Activity Record (ACTRE)	Self-report Paper-and-pencil form	Gathers information in half-hour intervals throughout the day Information includes a person's perception of competence, value of activity, enjoyment of activity, difficulty, pain, and rest
Occupational Performance History Interview 2nd Version (OPHI-II)	Semi-structured interview with three rating scales and a life history narrative	Provides measures of • occupational competence • occupational identity • occupational behavior settings Provides a format for interpreting the life history narrative and its implications for client's adaptation
Occupational Questionnaire (OQ)	Self-report Paper-and-pencil form	Gathers information in half-hour intervals throughout the day Information includes a person's perception of competence, value of activity, and enjoyment of activity
Role Checklist	Self-report Paper-and-pencil form	Provides information on what roles a person values and the client's view of role performance in the past, present, and future

Population	Psychometric Development	How to Obtain
Adults A version to be used with children is being investigated	A validity study with a diverse patient population with psychosocial deficits showed evidence of validity, inter- and intra-rater reliability	MOHO website AOTA
Adults Pediatric version available	Fully standardized, internationally and cross culturally on more than 12,000 individuals	Dr. Anne Fisher, Colorado State University
Adults	Several studies support reliability and concurrent validity	Virginia Commonwealth University OT Department Website
Adults	Limited psychometric data available	Department of Rehabilitation Medicine, National Institutes of Health
Mainly adults with physical disabilities	Studies support reliability	Gloria Furst at NIH — see MOHO website for instructions; computer version is available for downloading
Studied on persons from 18 years to old age Considered relevant for adolescents 15 and older Has been used and considered valuable with both physical disabilities and psychiatric populations	Instrument has been in development for 15 years Traditional studies of reliability and validity supported concurrent and predictive validity but revealed marginal reliability Revised 2nd edition has evidence of reliability and validity with a wide range of both physical and psychiatrically disabled populations	MOHO website AOTA
Adults	Original study provided evidence of retest reliability Instrument has been used in several studies, which indicate its ability to discriminate between populations with different adaptive status	MOHO website
Adolescents and adults	Several studies have indicated good reliability There is extensive evidence that this instrument captures role changes associated with disability	Fran Oakley at NIH — see MOHO website for instructions

(continued)

Table 4–1   **OUTLINE OF THE INSTRUMENTS** (*Continued*)

Instrument Name	Format	Purpose
Occupational Self Assessment (OSA)	Self-report Paper-and-pencil form followed by discussion, leading to treatment goals and strategies	Client-centered self assessment Yields measures of • values concerning self • values concerning environment • personal competence • environmental impact Allows comparison of what client values with how competent the client feels about his or her everyday activity
Volitional Questionnaire (VQ)	Observation assessment	Designed to evaluate volitional components through observation of persons with limited cognitive or verbal abilities
Worker Role Interview (WRI)	Semi-structured interview	Designed to have the client discuss various aspects of his or her job setting that have been associated with past work experiences The goal is to identify the psychosocial and environmental variables that may influence the ability of the person to return to work
Work Environment Impact Scale (WEIS)	Semi-structured interview with rating scale	Designed to assist the occupational therapist to gather information on how individuals with physical or psychological disabilities experience and perceive their work environments
Occupational Therapy Psychosocial Assessment of Learning (OT PAL)	Observational and descriptive assessment tool	Measures the psychosocial aspects of a student's performance within the classroom Addresses a student's volition (ability to make choices), habituation (roles and routines), and environmental fit within the classroom setting
School Setting Interview (SSI)	Semi-structured interview	Designed to assess student-environment fit and identify the need for accommodations for students with disabilities in the school setting
Model of Human Occupation Screening Tool (MOHOST)	Variety of ways of collecting data	Gathers information on a person's personal causation, values, interests, roles, habits, skills, and environment

Population	Psychometric Development	How to Obtain
Adolescents (ages 12 and up) and adults A children's version (ages 8–11) is currently under development	One validity study with a diverse international population provided evidence of validity and reliability Based on study results, revisions were made and a second study is underway	MOHO website AOTA
Adults Pediatric version available	Original study supports inter-rater reliability and content validity Two subsequent studies support internal validity and reliability	MOHO website AOTA
Adults	Two studies support internal validity and reliability Further research on predictive validity is underway	MOHO website AOTA
Adults	Two studies support internal validity and reliability Further research on the predictive validity is underway	MOHO website AOTA
School children	Original authors studied reliability Instrument was recently revised following pilot testing, and data collection on new version is underway	MOHO website AOTA
School children	Initial study supports reliability. Subsequent studies indicate instrument is effective in identifying needs for accommodation	MOHO website AOTA
Adults	Newly developed; in pilot testing phase	Monitor MOHO website for availability

TABLE 4-2 MODEL OF HUMAN OCCUPATION CONSTRUCTS AS ADDRESSED BY ASSESSMENT TOOLS

	Volition			Habituation		Skills			Environment		Method of Data Gathering			Population
	Personal Causation	Values	Interests	Roles	Habits	Motor	Process	Communication Interaction	Physical	Social	Observations	Checklist	Interview	Age Groups[a]
ACIS								✓			✓			Y, A, E
AMPS						✓	✓				✓			C, Y, A, E
AOF	✓	✓	✓	✓	✓	✓	✓	✓						A
Interest Checklist			✓									✓		Y, A, E
NIH Activity Record	✓	✓	✓		✓							✓		A, E

Assessment									Age
OPHI-II	✓	✓	✓	✓	✓	✓	✓	✓	A, E
OQ	✓	✓	✓	✓	✓	✓		✓	Y, A, E
Role Checklist		✓	✓	✓				✓	Y, A, E
OSA	✓	✓	✓	✓	✓	✓	✓	✓	Y, A, E
VQ	✓	✓				✓	✓		Y, A, E
WRI	✓	✓	✓		✓	✓	✓	✓	A, E
WEIS									A
OT PAL					✓	✓	✓		A, E
SSI									C

ªC, children; Y, adolescent; A, adults; E, elderly

from the Model of Human Occupation (personal causation, values, roles, habits, and skills).

The AOF includes two parts: (1) an interview schedule and (2) a rating scale. The interview consists of 24 questions. Although occupational therapists should use the questions as they appear, they are also encouraged to use probes and clarifications of questions as necessary. The questions are designed to elicit information regarding a client's perception of his or her occupational functioning. The interview takes approximately 30-40 minutes to complete. The occupational therapist then scores the rating scale which includes 20 items.

Interest Checklist

Although the *Interest Checklist* was developed before the introduction of the Model of Human Occupation, both the instrument and the theory have strong ties to the occupational behavior tradition. The Interest Checklist has been modified and used extensively over the years in studies based on the Model of Human Occupation because of this tool's utility in identifying clients' past and present interests and the degree of attraction clients express toward these interests.

Although a number of versions of the Interest Checklist exist, the revised version appears to be the one most commonly used by occupational therapists utilizing the Model of Human Occupation and will be the one referred to in this discussion. This version consists of 68 activities or areas of interest. The client is asked to place checks in each column to describe his or her level of interest (strong, some, or no interest) in each of the activities. Clients are asked to rate his or her level of interest in each activity over two time frames: the past 10 years and the past year. Further, clients are asked whether they actively participate in each activity now and whether they would like to pursue this activity at some point in the future. It is suggested that following completion of the checklist, the occupational therapist and client discuss the client's pattern of interests.

Activity Record

The NIH *Activity Record* (ACTRE) was developed as an outcome measure for a study of patients with rheumatoid arthritis. This instrument provides a 24-hour log of a patient's activities and is an adaptation of the Occupational Questionnaire (described later in this section). The ACTRE aims to provide details on the impact of symptoms on task performance, individual perceptions of interest and significance of daily activities, and daily habit patterns. Specific information gathered covers frequency and/or percentage of time spent in role activity and resting, frequency of rest periods during activity, frequency and/or percentage of time with pain and fatigue and time of day or activity with which it occurs, plus volitional concerns such as interests, meaning, enjoyment, and perception of personal effectiveness.

Occupational Performance History Interview

As a historical interview, the *Occupational Performance History Interview, 2nd Version* (OPHI-II) seeks to gather information about a patient or client's past and present occupational performance. The OPHI-II is a three-part assessment that includes (1) a semi-structured interview that explores a client's occupational life history; (2) rating scales that provide a measure of the client's occupational identity, occupational competence, and the impact of the client's occupational behavior settings; and (3) a life history narrative designed to capture salient qualitative features of the occupational life history.

As a semi-structured interview, it provides a framework and recommended questions for doing the interview to assure that the necessary information is obtained. However, the very idea of a semi-structured interview is that the therapist should improvise how best to conduct the interview with each individual client. What matters is not that the therapist ask a specific set of questions, but that the therapist obtain specific kinds of information. The semi-structured interview is organized into the following thematic areas: (1) Activity/Occupational Choices, (2) Critical Life Events, (3) Daily Routine, (4) Occupational Roles, and (5) Occupational Behavior Settings. Within each of these thematic areas a possible sequence of interview questions (with alternatives) is provided. Therapists can perform the interview by covering these thematic areas in any sequence or move back and forth between thematic areas. The interview is designed to be very flexible.

The second part of the OPHI-II is composed of the three rating scales. As already noted, they are Occupational Identity Scale, Occupational Competence Scale, and Occupational Behavior Settings Scale. The three scales provide a means of converting the information gathered in the interview into three measures. Occupational Identity measures the degree to which a person has internalized a positive occupational identity (e.g., having values, interests, and confidence; seeing self in various occupational roles; and having an image of the kind of life one wants). Occupational Competence measures the degree to which a person is able to sustain a pattern of occupational behavior that is productive and satisfying. Occupational Behavior Settings measures the impact of the environment on the client's occupational life.

The strength of the OPHI is that it provides a historical approach to interviewing and thereby lends itself to gathering information about the patient's life story. This aspect may be one of the important new directions for interview development.

Occupational Questionnaire

The *Occupational Questionnaire* (OQ) is a pen-and-paper, self-report instrument that asks the individual to provide a description of typical use of time and utilizes Likert-type ratings of competence, importance, and enjoyment during activities.

The OQ asks the client to complete the instrument in two parts. First, he or she completes a list of the activities he or she performs each half-hour on a typical weekday. After listing the activities, the client is asked to answer four questions for each activity. The questions ask the client to rate whether they consider the activity to be work, daily living tasks, recreation, or rest and to consider how well he or she does the activities, how important they are to him or her, and how much he or she enjoys doing them. The occupational therapist can use the scores to calculate the quality of waking activities in terms of value, interest, and personal causation, along with the actual number of half-hours spent in activity. While a variety of scores can be calculated, what matters most is what the client and therapist are able to deduce from them. The numbers obtained should provide insight into the person's pattern of occupational activity in daily life.

Role Checklist

The *Role Checklist* is a self-report checklist that can be used to obtain information about the types of roles people engage in and which organize their daily lives. This checklist provides data on an individual's perception of his or her roles over the course of his or her life and also the degree of value (i.e., the significance and importance) that they place on those roles. The Role Checklist can be used with adolescent, adult, or geriatric populations.

The Role Checklist asks the client to consider each of 10 roles described on the form. These roles are student, worker, volunteer, care giver, home maintainer, friend, family member, religious participant, hobbyist/amateur, and participant in organizations. There is also an "other" category in which clients may enter additional roles not listed. Each role is accompanied by a brief description and a reference to the frequency with which the role is enacted. Because the intent of the checklist is to identify roles that organize an individual's daily life, reference to frequency of performance is included for each role definition.

The Role Checklist has two parts. Part One asks the client to check those roles he or she has performed in the past, are currently involved in, and/or plan to perform in the future. For example, if an individual volunteered in the past, does not volunteer at present, but does anticipate volunteering in the future, he or she would check the role "volunteer" in both the past and future columns. "Past" refers to any time up to preceding week. "Present" includes the week prior, up to, and including the day of administration of the checklist. "Future" refers to tomorrow or any day thereafter. In Part Two of the checklist, the client is asked to indicate how much worth or importance (i.e., how valuable) each of the 10 roles is for him or her. Each role is rated as to whether the person finds it "not at all valuable," "somewhat valuable," or "very valuable." The Role Checklist takes approximately 15 minutes for a client to complete. The occupational therapist is encouraged to remain with the client to answer or clarify questions.

Occupational Self Assessment

The *Occupational Self Assessment* (OSA) builds on the work of the *Self Assessment of Occupational Functioning* (SAOF) (Baron & Curtin, 1990). Baron and Curtin first developed the prototype for the SAOF in 1985 for use with adolescents and adults. The OSA is an update of the SAOF and is designed to capture clients' perceptions of their own occupational competence and of the impact of their environment on their occupational adaptation. The OSA is designed to be a client-centered assessment, which gives voice to the client's view. The OSA is a two-part, self-rating form. Section one includes a series of statements about one's occupational functioning, to which the client responds by labeling each as an area of strength, adequate functioning, or weakness. The client then responds to these same statements, indicating the value he or she places on each item. Section two includes a series of statements about one's environments, to which similar responses are given. Once clients have had an opportunity to assess their occupational behavior and their environments, they review the items to establish priorities for change. In the last step, the client establishes priorities for therapy, which can be translated into therapy goals.

Volitional Questionnaire

Traditionally, it has been difficult to assess volition in clients who have communication and cognitive limitations due to the complex language requirements of most assessments of volition. The *Volitional Questionnaire* is an attempt to recognize that while such clients have difficulty formulating goals or expressing their interests and values verbally, they are often able to communicate them through actions. The client is observed in a number of occupational behavior settings, so that a picture of the person's volition and the environmental factors required to support the expression can be identified.

The Volitional Questionnaire is of most benefit when the client is observed over multiple sessions in a variety of occupational behavior settings. The author recommends that a person be observed in self-care, work, and leisure environments for a combined total of five sessions. The person's performance in each session is rated. Before beginning the evaluation, it is important to make adaptations to the setting if needed. Once the person arrives, he or she is invited to go in and explore the different alternatives for activity. Following this, he or she is invited to choose an activity. After the person has participated in the activity for some time, the occupational therapist starts to introduce novelty into the activity situation and to offer different levels of demands to evaluate personal causation indicators. When the activity is complete, the occupational therapist talks with the person about his or her feelings of competence, satisfaction, and personal goals related to the type of activities and environment. Following the session, the occupational therapist completes the rating form. The Volitional Questionnaire consists of 14 indicators in three areas: (1) intrinsic motivation, (2) personal causation, and (3) values/interests.

The person is rated in terms of the degree of spontaneity with which they demonstrate behavior reflective of the indicators. The ratings are on a four-point scale: 4 = spontaneous — the person engages in and responds to their environment with minimal support, structure, or stimulation; 3 = involved — the person engages in the environment with moderate support; 2 = hesitant — the person requires substantial support and structure to engage in the environment; 1 = passive — the person can engage in the environment only with a maximal amount of support or structure. The manual outlines specific examples of these ratings for each indicator.

The occupational therapist concludes by writing a brief narrative that details the person's interests and values; the amount and kind of support required for a person to accomplish a behavior; the influence of this person's values, interests, and personal causation on the person's motivation to engage in activities; and the influence of different environments on the person's volition.

Worker Role Interview

The *Worker Role Interview* (WRI) is a semi-structured interview designed to be used as the psychosocial/environmental component of the initial rehabilitation assessment process for the injured worker. The interview is designed to have the client discuss various aspects of his or her life and job setting that have been associated with past work experiences. The WRI combines information from an interview with observations made during the physical and behavioral assessment procedure of a physical and/or work capacity assessment. The intent is to identify the psychosocial and environmental variables that may influence the ability of the injured worker to return to work.

Administration of the WRI consists of five steps: (1) interview preparation; (2) conducting the semi-structured interview, which is completed at the beginning of initial assessment of the injured worker; (3) the usual physical/work capacity assessment procedures used in the rehabilitation setting; (4) scoring the WRI Rating Form following initial evaluation; and (5) re-scoring the WRI Rating Form at discharge from the treatment program.

The WRI has six content areas with subcontent areas. These subcontent areas were devised from an extensive review of the literature on factors that seem to affect return to work. The semi-structured interview includes 28 recommended questions covering the areas outlined below. The interview can be administered in approximately 30–60 minutes. The occupational therapist rates each of the subcontent areas on a scale of 1–4 depending on how strongly the interview findings appear to support the client returning to his or her previous employment or work in general, whichever is more appropriate for this client. The occupational therapist is encouraged to write brief comments to support each rating.

Work Environment Impact Scale

The *Work Environment Impact Scale* (WEIS) is a semi-structured interview designed to gather information about how individuals with disabilities experience and perceive their work settings. The focus of the interview is the impact of the work setting on a person's performance, satisfaction, and well-being. An important concept underlying this scale is that workers are most productive and satisfied when there is a "fit" or "match" between the worker's environment and the needs and skills of the worker. Hence, the same work environment may have a different impact on different workers. It is important to remember that the WEIS does not assess the environment. Rather, it assesses how the work environment impacts a given worker.

The scale allows therapists to translate the information gathered in the interview into quantitative ratings. The scale provides a measure of work environment impact on a continuum from negative to positive. In addition, scoring the individual items on the scale provides a profile of which aspects of the environment negatively or positively impact the worker.

The WEIS is designed to provide a comprehensive assessment of how the qualities and characteristics of the work environment impact a worker. The WEIS is organized around 17 environmental factors such as the physical space, social contacts and supports, temporal demands, objects utilized, and daily job functions. These 17 factors are reflected in 17 items on the rating scale. Each of the items is scored with a four-point rating scale that is used to indicate how the environmental factor impacts the worker's performance, satisfaction, and well-being (physical, social, emotional). After completing the rating scale, it is optional to complete a summary sheet to identify any environmental characteristics that facilitate successful employment experiences while highlighting those factors that inhibit worker performance and satisfaction and that may require accommodation. (The summary sheet may be a useful way to communicate the results and implications of the WEIS to other disciplines.)

Occupational Therapy Psychosocial Assessment of Learning

The *Occupational Therapy Psychosocial Assessment of Learning* (OT PAL) is an observational and descriptive assessment tool. It assesses a student's volition (ability to make choices), habituation (roles and routines), and environmental fit within the classroom setting. The observational portion consists of 21 items that address the major areas of making choices, habits/routines, and roles. These items are designed to facilitate the gathering of essential information in regard to the student's classroom and typical expectations within the classroom. In addition to the observation portion, there is a pre-observation form and interview guidelines. The pre-observation form is designed to gather environmental information as well as assist in determining an appropriate time to complete the observation. The semi-structured interviews of the teacher, the student, and the parent(s) are designed to have the teacher, student, and parent describe various psychosocial aspects of learning related to school. Different perspectives about the student's performance, behaviors, beliefs, and interests related to school are helpful in gaining a holistic view. The teacher's style of teaching and managing the classroom, the student's ability to meet these expectations, and the student's beliefs about his or her abilities as a learner within the environment are included. The OT PAL allows the occupational therapist to determine the effectiveness of the fit between the student and the classroom environment and how that match impacts the student's performance in the classroom.

The OT PAL targets students between the ages of 6 and 12 years, who are in elementary school, and who are experiencing difficulty meeting functional expectations and roles in the classroom which may affect learning. To minimize the effects of a new environment and allow the child an opportunity to learn what roles are expected of him or her, the OT PAL should not be administered until the student has been in the classroom for a minimum of 1 month. The observations are administered in the student's classroom during a minimum of a 40-minute period to complete the rating scale. The three interviews are administered after the observation and in private settings. Each interview should take approximately 15 minutes. The parent interview may be conducted as a written questionnaire or a telephone call. The OT PAL is composed of the following forms: pre-observation and environmental description worksheet, rating scale, teacher narrative, student narrative, parent narrative, and summary form.

School Setting Interview

The *School Setting Interview* (SSI) is a semi-structured interview designed to assess student-environment fit and identify the need for accommodations for students with disabilities in the school setting. The SSI is a client-centered interview intended to assist the occupational therapist in the planning of intervention by examining the student's interaction with the physical and social environments at school. The SSI provides the occupational therapist with a picture of the child's functioning in 14 content areas. This assessment is designed to be used collaboratively with the student and is therefore intended for students who are able to communicate adequately enough to discuss their feelings.

Students appropriate for the SSI are those who are able to communicate their needs and desires. Before beginning the interview, the therapist should stress to the student that this assessment is not designed to identify the student's weaknesses. The therapist should explain that the purpose of this assessment is to make the school setting less demanding for the student and to assist the student in functioning better at school. The SSI should be administered in a conversational manner to facilitate the student's sharing of circumstances in the school setting that are of importance to him or her. By using the everyday language of the questions to facilitate a conversation with the student, the student can begin to develop trust in the therapeutic relationship. The interview questions cover 14 content areas identified to be important in the school setting, including writing; reading; speaking; remembering things; doing mathematics; doing homework; taking examinations; going to art, gym, and music; getting around the classrooms; taking breaks; going on field trips; getting assistance; accessing the school; and interacting with staff. The questions consist of three sections: General Background, Need for Accommodations, and Environmental Accommodations and Interventions. The SSI is easy and quick to administer and takes only about 40 minutes to complete.

Model of Human Occupation Screening Tool

The *Model of Human Occupation Screening Tool* (MOHOST) was designed to be used in acute care settings. MOHOST, a new assessment based on the Model of Human Occupation, is currently being researched. It has completed several phases of pilot testing and is about to enter the first test of statistical properties. It has been developed with clinicians in response to their request for a comprehensive assessment that is quick and simple to complete. Its primary purpose is to screen for areas of occupational dysfunction requiring further assessment or intervention. It may also be useful for screening referrals to occupational therapy.

The MOHOST is fundamentally an observational therapist-rated tool. The data collection method, however, has been designed to be flexible to meet multiple needs. The criterion is "knowing your client's occupational life." This will usually be completed through observation; however, this may be achieved through discussion with the client, talking to ward/residential staff, and/or talking to relatives.

The assessment enables clinicians to gather knowledge about a client from many sources. It can be used at regular intervals to document baseline assessment and general progress thereafter. It aims to communicate the client's relative strengths, highlighting the impact of volition and habituation on occupational performance and thereby assisting clinicians in treatment and discharge planning.

The MOHOST seeks to objectify the observations an occupational therapist would make as part of regular practice. It is the most flexible assessment in terms of data collection. The MOHOST is not diagnosis specific. It is typically most useful in those circumstances in which client-centered practice is most challenged — when self-assessments may not be possible and lengthy interviews may not be appropriate, but where occupational therapists nevertheless build up an understanding of their clients' occupational functioning over time.

Published Articles and Videotapes

Case Illustrations Through Articles

There are a large number of published case examples and videotapes illustrating application of the model in assessment, treatment planning, and intervention. A selection of these are referenced below.

Affleck, A., Bianchi, E., Cleckley, M., Donaldson, K., McCormack, G., & Polon, J. (1984). Stress management as a component of occupational therapy in acute care settings. *Occupational Therapy in Health Care, 1,* 17–41.

Baron, K. B., & Littleton, M. J. (1999). The model of human occupation: A return to work case study. *Work: A Journal of Prevention, Assessment & Rehabilitation, 12,* 37–46.

Barrett, L., Beer, D., & Kielhofner, G. (1999). The importance of volitional narrative in treatment: An ethnographic case study in a work program. *Work: A Journal of Prevention, Assessment & Rehabilitation, 12,* 79–92.

Curtin, C. (1991). Psychosocial intervention with an adolescent with diabetes using the model of human occupation. *Occupational Therapy in Mental Health, 11,* 23–36.

DePoy, E., & Burke, J. P. (1992). Viewing cognition through the lens of the model of human occupation. In N. Katz (Ed.), *Cognitive rehabilitation: Models for inter-*

vention in occupational therapy (pp. 240–257). Stoneham, MA: Butterworth-Heinemann.

Froehlich, J. (1992). Occupational therapy interventions with survivors of sexual abuse. *Occupational Therapy in Health Care, 8*, 1–25.

Gusich, R. (1984). Occupational therapy for chronic pain: A clinical application of the model of human occupation. *Occupational Therapy in Mental Health, 4*, 59–73.

Helfrich, C., & Kielhofner, G. (1994). Volitional narratives and the meaning of occupational therapy. *American Journal of Occupational Therapy, 48*, 319–326.

Helfrich, C., Kielhofner, G., & Mattingly, C. (1994). Volition as narrative: An understanding of motivation in chronic illness. *American Journal of Occupational Therapy, 42*, 311–317.

Kavanaugh, J., & Fares, J. (1995). Using the model of human occupation with homeless mentally ill patients. *British Journal of Occupational Therapy, 58*, 419–422.

Mentrup, C., Niehaus, A., & Kielhofner, G. (1999). Applying the model of human occupation in work-focused rehabilitation: A case illustration. *Work: A Journal of Prevention, Assessment & Rehabilitation, 12*, 61–70.

Neville, A. (1985). The model of human occupation and depression. *Mental Health Special Interest Section Newsletter, 8*, 1–4.

Oakley, F. (1987). Clinical application of the model of human occupation in dementia of the Alzheimer's type. *Occupational Therapy in Mental Health, 7*, 37–50.

Pizzi, M. A. (1990a). The model of human occupation and adults with HIV infection and AIDS. *American Journal of Occupational Therapy, 44*, 257–264.

Pizzi, M. A. (1990b). Occupational therapy: Creating possibilities for adults with human immunodeficiency virus infection, AIDS related complex, and acquired immunodeficiency syndrome. *Occupational Therapy in Health Care, 7*, 125–137.

Series, C. (1992). The long-term needs of people with head injury: A role for the community occupational therapist? *British Journal of Occupational Therapy, 55*, 94–98.

Woodrum, S. C. (1993). A treatment approach for attention deficit hyperactivity disorder using the model of human occupation. *Developmental Disabilities Special Interest Section Newsletter, 16*, 1–2.

Case Illustrations Through Videotapes

Facilitating Empowerment and Promoting Self-Advocacy: ADA
Population: Disabled workers
Author: Renee Moore-Corner
Distributor: AOTA

Understanding the Work Hardening Client
Population: Injured workers
Authors: Clare Curtin and Trudy Mallinson
Distributor: AOTA

Work Environment Impact Scales
Population: Adult workers with recent/current work experience
Authors: Renee Moore-Corner, Linda Olson, and Gary Kielhofner
Distributor: AOTA

Worker Role Interview
Population: Injured workers
Authors: Craig Velozo, Gary Kielhofner, and Gail Fisher
Distributor: AOTA

Examples of Model of Human Occupation Programs

Manuals for Model of Human Occupation-based Programs

Work Readiness: Day Treatment for Persons with Chronic Disabilities
Population: Unemployed adults with chronic disabilities
Author: Linda Olson
Distributor: AOTA

Work Rehabilitation in Mental Health Programs
Authors: Trudy Mallinson, Dorianne LaPlante, and Jan Holmann-Smith
Population: Adults with mental illness
Distributor: AOTA

Wellness and Lifestyle Renewal: A Manual for Personal Change
Population: "Worried well" adults
Author: Mark S. Rosenfeld
Distributor: AOTA

Videotapes for Programs

Proud of Me
Work Readiness: Day Treatment for Persons with Chronic Disabilities
Population: Unemployed adults with chronic disabilities
Author: Linda Olson
Distributor: AOTA

Write Stuff
Work Rehabilitation in Mental Health Programs
Population: Adults with mental illness
Authors: Trudy Mallinson, Dorianne LaPlante, and Jan Holmann-Smith
Distributor: AOTA

Working it Out
Work Rehabilitation in Mental Health Programs
Population: Adults with mental illness
Authors: Trudy Mallinson, Dorianne LaPlante, and Jan Holmann-Smith
Distributor: AOTA

APPLYING THE MODEL THROUGH CASE STUDY

The above resources can be used to infuse the Model of Human Occupation into practice. The following section presents two case studies that will illustrate using the Model of Human Occupation constructs in practice. The volition, habituation, and mind-brain-body performance subsystems as well as the environment may all contribute to maladaptive function. When this is the situation, the occupational therapist uses the Model of Human

Occupation as a framework for understanding the interrelated factors that contribute to dysfunction. The therapist evaluating a particular client will discover the unique way in which these factors are involved in that person's function and dysfunction. In assessment, therapists seek out data to answer questions they generate from the theoretical perspective of the model. For example, therapists might ask how a person's habit pattern or personal causation is influencing a problem. Therapists then use the data they collect to make theoretically informed judgments about the answers to such questions and to create a theoretically based explanation of the client's circumstances. This explanation allows the therapist to engage in the process of deciding on and implementing strategies of intervention.

Gloria: An Illustration Using the MOHOST BY SUE PARKINSON

Gloria is a 73-year-old retired schoolteacher who has a longstanding history of agitated depression. She lives alone with her pet dog in the same house that she lived in as a child. Her husband died several years ago and her one child, a son, lives nearby but often works away. When unwell, Gloria becomes restless, unable to care for herself, and demanding of constant reassurance. Her presentation when she was last admitted to the hospital seemed to be no different from usual. She quickly became reliant on her fellow patients for support and could then be encouraged to participate in social activities. Her confidence did not improve, however, and she had difficulty retaining information. This was initially attributed to inattention, but a cognitive assessment carried out by the occupational therapist identified some memory problems and further testing confirmed the onset of multi-infarct dementia.

Gloria's mental state eventually stabilized but she became unsettled again whenever other patients were discharged. Although she was anxious about how she would manage in the future, she gradually became determined to return home herself. The occupational therapist was then involved in a series of domestic assessments and home visits in order to help Gloria and the team to determine the level of support that she would require. The observations were summarized using the MOHOST (Fig. 4-7) and are detailed below.

Motivation for Occupation

Gloria fluctuated between feeling highly overconfident and feeling hopeless — worried that she would "stay in the hospital forever." Her goal was to return home, but her anxiety often prevented her from working toward this goal, and she frequently felt unable to proceed with tasks that might have brought her closer toward achieving her objectives. She had clear interests that provided satisfaction in her home environment but insufficient interest or curiosity to afford her any pleasure while she stayed in the hospital. Here, she remained dependent on the company of her peers for motivation to participate in any new activities, whereas at home she described a fulfilling lifestyle, centered around her church and voluntary work at a charity shop.

Pattern of Occupation

Gloria's sleep pattern was good and she could remember her weekly schedule of main activities perfectly. However, it became clear that for some time before being admitted to the hospital she had had difficulty organizing her everyday routine. She had a history of not keeping appointments with her community psychiatric nurse, and on her first home visit a large quantity of medication was found, indicating that she had not been taking any for a long time. It also became apparent that her eating habits had been irregular. She stated that she had been eating her main meal each day at a supermarket café and making ham sandwiches for her tea,

(Continued)

SUMMARY OF MODEL OF HUMAN OCCUPATION SCREENING TOOL (MOHOST)

Client: *Gloria*

Date of birth: ____/____/____

Date of assessment: ____/____/____

Assessor: _____

Dsignation: _____

Signature: _____

The assessment of occupational function offers a tool for occupational therapists to highght client's needs, aiding documentation and communcation. It is a record of occupational behaviour that has been observed consistently over a period of time. The ratings exist to provide an indication of progress on repeat assessments.

Competent [4]	Competent performance that supports independent functioning and leads to positive outcomes. Assessor observes no evidence of a deficit.
Questionable [3]	Questionable performance that places independent functioning at risk and leads to uncertain outcomes. Assessor questions the presence of a deficit.
Ineffective [2]	Ineffective performance that interferes with independent functioning and leads to undersirable outcomes. Assessor observes a mild to moderate deficit.
Deficient [1]	Deficient performance that impedes independent functioning and leads to unacceptable outcomes. Assessor observes a severe deficit.

ANALYSIS OF STRENGTHS & LIMIITATIONS

Gloria is easily confused and can become anxious and despondent, although she routinely overestimates how well she will be able to cope. In addition, she has great difficulty coping with change. Her strengths can be seen in her commitment to her previous lifestyle and roles and her good physical health, but her process skills are undoubtedly poor and she will need much assistance to organise her routine and responsibilities.

SUMMARY OF RATINGS

Motivation for Occupation				Pattern of Occupation				Communcation & Interaction				Process Skills				Motor Skills			
Self-belief	Goals	Interest	Values	Routine	Flexibility	Responsibilities	Role behavior	Body language	Conversation	Expression	Co-operation	Knowledge	Planning	Organisation	Problem-solving	Posture & mobility	Co-ordination	Strength & effort	Energy
4	4	4	[4]	4	4	4	4	4	4	[4]	4	4	4	4	4	[4]	[4]	4	4
3	3	[3]	3	3	3	3	[3]	3	3	3	3	3	3	3	3	3	3	[3]	3
2	[2]	2	2	[2]	2	2	2	[2]	[2]	2	[2]	[2]	2	2	2	2	2	2	[2]
[1]	1	1	1	1	[1]	[1]	1	1	1	1	1	1	[1]	[1]	[1]	1	1	1	1

Figure 4-7. Model of Human Occupation Screening Tool (MOHOST). Reprinted with permission from Kielhofner, G. (1995). *A model of human occupation: Theory and application* (2nd ed.). Baltimore, MD: Williams & Wilkins.

but her fridge contained a series of packets of butter and sliced ham that she had bought on successive weeks but never opened. There was no other food in the house.

Gloria's identity evidently hinged on being able to fulfill her previous roles, including looking after her small dog and socializing with her neighbors. Thus, the prospect of encouraging Gloria to review her lifestyle was fraught with problems, particularly as she found it so difficult to tolerate change. She also had difficulty accepting that any risks might be involved. For example, her house was situated on a busy road with a blind bend close by, which Gloria was used to crossing each day to catch the bus into town. On her first visit home Gloria showed a significant lack of road safety awareness. Although she acknowledged that she had not seen an approaching car, Gloria ignored the concerns expressed by the staff. Fortunately, this incident was not repeated on further visits.

Occupational Communication Skills

When distressed, Gloria had difficulty controlling her agitation. However, this was more congruous than when she presented with complete calm, despite having been unable to manage everyday tasks. Her conversation was also very changeable, and she would repetitively either request reassurance or become sharply abrupt when she disagreed with feedback. Her vocal expression, however, was unerringly clear, often assertive, and would sometimes serve to remind others that she had once been a schoolteacher. The overall effect was one of unpredictability, with Gloria appearing dependent one moment and independent the next, making it difficult at times to establish a collaborative relationship.

Occupational Processing Skills

Gloria had problems retaining information and relied heavily on her previous knowledge of activities. She could manage personal activities of daily living independently, but her inability to plan, organize, and problem-solve interfered with her ability to manage more complex tasks. She was disoriented on the ward but could easily find her way around her own home. Once in her familiar surroundings, she could use tools safely, but she did not always select the most appropriate tool. For example, she might state her intention to make a cup of tea but made a cup of coffee instead, and she might select the washing-up liquid (dishwashing liquid) when she was looking for shampoo. She also had enormous difficulty deciding which clothes to pack to take back to the hospital and would forget what she had already packed, causing her to repeat her actions over and over. In addition, there was some evidence that she had forgotten where a few items were located in her house, so that she had to search for the tea and coffee even though they were clearly situated on the kitchen worktop. Finally, there was the question of her poor judgment when crossing the road and the risk that she would make inappropriate decisions.

Occupational Motor Skills

Happily, Gloria was not troubled by many of the physical signs of getting older. She was not as strong as she used to be and could of course be restless at times, but she was otherwise very nimble and could move easily without awkwardness or stiffness. She had sufficient strength to manipulate a kettle safely, sufficient coordination to manage her door key, and sufficient mobility to reach for all necessary household objects (Fig. 4-7).

Completing the MOHOST helped the occupational therapist to analyze Gloria's relative strengths, placing her skills into the wider context of volition (motivation for occupation) and habituation (pattern of occupation). In particular it helped to communicate Gloria's strongly held values and served to highlight the importance of her roles in maintaining good mental health. The difficulties that she would have in coping with change and developing new interests were also made clear.

(Continued)

The team agreed that despite Gloria's limitations, it would be in her best interests and would afford her a better quality of life if she could return home. It was also considered that Gloria's distress when she became confused might have been made worse by being in an assessment situation, and that this may indeed have been the underlying cause of some of her confusion. Gloria's son was naturally concerned about the increasing risks as Gloria's dementia progressed, but was equally convinced that Gloria would be unable to function in a new environment. He acknowledged that although she might become muddled, there was little evidence of actual risk.

The plan was therefore to arrange a period of home leave to assess whether Gloria could settle back into her old routine with increased support to help organize her meals and medication. The main concern was that Gloria might not cooperate with increased intervention, but by planning visits around Gloria's set routine, the team was able to maximize the chance of success. Gloria was discharged home and, as hoped, her confusion was much less apparent once she was reintegrated in her previous lifestyle.

Laurence: An Illustration of the Use of the AMPS BY JANE MELTON

Laurence is a 65-year-old man with mild intellectual impairment. He has had ulcers on his lower legs for many years which have never healed, despite treatment. As a consequence of the dressings required, he owned no shoes that fit. In addition, he has marked kyphoscoliosis, poor circulation to his extremities, and visual difficulties. Laurence is of slight built, is quietly spoken, and often stutters when he converses with people. He was referred to the occupational therapist and other members of the specialist multidisciplinary team by his family physician following concern that he was refusing to leave his bedroom and that there appeared to be a volatile relationship between him and his brother with whom he lives.

Laurence had lived with his family all his life. Most of his relatives had passed away, and for 10 years he has shared a rented house in the British countryside with his older brother. Laurence attended school infrequently and had never worked. His brother had inherited the role of care-giver for Laurence but admitted finding this difficult due to his own physical ill health and his frustration when Laurence failed to "do as he was told." Laurence had not developed a sense of responsibility for himself and presented as passive, waiting for instructions and having difficulty with the concept of choice.

Both Laurence and his brother were very anxious about being offered help or support from welfare services, but were burdened by the pressures of household management — their living conditions were marginal. Laurence had survived on sandwiches, cereals, and potatoes — a diet that contributed to his general poor health. He had no awareness of his income or the value of the money that he had accumulated from his state benefit. He had been isolated from general society most of his life, having no contact with people beyond his family and visits from the district nurse. The only weekly excursion from his home to a luncheon club for older people had recently ceased because the organization closed. Therefore, Laurence's opportunities for learning skills, developing self-esteem, and socializing were negligible and he was becoming increasingly frustrated at his lack of opportunities.

Laurence found it difficult to identify his problem areas with regard to function around his home. He had very little experience from which to draw about community life but expressed a great desire to be exploring his community. The occupational therapist concentrated on this aspect in the first instance to build rapport and provide an opportunity to ease tension within the household. Weekly visits to the nearby town were established, and the exploration involved offering choices to Laurence of public places to visit. These included shops, leisure facilities, cafes, museums, and the occupational therapy department at the local hospital. Laurence was gradually introduced to many life and leisure activities including use of the telephone, light meal preparation, shopping, and laundry. He expressed a great motivation toward the intervention and learned new skills quickly. His achievements were reinforced by the development of a photographic portfolio. Laurence demonstrated the ability to recognize but not count numbers. He is unable to read but can identify items from company logos on packaging (e.g., he knows a particular brand of baked beans).

Choice and Use of the AMPS

Because Laurence had both intellectual and physical impairments, the occupational therapist identified the AMPS as well suited to gather information on his motor and process skills. This assessment would also highlight his strengths and weaknesses in performing daily living tasks necessary for greater independence in community living, which he desired to improve.

The therapist identified five tasks of appropriate challenge for Laurence from the standardized tasks available in the AMPS. From these, Laurence chose to perform two tasks: preparing a cheese sandwich and preparing a fresh fruit salad. He considered these occupational forms to be meaningful in his life.

The evaluation was carried out in Laurence's own home following the preparatory work highlighted above. He engaged in a few practice sessions of the specific tasks before the formal AMPS administration to allow him to become familiar and practiced in the activities. The occupational therapy kitchen was used for practice sessions to limit the intrusion caused by the therapist in the family environment.

Results of the Evaluation

Laurence scored 0.9 on the motor skill scale, which is below the cut-off point. He scored 0.5 on the process scale, which is also below the cut-off point. These scores indicate that Laurence does have skill deficits that negatively impact on his performance of daily living tasks and highlight Laurence's difficulty with independent living. Laurence demonstrated some areas of adequate motor and process skills. AMPS also identified very specific areas of difficulty during task performance.

Laurence demonstrated ineffective motor skill across all his performance in the following areas:
- Aligning his body in a vertical position
- Walking around the task environment
- Positioning and bending the body appropriately to the task
- Coordinating two body parts to securely stabilize and grip task objects
- Transporting and lifting objects used in the task
- Enduring and pacing himself during the task performance

In the area of process skills, Laurence experienced difficulty in:
- Choosing appropriate tools and materials
- Using objects according to their intended purpose
- Knowing how to handle objects
- Heeding (attending to the purpose) of the specific occupational form he was doing
- Inquiring about necessary information
- Initiating actions or steps without hesitation and terminating actions at the appropriate time
- Gathering tools and materials into the task workspace
- Organizing tools and materials in an orderly, logical, and spatially appropriate fashion
- Accommodating his actions to overcome problems
- Benefiting from experience to prevent recurrence of problems

(Continued)

Finally, skills in noticing and responding to nonverbal task-related environmental cues, benefiting from experience to prevent recurrence of problems, and adjusting to changing workspace to overcome problems were significantly deficient.

Interpretation of the Results

In the area of motor skills, Laurence's kyphoscoliosis, which combined with his difficulty with walking, limited his ability to effectively mobilize, bend, lift, or transport objects over any distance. His poor circulation and his sight problems seemed to affect his ability to use his hands effectively. These problems were exacerbated by the fact that Laurence was not well practiced at the tasks, despite being highly motivated to participate. Because of his misaligned physique, his body and arm positioning in relation to work surfaces and objects made performance more difficult for him.

In the area of process skills, it was clear that Laurence had problems in initiating the newly learned tasks and making independent decisions about the task progression. For example, when preparing the fruit salad, he incorporated some extra ingredients that were not part of the agreed task. When asked about this following the evaluation, Laurence said that he had "forgotten" which fruit were decided upon. This exemplifies Laurence's general inexperience at being engaged in self-care tasks and his difficulty with completing all the steps or components of an occupational form. This same problem is echoed within other skill areas, such as the areas of adaptation to the task environment where he demonstrated marked difficulty in noticing and responding to the changing circumstances of the task.

Laurence hesitated at the beginning and during familiar tasks. He organized his workspace so that it was crammed. He used some tools in such a way that he could have injured himself. He generally had difficulty adapting to his environment and responding to environmental changes.

Despite Laurence's problems in both motor and process skills, he did have many adequate skills. These strengths indicate that he does not require assistance at all times during performance, but would benefit from specific support to ensure that he has the opportunity and confidence to engage safely in routine occupational performance.

Usefulness of the Information for Therapeutic Reasoning

The recommendations highlighted by the AMPS were introduced to Laurence and his brother sensitively and over time so that they would be accepted and integrated into daily life.

With the information provided by the motor scale, the occupational therapist was able to make specific recommendations that Laurence's environment be suitably adapted to accommodate his motor needs. His home was modified with consideration to his unsteady mobility. For example, attention was given to suitable flooring with the removal of obstacles (such as rugs) that might cause a fall. Household equipment was rearranged at a height to limit difficult bending or lifting. His bathroom was altered to incorporate a perching stool. Alterations to the decoration of the house incorporated a greater degree of light being available when carrying out tasks. His armchair was adapted to accommodate his back deformity, and a referral was made to physiotherapy for advice on suitable footwear.

The process scale yielded information that highlighted Laurence's need for regular practice at learning some tasks (e.g., light meal cooking) and assistance with other tasks (e.g., household cleaning). In addition, the need for support to solve problems when faced with difficult or novel situations was evident. The following resources were developed to address these ongoing needs. The occupational therapist and community support worker developed protocols for empowering Laurence to carry out tasks as independently as possible but within his skill capacity. For example, they created pictorial shopping lists, recipe cards, diary charts, and telephone number lists.

Opportunities to participate in routine tasks of meaning to Laurence were developed to consider his process skills. The information generated about process skills identified strengths and weaknesses that Laurence would bring to performance and, therefore, likely supports he would need. For example, attending to his laundry was split into component parts. Laurence does what he can safely complete, some aspects with verbal guidance, and his care worker does the other parts. Aspects of tasks have also been adapted to compensate for Laurence's inability to read. For example, the washing machine programs were coded by color.

Laurence also attended a community group run by the occupational therapist and community nurse to address issues of safety at home. Furthermore, Laurence enrolled in a basic literacy college course and has discovered a new hobby, playing cards with some people that he met at college. Laurence's awareness of his own capacities and his sense of efficacy improved significantly and with the regular support he received at home, he is able to function safely and with a reasonable degree of independence. His relationship with his brother improved, and he has become less dependent for physical care from him. Laurence has also achieved his ambition to own and care for a cat, a role and responsibility in which he takes great pride. As Laurence and his brother have developed trust in the therapist over time, additional workers and services have been possible to introduce. He has regular contact with a specialist community nurse, his family physician, and other health care workers.

In summary, the AMPS provided critical, objective information concerning Laurence's occupational performance, which guided the therapist in making decisions about Laurence's therapy. Importantly, it also allowed the therapist to document the need for the resources that Laurence received in the community. The comprehensiveness and precision of the AMPS in providing detailed and research-based information makes it an important asset in understanding and meeting a client's performance needs.

STUDY QUESTIONS

4-1. This chapter focuses on reclaiming occupational as a process as per Reilly. Explain.

4-2. Explore the concepts of activity choice and occupational choice. Apply them to your daily life and provide examples.

4-3. Judge or rate your own performance regarding how effective you are in the world. What do you view as important and what do you find enjoyable and satisfying? Find a classmate to share with and compare your two sets of responses. What are the similarities and what are the differences? To what can you attribute the similarities and differences?

4-4. Think about your life. What did you value as a child? What did you value as an adolescent? What did you value as a young adult? If appropriate, what do you value as a middle-aged adult? How have your values changed over time? How might you anticipate them to change in the future?

4-5. Compare your values to the values of those who raised you. How are they the same or different? How do you explain this?

4-6. In this chapter, the authors refer to Csikszentmihalyi's concept of flow. Speculate about antonyms to flow.

4-7. Differentiate habituation from habits.

4-8. Compare habits and roles.

4-9. Define role strain. Give examples of it from your own life.

4-10. Differentiate occupational form from occupational participation.

References

Ayres, A. J. (1972). *Sensory integration and learning disorders*. Los Angeles: Western Psychological Services.

Ayres, A. J. (1979). *Sensory integration and the child*. Los Angeles: Western Psychological Services.

Ayres, A. J. (1986). *Developmental dyspraxia and adult onset apraxia*. Torrance, CA: Sensory Integration International.

Baron, K., & Curtin, C. (1990). A manual for the use with the self-assessment of occupational functioning. Unpublished manuscript. Department of Occupational Therapy, University of Illinois at Chicago.

Bernspang, B., & Fisher, A. (1995). Differences between persons with right or left cerebral vascular accident on the assessment of motor and process skills. *Archives of Physical Medicine and Rehabilitation, 76*, 1144–1151.

Bruner, J. (1990). *Acts of meaning*. Cambridge, MA: Harvard University Press.

Bundy, A. C., Lane, S. J., & Murray E. A. (Eds.). (2002). *Sensory integration: Theory and practice*. Philadelphia: F. A. Davis.

Csikszentmihalyi, M. (1990). *Flow: The psychology of optimal experience*. New York: Harper and Row.

Dewey, J. (1922). *Human nature and conduct*. New York: Henry Holt & Company.

Doble, S. (1991). Test-retest and inter-rater reliability of a process skills assessment. *Occupational Therapy Journal of Research, 11*, 8–23.

Fisher, A. (1998). Uniting practice and theory in an occupational framework. *American Journal of Occupational Therapy, 52*, 509–520.

Fisher, A. G. (1993). The assessment of IADL motor skills: An application of many-faceted Rasch analysis. *American Journal of Occupational Therapy, 47*, 319–329.

Fisher, A. G., & Kielhofner, G. (1995). Skill in occupational performance. In G. Kielhofner (Ed.) *A model of human occupation: Theory and application* (2nd ed.). Baltimore, MD: Williams & Wilkins.

Forsyth, K., Lai, J., & Kielhofner, G. (1999). The assessment of communication and interaction skills (ACIS): Measurement properties. *British Journal of Occupational Therapy, 62*, 69–74.

Forsyth, K., Salamy, M., Simon, S., & Kielhofner, G. (1997). *A users guide to the assessment of communication and interaction skills (ACIS)*. Bethesda, MD: American Occupational Therapy Association.

Grossack, M., & Gardner, H. (1970). *Man and men: Social psychology as social science*. Scranton, PA: International Textbook Co.

Hahn, H. (1985). Toward a politics of disability: Definitions, disciplines, and policies. *Social Science Journal, 22*, 87–105

Hahn, H. (1993). The political implications of disability definitions and data. *Journal of Disability Studies, 4*, 41–52.

Husserl E. (1962). *Ideas: General introduction to pure phenomenology*. Translated by WRB Gibson. London: Collier Books.

Kalish, R. A., & Collier, K. W. (1981). *Exploring human values*. Monterey, CA: Brooks/Cole.

Kielhofner, G. (1975). The evolution of knowledge in occupational therapy: Understanding adaptation of the chronically disabled. Unpublished Master's Thesis, University of Southern California, Los Angeles.

Kielhofner, G. (1980a). A model of human occupation, part three: Benign and vicious cycles. *American Journal of Occupational Therapy, 34*, 731–737.

Kielhofner, G. (1980b). A model of human occupation, part two. Ontogenesis from the perspective of temporal adaptation. *American Journal of Occupational Therapy, 34*, 657–663.

Kielhofner, G. (1985). *A model of human occupation: Theory and application*. Baltimore, MD: Williams & Wilkins.

Kielhofner, G. (1995). *A model of human occupation: Theory and application* (2nd ed.). Baltimore, MD: Williams & Wilkins.

Kielhofner, G. (1997). *Conceptual foundations of occupational therapy* (2nd ed.). Philadelphia, PA: F.A. Davis.

Kielhofner, G. (2002). *A model of human occupation: Theory and application* (3rd ed.). Baltimore, MD: Lippincott Williams & Wilkins.

Kielhofner, G., & Burke, J. (1980). A model of human occupation, part one. Conceptual framework and content. *American Journal of Occupational Therapy, 34*, 572–581.

Kielhofner, G., Burke, J., & Heard, I. C. (1980). A model of human occupation, part four. Assessment and intervention. *American Journal of Occupational Therapy, 34*, 777–788.

Kielhofner, G., Tham, T., Baz, T., & Hutson, J. (2002). Performance capacity and the lived body. In G. Kielhofner (Ed.), *A model of human occupation: Theory and application* (3rd ed.). Baltimore, MD: Lippincott Williams & Wilkins.

Klavins, R. (1972). Work-play behavior: Cultural influences. *American Journal of Occupational Therapy, 26*, 176–179.

Lee, D. (1971). Culture and the experience of value. In A. H. Maslow (Ed.), *Neural knowledge in human values*. Chicago, IL: Henry Regnery.

Matsutsuyu, J. (1969). The interest checklist. *American Journal of Occupational Therapy, 23*, 323–328.

Merleau-Ponty, M. (1962). *Phenomenology of perception*. Translated from the French original version, *Phénoménologie de la perception*, by Colin Smith. London: Routledge & Kegan Paul, Ltd.

Murphy, R. F. (1987). *The body silent*. New York: W. W. Norton.

Price, R. (1994). *A whole new life*. New York: Atheneum.

Reilly, M. (1962). Occupational therapy can be one of the great ideas of 20th century medicine. *American Journal of Occupational Therapy, 16*, 1–9.

Reilly, M. (1969). The educational process. *American Journal of Occupational Therapy, 23*, 299–307.

Sachs, O. (1993). *A leg to stand on*. New York: Harper Collins Publishers.

Sarbin, T. R., & Scheibe, K. E. (1983). A model of social identity. In T. R. Sarbin, & K. E. Scheibe (Eds.), *Studies in social identity*. New York: Praeger.

Smith, M. B. (1969). *Social psychology and human values*. Chicago, IL: Aldine.

Trombly, C. A., & Radomski, M. V. (2002) *Occupational therapy for physical dysfunction* (5th ed.). Baltimore, MD: Lippincott Williams & Wilkins.

5

Occupational Form, Occupational Performance, and a Conceptual Framework for Therapeutic Occupation

David L. Nelson and Julie Jepson-Thomas

OBJECTIVES

This chapter will help you to:

- Characterize occupation, according to the Conceptual Framework for Therapeutic Occupation, using the following key phrases: occupational form, developmental structure, meaning and purpose, occupational performance, and dynamic relationship.
- Define and contrast therapeutic occupation and naturalistic occupation.
- Explain the roles of adaptation, compensation, and prevention in therapeutic occupational synthesis.
- Apply the Conceptual Framework for Therapeutic Occupation to practice situations.
- Identify various sources of Conceptual Framework for Therapeutic Occupation ideas.

⌐ABOUT THE AUTHORS

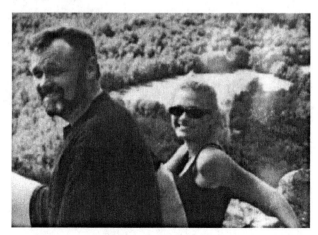

David hiking with his daughter in Vermont.

David Nelson is a man who is highly enthusiastic about the profession of occupational therapy. He believes strongly in the profession; he thinks it is a good thing for people and should be a much larger part of our civilization. "I guess I feel a personal responsibility to try to help make that happen as much as I can... that's what my job is about... to try to enlarge the applications of occupational therapy."

David describes himself as someone who is interested in living a good life, and he bases the idea of a good life in terms of relationships. Most important to him are his wife Ingrid, his children, and his sisters. Caring about others, being involved with them and their lives, and establishing good friendships enhance life.

His occupational therapy career began at New York University with Frieda Behlen and Anne C. Mosey. Both had a strong influence on him. Mosey convinced him that there was a role in occupational therapy for someone who kept questioning what he saw around him. She let him know that while the profession was practical, there was also room for someone who was less practical, who wanted to be theoretical, and who wanted to develop ideas that might have a long-term effect on the profession and practice. His initial work with autistic children stimulated his thoughts on meaning and purpose as well as the connections between perception, symbolic interpretation, sensory motor abilities, language, and the way in which people take on a social identity in life.

During his doctoral work, David spent time working with A. Jean Ayres, and although he never became a proponent of sensory integration, he was impressed with Ayres' "total dedication to the integration of theory, practice, and research. The integration of those three things was a model of how to be a professional; that influenced me a lot." He also was influenced by the writings of many other leaders in the profession. David moved on to a teaching position at Boston University that he credits with helping him to begin to tie science together with theory and practice. "We were all trying to figure out how to do that, how to develop a scientific methodology, identify scientific methodologies and how they would fit to explore questions about occupational therapy." The germination of ideas from this stage served as the basis for some of his work for the next 10–15 years.

David feels strongly that students need to understand that along with developing an appreciation for research, they must recognize the critical nature of active doing, how this defines a person and helps him or her develop for the future. Once there is an understanding of occupation, one should focus on how occupation is presented in all models of practice, whether the term occupation is specifically used or not. Then students should compare and contrast all models to get a sense of the profession as a whole. Finally, students can apply these constructs in fieldwork, which is critical to the learning process, and it is hoped, see the potential for using that understanding in research.

Whereas David acknowledges that the Conceptual Framework for Therapeutic Occupation is only one perspective, it is one to which he committed. He views occupation as not just a long-term role for people but a method that can be used in a therapeutic manner with an individual. Although his fundamental ideas have not changed since the original publication of this perspective, they have become more detailed and in-depth. He hopes that in the future it will become a practical way for analyzing clinical situations, for guiding clinical reasoning, and for developing additional models of practice and frames of reference that people will use.

From David's perspective, it is critical for students and future practitioners to become more concerned about the core of the profession and its theory as well as about research, interpreting research, and applying research to their practices. Even if they do not agree with his theoretical orientation, he hopes that he has served as a role model, to see that there is a place for someone who wants to develop theory, even if it takes much time and effort to move the profession forward.

David's long-term hope for the profession is that it will grow dramatically and in many different areas, such as in the areas of community and wellness, all incorporating occupation. This would apply to people with noted impairments and those who are out in the community with real impairments that have not been identified through illness or an acute hospital experience. "There's a great need . . . I think there's a tremendous growth opportunity."

David continues to develop, refine, and embellish this theoretical model at the Medical College of Ohio along with his colleague Julie Jepson-Thomas.

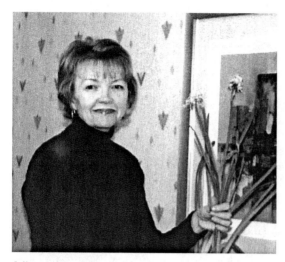

Julie arranging flowers in her home.

Julie Jepson-Thomas began her career as an occupational therapist in the Navy during the early 1970s. She was expected to take an active role in teaching fieldwork to students, residents, and therapy technicians as well as working with the patients seen daily. The role of teacher was particularly suited to her interests. She participated in research, which she found fascinating, and realized that she wanted to be part of academics.

A combination of continued practice, a master's degree, and a doctoral degree provided the depth of experience and tools she needed to begin conducting research and teaching future therapists. She found great joy and personal satisfaction in the academic role. Conveying to students the thrill of our practice and instilling in them a thirst for new knowledge is something that she hopes to provide on an ongoing basis.

She has benefited by the mentorship of many people (too numerous to list here) during every stage of her career. Currently, David Nelson provides a lexicon for our discipline and models for research. She is very grateful for the knowledge and passion shared with her by many colleagues. Collaboration with talented colleagues fuels her belief in the valuable contributions occupational therapy makes to society.

She is blessed with a wonderful and supportive family who understands that the academic life is not confined to regular working hours. Together with her husband Stephen, she balances their professional lives with intense and therapeutic gardening, experimenting with novel restaurants, traveling to foreign cities near warm beaches, visiting extended family, and community service. Their children, Jeffrey and Elliot, help her realize that true fulfillment comes from closely connected lives. She continues to foster close family bonds, even as the children move on in their lives, away from home.

Julie feels that it is an exciting time to be an occupational therapist, with so many possibilities. With careful consideration of different viewpoints, she believes that occupational therapists are better off "not only when we stand on the shoulders of those who have come before us, but because collectively, we are boldly stretching our understanding into the future."

DEFINING OCCUPATION

Occupation is the central concept in our profession of occupational therapy. The reason for the founding of the profession was the use of occupation as a method to enhance human lives (National Society for the Promotion of Occupational Therapy, 1917; Meyer, 1922; Slagle, 1922). (The reader is referred to a discussion of the history of therapeutic occupation in the 1996 Eleanor Clarke Slagle lecture [Nelson, 1997].) Our profession's focus on occupation as a method of therapy is what makes the profession unique and valuable to society.

Given the critical importance of the term "occupation," it is remarkable that this term was seldom discussed in the professional literature of occupational therapy in the 1950s and 1960s. A growing profession called "occupational therapy" seldom used the term "occupation." No wonder our fellow health professionals and the public often did not understand why occupational therapy was called occupational therapy. Christiansen (1990,

p. 262) stated that it was "startling" that the profession long went without developing a workable definition of occupation.

Much of this chapter is devoted to a definition of occupation. This definition is essentially the same as published previously (Nelson, 1988, 1994). Changes in wording reflect what we have learned over the years in trying to communicate the essence of occupation as we see it. Sometime around 1995, we started using the phrase "Conceptual Framework for Therapeutic Occupation" to label these definitions and their relationship with the profession of occupational therapy.

Occupation is a complex construct consisting of many interrelated concepts, each of which is complex in its own right. Each time we define a term we then have to go on to define the terms used in the original definition. Defining a complex construct like occupation is a little like opening a box only to find out that the box contains a series of ever-smaller boxes to be opened. If you see those ever-smaller boxes as having a kind of logical beauty, you have the main prerequisite for being a theoretician! Later in the chapter, it is shown how this definition is useful in understanding how to analyze and use occupation in therapy.

It is not the goal of this chapter to cite references for each of the ideas found here. Rather, the attempt is made to make the reading as smooth and conversational in tone as possible, given the complexity of the ideas. This attempt is made at the explicit request of students and others who have tried to read our past writings without the benefit of supplemental verbal discussions. Past publications (Nelson, 1988, 1996, 1997) provide substantial references. Toward the end of this chapter there is a section on the sources of ideas influential in the development of the Conceptual Framework for Therapeutic Occupation. Future scholarly work will continue to identify the relationships between Conceptual Framework for Therapeutic Occupation and the works of other occupational therapists as well as the works of philosophers, anthropologists, linguists, sociologists, psychologists, and scientific methodologists. A final word before the definitions begin: We do not think that this is the only possible definition of occupation, and we recognize that many others are taking different approaches. We only hope that the Conceptual Framework for Therapeutic Occupation contributes to the dialogue and to the development of the profession.

> **A Definition of Occupation:** *Occupation is a dynamic relationship among an occupational form, a person with a unique developmental structure, subjective meanings and purposes, and a resulting occupational performance.*

This very abstract definition requires much explanation. What is an occupational form? What is meant by developmental structure? What is an occupational performance? We begin by defining and discussing the term *occupational form*. One point to make first is that occupation, as here defined, is the actual doing of a real person at a particular time. When we speak of occupation, we are not just talking about the types of things that people do; we are talking about the real life of an individual human being. Each occupation is unique and actual.

OCCUPATIONAL FORM

> **A Definition of Occupational Form:** *Occupational form is the objective set of physical and sociocultural circumstances, external to the person, at a particular time. The occupational form guides, structures, or suggests what is to be done by the person.*

To understand this definition, let us first discuss the phrase "external to the person." Everything surrounding the person is part of the person's occupational form, and everything that is a part of the person is not the occupational form. Therefore, the objects around the person are parts of the occupational form, and even the person's clothes are parts of the occupational form; however, the person's body, capabilities, and actions are not parts of the occupational form.

The occupational form is objective. Objectivity implies that scientists and other careful observers can independently come to some agreement about a person's occupational form (they can have inter-rater reliability). In contrast, the person's thoughts and feelings are not objective. Thoughts and feelings are subjectively experienced by the person, and no one else has direct access to them. Thus, we can say that a table set for dinner is part of the occupational form, but the person's thoughts and feelings about the dining situation are not parts of the occupational form.

An occupational form has a *physical* dimension and a *sociocultural* dimension. Box 5-1 shows the components of these dimensions (Nelson, 1994).

Physical Dimension

A physical scientist or engineer can measure and describe the physical dimension of an occupational form. The physical dimension of an occupational form includes the objects present, their spatial characteristics (height, width, and depth), their relative positions in relation to each other, their weights, the textures of their surfaces, the sounds they make, and background features such as lighting and air temperature. For example, let us take the occupation of putting a load of laundry into the dryer. Important factors to consider are the physical features of the dryer (size? type of door? types of controls? type of mechanical action?), the physical nature of the clothes (amount? weight when wet and weight when dried? colors? fabrics?), and other features of the surrounding environmental (Laundromat, kitchen, or basement? lighting? odors? operation of adjacent washing machine?). All these physical features might well affect the occupation of an individual.

Persons are quite sensitive to the physical features of their occupational forms. The height of a work desk can affect productivity. The contour of a car seat can spell the difference between frequent use and abandonment. Adequate lighting and temperature are necessary for most human occupation. A principle of many restaurants is "Presentation is everything." When we analyze occupational forms, sometimes we must be very precise

---

Box 5-1 DIMENSIONS OF OCCUPATIONAL FORM

Physical Dimension		Sociocultural Dimension	
Shapes	Temporal Aspects	Symbols	Social Levels
Sizes		Norms	Universal
Distances	The moment-by-	Sanctions	Cultural
Relative positions	moment changes	Roles	Subcultural
Weights	in all physical	Typical uses	National
Textures	factors	Typical variations	Regional/community
Colors		Language rules	Institutional
Lighting		etc.	Organizational
Sounds			Neighborhood
Physical presence			Family
of others			Other groups
etc.			

about physical issues, such as the height, firmness, and support of a chair, or such as the glare and color contrast within a frequently traversed hallway. The physical arrangements of toys can make the difference between productive play and random, exhausting trials with error.

Another aspect of the physical dimension of an occupational form involves the *physical presence of others*. Whenever we analyze an occupational form, we look at the people in the surroundings of a particular individual. The locations, postures, clothes, movements, facial expressions, and speech of others in the individual's occupational form can be critical aspects affecting the individual's occupation. For example, in a tennis game, one's opponent's movements, location, and speech can become critical factors influencing the individual's occupational performance. Social situations involve reciprocity: One person's physical presence is part of the other person's occupational form, and vice versa.

Another facet of the physical dimension is its *temporal aspect,* that is, the moment-by-moment changes in the materials over the course of the occupation. In the course of a tennis match, the occupational form encountered by the player is continuously changing. The ball moves from place to place at different velocities and trajectories, one's opponent moves into different locations, and even the temperature changes as the hours pass. In contrast, some things remain relatively stationary or unchanged over the course of the game (the net, the boundary lines, and the fence surrounding the court). All the physical features listed in the left-hand column of Box 5-1 (e.g., shape, size, weight) are subject to temporal change over the course of an occupation. In some occupations, key moment-to-moment changes involve physical transformation of materials (as in the making of a craft or a dinner). In other occupations, the most important moment-to-moment changes involve the movements of others (e.g., ballroom dancing) or the speech of others (e.g., attending a lecture).

This concept of temporal aspects is often difficult for students of the Conceptual Framework for Therapeutic Occupation to understand. One way of picturing the temporal aspects of an occupational form is for students to imagine themselves to be ghosts. Students can then mentally picture the changes in the objects that surround them. The trick is to separate the changes in the occupational form from the reactions of the person (we will see that the reactions of the person are occupational performances, not occupational forms). The occupational form around a person is continuously changing and providing new challenges.

Sociocultural Dimension

The other major part of an occupational form is its sociocultural dimension. Cultural and social issues pervade most situations. For example, in a cooking occupation, there are issues of ethnicity, finances, and role expectations (e.g., the expected role of a parent in food preparation for children). The culture of the country club golfer is different from the culture of the football player, and the social expectations for a business executive are different from those of a bus driver. Sociocultural issues are so pervasive and familiar in our everyday occupational forms that healthy adults are often unaware of them. Observations of healthy parent-child interactions can help us be more conscious of the sociocultural webs in which we live. The parent of a toddler points out the rules for appropriate dress and speech. The parent of an 8-year-old communicates the importance of school as an occupational form. The parent of a teenager persistently (and with great patience) points out rules regarding curfew, transportation, substance ingestion, and courtesy.

In this Conceptual Framework for Therapeutic Occupation framework, the sociocultural dimension of an occupational form is inseparable from its physical dimension. As in Box 5-1, we can make columns of words on the left that list physical features and columns on the right that list sociocultural features, but in the real world the two dimensions are mutually dependent on each other. The sociocultural aspects of an occupational form always have a physical manifestation. Let us consider a simple symbol: a stop sign. Physically, the sign is metallic, octagonal, flat, approximately 2 feet in diameter, mounted on a metal pole at a height of about 7 feet, and located at an intersection in such a way that its red and white face is perpendicular to the road. Socioculturally, what is the message of this physical object in its proper context? The rule is that the driver of a vehicle should stop at the appropriate place; look both ways; and proceed with caution after ensuring that the path is safe. Implicit in the occupational form is a set of punitive sanctions that the driver can expect if the rules are not followed (police enforcement, the potential of injury to self or others, and potential changes in insurance rates). The point here is that the sociocultural significance of the stop sign is embedded in its physical nature. Society has decided that red and white should be the colors of the stop sign. Without the red and white pattern (and without all the other essential physical features of the occupational form), the message to stop and all the other messages in the stop sign could not be communicated effectively. Transmission of culture depends on the physical world, whether through signs, artifacts, the printed word, electronic transmissions, or the sound waves made by human speech. Although the sociocultural dimension of the occupational form depends on the physical dimension, the sociocultural dimension cannot be reduced to physical characteristics.

At this point, it is important to point out that we are still discussing the world that is external to the individual. When we discuss the sociocultural aspects of occupational form, we are *not* describing the experience of an individual person. We are describing the sociocultural reality that surrounds an individual and that exists independently of the individual. Just as a physical scientist can measure and describe the physical aspects of occupational forms, a social scientist can measure and describe the sociocultural features of occupational forms. The sociocultural aspects of an occupational form can be identified by finding out what healthy adults in the culture have to say about the occupational form. What is the typical interpretation of this situation? What do the physical materials hint at as to what is supposed to be done? Do the physical materials suggest that this is a party place, a work place, or a worship place? Whether or not the individual lives up to the social expectations in the occupational form, the form is objectively present (it is assumed that two or more independent observers who are familiar with the culture could agree as to the sociocultural situation).

Symbols

To provide examples of each of the factors listed under the sociocultural dimension in Box 5-1, let us consider the occupation of a person driving a car to work. We have already described the stop sign as a symbol, with its sociocultural rules embedded in its physical characteristics. Other symbols to be encountered are the advertisements that fill up the periphery of the occupational form. Signs on stores and trucks, billboards, and radio messages not only advertise wares but lifestyles. Communications experts make excellent salaries in designing messages that define the American landscape. Advertisements are powerful examples of how important it is to shape the physical aspects of the occupational form into a coherent whole that suggests a message: "Buy this and enjoy happiness/pleasure/prestige." Generally, one does not sell a car by discussing its mechanical properties, and one does not sell a hamburger by analyzing its nutritional qualities. Symbols, carefully designed integrations of physical materials and sociocultural messages, lead to sales.

Norms

A norm is a socioculturally regulated expectation. A norm reflects something we are supposed to do. For example, a driver on the way to work should stop at a red light and conform to all the other norms of driving. Norms pertain not only to legalities, but also to other kinds of social expectations. For example, it might not be illegal for a driver to make obscene gestures at other drivers, but it would be considered improper in most communities. It is important to distinguish between the word "norms" as it applies to professional measurement and the word as it applies to the sociocultural aspects of occupational forms. A measurement norm simply summarizes typical performance of persons that have been measured in the past. A social norm is an expectation for future occupation.

Sanctions involve the socially administered benefits or punishments associated with adhering or not adhering to norms. For example, going through a red light might result in a traffic ticket and a fine. Violation of a taboo leads to negative sanctions. On the other hand, positive sanctions can be experienced if the driver is consistently on time and ready for work. On a larger scale, pay for work can be thought of as a positive sanction administered by the work organization. Sanctions might be formal (codified) or informal. Legal sanctions and workplace sanctions are written down, but informal sanctions, such as the approval or disapproval of friends and family, are also important aspects of the occupational form.

Roles

A social role is a set of expectations involving others. For example, the person behind the wheel of a car is carrying out the role of driver. The driver, as in the prior example, is also trying to live up to the demands of having a role as a worker (being on time for work). There are many different types of roles; some are temporary and some are enduring. The driver might be dealing with family roles (as spouse, parent, child, sibling) as well as with a variety of other roles (citizen, friend, club member, money lender). Associated with each are sociocultural expectations. It is important once again to point out that we are not yet talking about how a particular individual accepts or rejects a role or social responsibility; we are still talking about the occupational form external to the individual.

Typical Uses and Variations

Most physical objects encountered in everyday life have typical or intended uses. For example, the windshield wipers, the brakes, and the steering wheel have clearly designed uses and specifications. Culture even defines the natural environment for typical uses (e.g., the ideal spot for a picnic). Tools constitute a special class of objects to be used instrumentally in the modification of other objects. However, socioculturally defined objects sometimes have multiple and/or alternative uses. Typical variations in object use are common, even in basic self-care. In a class of approximately 30 occupational therapy students, 11 distinctly different ways of donning a pullover shirt were identified from the everyday lives of the students. Another example of typical variations of expected use in an occupational form can be seen in handwriting. Some people in U.S. culture maintain that the dynamic tripod grasp is the preferred method for handwriting, but the fact is that many Americans habitually and effectively grasp pens in different ways. Consider the many forms of handwriting, dancing, or home management. Hence, occupational forms are not always rigidly structured — they often present alternatives and options.

Sometimes the culture positively sanctions various alternatives, and sometimes the culture draws clear lines as to what is appropriate and what is not. Whenever we talk about what is appropriate, we are talking about the sociocultural aspects of an occupational form. All cultures draw some clear lines concerning what is appropriate and what is not. When the use of an object infringes on the rights of others, a negative sanction can be expected.

Language

Language is the ultimate set of symbols for a culture, and it is often a critical part of a person's occupational form. Language involves a complex set of rules for vocabulary, grammar, and syntax. One set of rules governs written language, and a related set of rules governs speech, including rules for pronunciation. Many of the rules are arbitrary. For example, in a vocabulary, there is often no inherent relationship between the physical object and the proper label. Through consensus built over time, the culture decides to call a rose a rose, even though another label might have worked just as well. Because of the complexity and arbitrariness of language rules, it takes many years to master a language. Like other culturally defined symbols, a special power of language in an occupational form is to communicate complex relationships in representative forms, such that the actual physical objects under discussion need not be present. Still, language as part of the occupational form always involves a physical manifestation: sounds waves in speech, squiggles on paper or a computer screen in written communications, or the hand movements used in sign language. As stated previously, the sociocultural aspects of the occupational form always have a physical manifestation.

Cultural Changes

Humans construct culture and society, and each culture is in a constant state of change (some at more rapid rates than others). In our age, cultures throughout the world are rapidly adopting each other's menus, music, communications technology, business practices, and lifestyles. Only a few generations ago, most people throughout the world had very limited access to the cultural norms of other groups. An example of cultural change within the authors' lives has been a radical reconstruction of gender relationships. The rules have changed for male and female roles. Culture as a whole must not be looked on as static or unchangeable, even though certain values within the culture can be enduring.

The individual, through occupation, can have an effect on one's culture (later we will label this kind of effect as an "impact" in Conceptual Framework for Therapeutic Occupation terms). Therefore, although culture is powerful and omnipresent in occupational forms, the individual can contribute to culture in many ways. For example, an individual can write a novel that influences others, make a contribution to science, or live an exemplary life affecting many others with whom that person comes into contact. Working with others, the person can write laws, go to the moon, or put a new technology into the hands of billions of people. On a smaller scale, all work involves some sort of social impact. The potential contributions of an individual's occupations to occupational forms will be especially clear in the next section, in which smaller and smaller levels of cultural organization are discussed.

Social Levels

The right-hand column of Box 5-1 suggests that the sociocultural dimension of the occupational form must be interpreted at many different levels within culture and society. Symbols, norms, sanctions, roles, typical uses, and typical variations in uses of objects all depend in part on the social level. Cultural influences are pervasive, and few things are interpreted the same way from culture to culture.

The highest social level depicted in Box 5-1 is the *universal* level. One can argue that certain aspects of the occupational form are interpreted universally across cultures. For example, across all cultures, fresh water is for drinking, fresh air affords breathing, the sun provides warmth and light, and the earth supports edible plant growth. The universality of basic, survival-oriented symbols such as water, air, the sun, and the earth seems clear. However, even these most basic symbols will be colored by culture. One culture will develop a unique set of rituals centered on water, and another culture will deify the sun. For another example, it can be argued that all cultures universally place a special importance on kinship. However, one culture will emphasize the extended family, while another focuses on the nuclear family.

At the *subcultural level*, social expectations as defined by the culture are modified for people in a defined minority. For example, many Mexican Americans are often expected to adhere to the language rules of American-style English in work and public settings but are also often expected to use Mexican-style Spanish in leisure and private settings. Because members of a minority subculture are expected to be able to live according to two different sets of rules, ambiguities and conflicts can be expected. Does the Mexican norm of remaining in close proximity to a large extended family prevail for someone who is newly married, or does the American norm of mobility apply? Is a midwife preferable to an obstetrician, and under what circumstances? As stated above, the cultural level is always in flux and is under the constant influence of many people making decisions. Change at the subcultural level is often even faster.

At the *national* level (and at other governmental levels), norms and sanctions are often codified in law. A relevant example is that the legal rights and resources of older persons vary considerably from one political jurisdiction to another. In Sweden, the older person has a legal right to home modification if the person's home has architectural barriers and lacks supports. In contrast, current law in the United States does not guarantee this type of assistance. National laws often codify negative sanctions (punishments). For example, capital punishment is not a legal sanction in many countries. Laws can be seen as inherent parts of the occupational form. Once again, there is a necessary relationship between the sociocultural aspects of an occupational form (law in the abstract) and the physical aspects of an occupational form (e.g., physical evidence).

The sociocultural dimension of an occupational form often varies by *region* and by *community*. For example, there are regional specialties in most large countries concerning food and regional differences of spoken accent. We can also recognize symbols that have special resonance to members of a particular community (e.g., the "Big Apple" or the county fairgrounds).

Institutions and *organizations* have their own ways of interpreting situations in the social world. Religious institutions often provide detailed mandates concerning symbols, norms, sanctions, and roles. A particular university will argue the special benefits of its unique curriculum. We can identify social expectations that are particular to a specific professional organization: Everyone who is "wise" to the profession of occupational therapy interprets a class period devoted to a craft such as woodworking in a special way that is different from the interpretations of those who are unfamiliar with the history and traditions of occupational therapy. A sorority has complex rules and expectations, some of which are deliberately kept secret as a way of emphasizing the unique nature of the association.

Social levels with their own special symbols and norms can be localized and quite small. In a *neighborhood*, a particular postal worker might be known for her kindness, a store might be known as valuable for certain items but overly expensive for others, and a section of a park might be known as a gathering place for mothers of small children. Most importantly, there is the *family* level to consider. A particular family might have a special joke that everyone is expected to understand and remember. An extended family might have an accepted way of conducting family reunions. Role expectations for various family members can vary tremendously from family to family, even in the same neighborhood. For example, in one family, mother can expect breakfast in bed on Sunday, and in another there is a unique way of celebrating the Fourth of July. At the intimate level of the family, it often seems difficult to separate the occupational form from the individual. However, by definition, the occupational form is always external to the person. A way of making the distinction is to note what happens to the social unit of the family when an individual becomes unable to live up to family norms or unable to interpret family symbols (e.g., the family joke) in the predicted way. Sometimes it is easier to see what is embedded socioculturally in an occupational form when norms are violated than when they are followed routinely.

Finally, the norms and symbols of *other groups* making up the individual's world must be considered. As opposed to formal organizations, informal groups have no written rules, but expectations can still be very robust. One's roommates, one's regular bowling buddies, classmates in school, or married couples who regularly get together for dinner parties constitute important social groupings making up the context of a person's life. Each of the groups has its own symbols, norms, sanctions, and roles. A group is not just a collection of individuals — over time, it takes on an identity of its own. Even a short-term group, such as a platoon in basic military training, can evolve quickly into a powerful occupational form.

Conflict across Levels and Ambiguities in the Occupational Form

We have already stated that the cultural aspects of occupational forms are often in flux, as individuals have effects on their culture. We have also stated that occupational forms frequently present the individual with options among various sanctioned alternative courses of action. Now we need to discuss the fact that an occupational form sometimes is ambiguous and even contradictory in the messages it delivers to the individual. Different social levels often account for these ambiguities and contradictions.

One social level might prohibit what another social level encourages. For example, American movies and television shows are fascinated by the family lives of gangsters. At the governmental level, of course, the gangster lifestyle violates basic norms in egregious fashion. However, at the small-group level and at the family level, the rules are codified quite differently (the murder of an uncle is "only business"). This tension between cultural norms at the upper levels of the hierarchy depicted in Box 5-1 and the lower levels is common grist for the narrative arts as well as the source of much conflict in the lives of individuals. For example, the child can learn the evils of racism at school but experience a neighborhood norm of racial discrimination. For another example, the immigrants to a Western country might be confounded by laws governing divorce and the rights of women to make their own decisions. These ambiguities across social levels can be particularly confusing when combined with the fact that the larger culture and subcultures are continuously in transition. In our culture, exactly what is appropriate dress? In later sections, we will see that questions like this pose special problems to persons with disabilities.

Occupational Form as a Complex Unity

Despite the sometimes conflicting demands of different social levels, and despite the culture's changing interpretations of physical reality, most of the occupational forms we encounter in everyday life are quite clearly structured in predefined ways. Each room in the typical home has a recognizably clear set of typical uses (two or more independent observers would come to similar conclusions). Restaurants are for dining out (or for working). Cars are for transportation according to carefully codified rules. Gardens, classrooms, synagogues, courts, party rooms, offices, and cruise ships are more or less structured to elicit fairly predictable occupational performances. Of course, the individual will put a personal "spin" on any given setting (depending on the person's meanings and purposes, as we will see), but the world of occupational forms is quite well structured. Generally, the physical and sociocultural aspects of the occupational form call for a unified response.

This idea of occupational form as a relatively organized, structured entity is different from the idea that the environment is made up of isolated physical features (e.g., objects or stimuli). A culture does not organize stimuli in isolation from other stimuli. Naturalistic occupational forms consist of *integrated* materials and norms. For example, the chair, the table, the floor, and the lighting make an integrated statement: This is a place for doing things in a sitting position. When we analyze the parts of an occupational form, we must be careful not to see the parts in isolation from the whole. The height of the chair seat is integrally related to the height of the table, the flatness of the floor, and the types of things one can be expected to do while seated at the table. Although the occupational form frequently presents options (no one is forcing us to sit at the table, as opposed to walking out of the room), the options are not at the level of isolated stimuli.

In Conceptual Framework for Therapeutic Occupation terminology, the unity of the occupational form is communicated through labeling the form before analyzing its details. For example, a label could be, "A night game of baseball," or "Dinner at Sister's house," or "Lecture on kinesiology of the hand." Once again, it is important to point out that the occupational form is separate from what the person actually does or feels. Hence, the occupational form could be "Dinner at Sister's house," but the person could be too ill or upset to eat anything, despite the sociocultural expectations in the situation. The label simply implies what is expected or what options are expected (as judged by objective observers familiar with the culture). The objective observers must view the physical reality encompassing the person and make an interpretation. The importance of this reflects the Conceptual Framework for Therapeutic Occupation principle that all cultures provide integrated, complex occupational forms to support human performance. To see the parts of the occupational form only in isolation from the other parts is a pathologic and dysfunctional condition for a human being. Therefore, even when we analyze an occupational form in great detail, we must never forget each potential for eliciting a unified occupational performance.

THE PERSON'S DEVELOPMENTAL STRUCTURE

The reader is referred once again to the Conceptual Framework for Therapeutic Occupation definition of occupation (page 90). The next major concept in that definition, after "occupational form," is "a person with a developmental structure." Occupation depends not only on the occupational form external to the person, but also on the uniqueness of the person.

A Definition of Developmental Structure: *A person's developmental structure consists of sensorimotor, cognitive, and psychosocial abilities and characteristics. The term "developmental" implies that the structure is the end product of a long-term process influenced both by maturation (genetically unfolding physical changes) and by past occupational adaptations (personal experiences).*

Concept of Developmental Structure

The term "structure" implies that the person is not just a "blank slate" that is "written on" by the occupational form. The person is not under the "control" of the occupational form. Occupational performance depends both on the occupational form and on the unique abilities, or *structure*, that the individual brings to the situation. No two people are exactly alike in the way that they do any complex thing, even if the occupational form (in the environment) is approximately the same for the two people.

A human being is incredibly complex. How can we analyze what a person brings to an occupation? One way to begin to analyze the complex unity and adaptability of the human being is to use *Uniform Terminology for Occupational Therapy, Third Edition* (UT III) (American Occupational Therapy Association, 1994). This document describes three main categories of human abilities: (1) sensorimotor components, (2) cognitive integration and cognitive components (simply called "cognitive components" here), and (3) psychosocial skills and psychological components (simply called "psychosocial components" here). Within each component there are subcategories, and within the subcategories are lists of specific abilities and characteristics.

Sensorimotor, Cognitive, and Psychosocial Abilities and Characteristics

To give examples of specific *sensorimotor* abilities used in occupation, let us imagine a person (with a 14-year-old boy's developmental structure) playing soccer. In terms of *sensory processing*, he uses his *vestibular* and proprioceptive organs when correlating *visual* stimuli with his own running and pivoting (*gross motor coordination*). Let us assume that his *position in space perception* and *depth perception* are superior compared with most children his age; therefore, he is able to time the kicking of the ball with great precision to positions unoccupied by the opposition. Let us also assume, however, that his cardiovascular *endurance* is such that his performance tails off somewhat toward the end of the game because of fatigue. He utilizes *praxis* when he is able to adapt to an unusual situation (a ball is kicked toward his hands, and rather than breaking the rules of the game by reaching for the ball, he moves his head to an awkward posture and successfully "heads" the ball).

In the *cognitive* area of abilities, he has to use his long-term *memory* to recall his training regarding strategy as the score shifts, and his short-term *memory* to keep track of the score and opponents' positions. *Problem solving* is required to adopt the appropriate strategy under changing game circumstances. *Generalization* of *learning* is evident in his being able to apply what the coach taught him in the past. After the game, synthesis of *learning* and *concept formation* are required when the coach and team discuss possible new strategies when playing again against a similar team in the future.

In terms of *psychosocial* skills, the boy has long exhibited a strong *interest* in soccer as a sport, and the challenges faced through playing soccer over the years has contributed to his *self-concept.* He knows how to take on the *role* of being a teammate, and he draws on his ability to sustain appropriate *social conduct* in that role. *Values* in regards to fairness and respect for members of the other team are shown. *Self-control* and *coping skills* are exhibited when the boy's team loses a match.

In most occupations many different abilities are exhibited. Indeed, the sensorimotor, cognitive, and psychosocial areas are almost always involved in every occupation. A more detailed analysis of the boy's occupation than given above would reveal that he used additional abilities listed in Uniform Terminology III (UT III). It would also reveal that UT III does not always give us the detail we need when we are trying to describe the abilities used in occupation. For example, UT III does not deal adequately with the skills involved in human language, nor does it begin to deal with the full range of emotional expression that a human being needs to exhibit.

We will see later that specific models of occupational therapy practice have their distinct ways of emphasizing different facets of the human being, and each model of practice has its unique terms. For example, models of occupational therapy for persons with cognitive deficits specify many more component abilities than those listed in UT III. Therefore, a detailed analysis of actual occupation requires much more detail than can be given through UT III. For now, UT III gives us a starting point toward understanding the relationships between the person's developmental structure and the occupational form in which the person finds himself or herself.

Body Systems and the Developmental Structure

Students of Conceptual Framework for Therapeutic Occupation, particularly those interested in neurologically based models of occupational therapy, frequently ask, "Where does the nervous system and other body systems fit into Conceptual Framework for Therapeutic Occupation?" The answer is that the body systems make up the developmental structure. These systems constitute the structure. The sensorimotor, cognitive, and psychosocial abilities and characteristics of the developmental structure reflect the physiologic organization of the person. At any given point in the life of the person, all those characteristics are present in body systems. The neurologic system is perhaps the most important source of these abilities (e.g., sensory, perceptual, cognitive, and psychosocial abilities), but other systems such as the musculoskeletal and connective tissue systems are also very much involved.

From a Conceptual Framework for Therapeutic Occupation perspective, it is not technically correct to say that the body systems *cause* abilities. In the Conceptual Framework for Therapeutic Occupation, the body systems *are* the abilities. An ultimate goal of the science of body systems is to explain the physiology of human abilities. For many ethical and technical reasons, progress is slow. For each ability, there must be a physiologic representation of some kind. However, simplistic models of brain–behavior relationships have proven inadequate. Even the physiology of simple memory storage and retrieval is still not fully understood, although much progress has been made. It will take many years to develop a coherent physiologic theory of complex human abilities, such as a person's proclivity to be interested in certain kinds of occupational forms. As time goes by, however, it can be expected that the abilities characteristic of the developmental structure will be discussed increasingly in neurologic and physiologic terms.

Does this mean that human occupation can be reduced to physiology? Here the answer is "No." The developmental structure of the person reflects physiology, but other aspects of occupation cannot be reduced to physiology. In the following section, we will begin to discuss the experiential aspects of occupation. When a person with a unique developmental structure (organized physiologically) encounters an occupational form, *experience* occurs. In the Conceptual Framework for Therapeutic Occupation, human experience cannot be reduced to physiology, although the physiology of the developmental structure makes experience possible.

MEANING AND OCCUPATION

Meaning is the next major part of the definition of occupation. Please consider the abstract definition given below.

A Definition of Meaning: *Meaning is the entire interpretive experience engaged in by an individual encountering an occupational form. Meaning involves perceptual interpretation, symbolic interpretation, and affect.*

Meaning has to do with interpretation, that is, figuring things out or making sense out of the occupational form. It also has to do with feelings elicited in the context of the occupational form (affective meanings). Meaning is an active process of the individual, and the type of meaning assigned to the occupational form depends on the individual's unique developmental structure.

Figure 5-1 shows a graphic depiction of the relationships between occupational form, the person's developmental structure, and meaning. At a given time and in a given space, a real person with a real developmental structure encounters an occupational form. The result of this encounter is the experience of meaning. The person assigns meanings to the occupational form. This is an active process. The occupational form does not determine the meaning, but in conjunction with the unique developmental structure, the occupational form contributes to the meanings. The same occupational form will lead to different meanings in different persons. In addition, the same person will experience different meanings in different occupational forms. Hence, meaning is depicted in Figure 5-1 as an interaction between form and person.

For example, let us consider the meanings of a 6-year-old girl at a professional hockey game. Meanings include the girl's perceptions of the players, the rink, the fans, the stands, the vendors, and her family members. Part of the meaning for the girl is to grow bored with the big men in floppy outfits skating up and down the ice, which she cannot

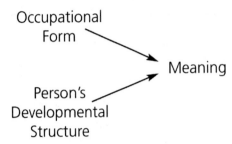

Occupational
Form

Person's
Developmental
Structure

Meaning

Figure 5-1. Meaning.

see so well anyway because of the large people in front of her. Another part of the meaning is that she becomes interested in the coloring book her father brought for her. The meaning of the situation is an opportunity to color while waiting for the silly hockey game to be over. Every once in a while she must cope with her father's attempts to interest her in the game, but the only other thing that has much meaning to her is the opportunity to eat foods forbidden at home.

As can be seen from the example, meaning is a personal matter. One person will make one kind of meaning out of the occupational form (e.g., the father loves to watch a penalty play), while another person (e.g., the 6-year-old girl) does not understand what a penalty play is and does not care. As stated above and as depicted in Figure 5-1, meaning depends on the interaction of the person's developmental structure and the occupational form. The father's developmental structure includes memories of past hockey games and a long attention span with an appreciation for fine detail, whereas the little girl's developmental structure is action-oriented without the cognitive abilities to appreciate the trickery taking place among the players on the ice.

Perceptual Meanings

Perceptual meaning involves interpreting the physical aspects of the occupational form. Any or all of the sensory systems within the developmental structure might be called on in the interpretation of an occupational form. For example, the perceptual meanings of a male assembly line worker include mental representations of the sizes, shapes, and numbers of objects on the assembly line as well as their velocity (perceptually, the worker must be able to predict where the fast-moving object will be located in the next moment so that he can grasp it). Other perceptual meanings involved include the worker's sense of position in space and the relationships between his own body parts and the moving objects. So, the experience of proprioception in his somatosensory receptors is part of his meaning, as defined in the Conceptual Framework for Therapeutic Occupation. His perception of vibration is also part of his perceptual meaning. The noises from the machinery and tools contribute to his auditory meanings. In summary, his perceptual meanings include visual, auditory, and somatosensory processing, all made possible by intact sensory systems in his developmental structure. Gustatory and olfactory experiences also contribute to the overall interpretation of many situations (the meanings assigned to many situations).

Perceptual meaning is an active process in which the individual seeks out elements of the occupational form in a selective way, not in a passive way. Some part of the occupational form might be objectively present, but the person might ignore it because of its perceived irrelevance (its lack of meaning). For example, the movement of the hockey puck was objectively the same for the girl and her father, but the father was able to discern details (find meaning in them) that were ignored as irrelevant by the girl.

Symbolic Meanings

Symbolic meanings, on the other hand, involve interpretations of the *sociocultural* aspects of the occupational form. Symbolically, the worker sees the assembly line as providing work challenges and as an opportunity to earn an income. The observer at a hockey game understands (finds symbolic meaning in) the rules as applied in various situations. Symbolic meaning also has to do with interpreting spoken or written words according to the rules of a language system. We are surrounded by signs and symbols that must be interpreted for us to be successful. Verbally or nonverbally, each of us needs to "read" the situation confronting us. This reading of sociocultural cues is symbolic meaning. This might be a creative process, as when interpreting fine art, or it might be the relatively mundane process of figuring out how to remove a window for routine maintenance.

In English, some common words for describing the experience of symbolic meaning include understand, comprehend, think about, recognize, and make sense of. We will see that the Conceptual Framework for Therapeutic Occupation has its own grammar. For example, in the sentence, "He understood the rules of the game," "he" refers to developmental structure, "understood" refers to symbolic meaning, and "the rules of the game" refer to occupational form. In everyday English, sometimes the same word can refer to symbolic meaning in some contexts and to perceptual meaning in other contexts. For example, in the sentence, "She sees the sky," perceptual meaning is implied by the word "sees." However, in the sentence, "She sees the point of the speech," symbolic meaning is implied by the word "sees." The verb "perceive" can also refer to perceptual meaning or to symbolic meaning, depending on the context. A further complication can be seen in the sentence, "He listened carefully to the speech." Here, the word "listened" probably refers both to perceptual meaning (hearing the sounds) and to symbolic meaning (understanding the social importance of the speech). In the Conceptual Framework for Therapeutic Occupation, it is not so important to distinguish between perceptual meaning and symbolic meaning. What is important is to try to understand the experience of the person.

Affective Meanings

Affective meaning is the emotion experienced by the person when he or she encounters an occupational form. For example, we said the little girl felt bored by the professional hockey game but felt interested in her coloring book. The experience of boredom or interest involves affective meaning. Affective meanings span the entire range of human emotion, from joy to sorrow, from love to hate, and from elation to depression. Affect colors all human perception and symbolic interpretation, sometimes more than at other times. The developmental structure is made to experience intense affect, depending on the occupational form. Indeed, we continuously experience feelings, positive or negative, that are typical of human existence.

Affective meanings accompany perceptual and symbolic meanings (affective meanings are not separate or independent from perceptual and symbolic meanings). For example, for most people the experience of being touched without warning (a tactile perceptual meaning) is tied to an affective meaning of fear or the feeling of being startled. For another example, the perception of warmth on a cold day will usually be tied to positive affective experience. Pain is a perceptual meaning that is almost always accompanied by negative affect. Symbolic meanings are also frequently accompanied by affective meaning. For example, a particular person might be outraged by reading a political essay (the affective meaning of outrage accompanies the person's symbolic interpretations). Symbols can inspire awe, anger, ennui, or joy, depending on the person's developmental structure. Powerful symbols (in the occupational form) engender powerful thoughts (symbolic meanings) and powerful emotions (affective meanings).

Difference Between Meaning and Developmental Structure

In Conceptual Framework for Therapeutic Occupation terminology, the developmental structure of the person encounters an occupational form, and meaning is created. Meaning is a lived, felt experience at a particular time. The developmental structure of a person makes meaning possible, but meaning is different from the developmental structure. The developmental structure consists of the abilities and characteristics that make up the person. These sensorimotor, cognitive, and psychosocial abilities and characteristics can be thought of as potentials, not as actual experiences. For example, in the skin of the person there are many pain receptors, and these pain receptors make up part of the person's developmental structure. Actual pain is not experienced (meaning does not occur) until some stimulus provokes the pain receptor. For another example, a person can have a memory of her grandmother in her developmental structure, but the memory does not result in a lived experience of meaning until something in the occupational form (e.g., a photo, a dinner, or a garden) triggers the memory. The experience of remembering the grandmother, with all accompanying feelings, is different from the stored potential for memory in the developmental structure. The human experience of meaning, as depicted in Figure 5-1, results from an interaction of the occupational form and the developmental structure. In Conceptual Framework for Therapeutic Occupation, meaning is not something stored in the person, like a memory; meaning is an active experience that is felt.

Difference Between Meaning and Occupational Form

Among students of the Conceptual Framework for Therapeutic Occupation, a common error is to confuse the idea of meaning with the sociocultural aspects of the occupational form. For example, the student can confuse a picture of a pond with the perception of the picture of the pond, or the student can confuse the expectations for action in an assembly line with the worker's understanding of those expectations. This error is particularly common when describing the occupation of healthy adults, because healthy adults within a particular culture tend to be competent interpreters of occupational forms. Indeed, that is part of what it means to be a healthy adult: to make sense out of cultural expectations. The healthy adult is typically able to see what needs to be done, so there is a good match between the expectations in the occupational form and the healthy adult's understanding of those expectations. A good match between the occupational form and meaning does not mean that they are the same thing, however. All human attention is selective. The picture we have of the world in the "mind's eye" does not account for details in the actual world that are deemed irrelevant by the person.

Although healthy adults will tend to interpret a common occupational form in similar ways, each unique person will bring a different slant, or meaning, to the situation. For example, the person who loves another will see something in the loved one that is not seen by others. For another example, healthy adults in our culture will understand in broad terms what is supposed to be done in a clothing store, but each person will see the potentials in the store differently. It is also important to point out that even healthy adults sometimes make perceptual or symbolic errors. For example, a common perceptual error is to guess incorrectly that a large box is heavy when it is actually quite light. Slips and trips reflect perceptual errors of proprioceptive, tactile, vestibular, and visual meanings. In the area of symbolic meaning, testing situations (occupational form) usually involve some test questions that are not properly understood by all the students in the class. Even for healthy adults, it is important to point out the difference between what is right or wrong objectively and what is experienced by the person.

Another reason that the Conceptual Framework for Therapeutic Occupation emphasizes the difference between meaning and occupational form is that certain groups of persons tend to misinterpret common occupational forms. Not everyone is a healthy, well-enculturated adult. Three groups can be identified: persons with immaturities, persons who are not enculturated, and persons with disabilities.

Children frequently make errors of perceptual meaning and symbolic meaning. The toddler frequently misinterprets the objective reality of gravity and makes errors of perceptual meaning (the toddler falls). The 4-year-old frequently does not find a meaningful difference between a "p" and a "q," although there is an objective difference in the occupational form. In the area of symbolic meaning, children frequently do not understand what is considered polite in common occupational forms. In addition, depending on their ages, they have trouble understanding and applying rules in fair ways. We expect children to make errors of meaning, and we look on them as engaged in a long period of enculturation whereby they learn about the occupational forms characteristic of their culture.

One does not have to be young to be poorly enculturated. Adults who are unfamiliar with the cultures of others also tend to make errors of meaning. For example, the driver from Toledo, Ohio, will probably make errors of meaning when trying to negotiate the streets of Toledo, Spain, where the streets are narrow, traffic signs are different, pedestrians walk in the middle of the street, and fellow drivers have their own concept of right-of-way. The rules of the road for Toledo, Spain, are objective, whether or not the American tourist can make sense of them. Language, one of the most important expressions of culture, has definite rules, but the non-enculturated person will only hear noises (often the language-naive person is not even able to perceive the sounds accurately). Problems of enculturation can occur at all the social levels discussed earlier. The person who is not "wise" to occupational therapy might well misinterpret the occupational therapy class involving a craft. The person who is not a family member might not understand the family's joke and might misinterpret why everyone is laughing.

The third group likely to make errors of meaning consists of persons with disabilities. People with sensory disabilities will find different perceptual meanings than those found by others in the same occupational form. For example, the person with tactile defensiveness might feel threatened by a common fabric, or the person with hemi-inattention because of a stroke might not see large, relevant objects on the left side of space. People with cognitive disabilities often do not assign the same symbolic meanings that others do. For example, the person with frontal lobe damage secondary to a traumatic brain injury might not understand the rules regarding touching others or appropriate speech. The person with organic brain syndrome might not recognize family members. People with psychosocial disabilities often tend not to experience the same affective meanings as others encountering the same occupational form. For example, a friendly gesture could be interpreted as sinister by a person with paranoid schizophrenia. We will see later in the chapter that the mismatch between culturally sanctioned interpretations of occupational forms and the actual meanings assigned to the forms by people with disabilities is often the focus of occupational therapy intervention.

Occupational therapists are particularly concerned with people with disabilities, with immature people, and with people disenfranchised from their cultures. Occupational therapists are also very concerned with the uniqueness of the individual and the lived experience of the individual. Therefore, it is critical to distinguish systematically between occupational forms (objective physical reality and socioculturally defined expectations) and the experience of meaning.

PURPOSE AND OCCUPATION

A Definition of Purpose: *Purpose is the felt experience of desiring an outcome (having a motive). When a person with a unique developmental structure interprets the occupational form (meaning), he or she often wants to do something about it (purpose).*

Once a person finds meaning in an occupational form, a sense of purposefulness is possible (Fig. 5-2). In other words, the person first makes some kind of sense out of the situation and then wants to do something about it. Verbs implying purpose include desire, want, try, and seek. Nouns implying purpose include motive, intention, reason, and goal orientation. The infinitive phrase that begins with "to" in the English language (e.g., to achieve some goal) is another way of expressing purpose. English also has many other ways to express purpose. When we say that someone is highly or poorly motivated, we are talking about the person's level of purpose.

Purpose provides the energy for occupational performance. Similar to meaning, purpose is a felt experience characterized by emotion. Also, like meaning, purpose is subjective and not objectively observable by others. Meaning and purpose take place inside the person. Although the person might do or say things that indicate meaning and purpose to others, the meaning and purpose of a person cannot be experienced directly by anyone except that person.

For an example, let us consider a student taking a test who suspects that a classmate is cheating by looking at her answer sheet. Symbolic meanings of the student include the suspicion that cheating is taking place; the judgment that, if cheating is really taking place, the rules of fairness are being violated; the awareness that her reading of the situation might be wrong; feelings toward the other student and consideration of the possibility of

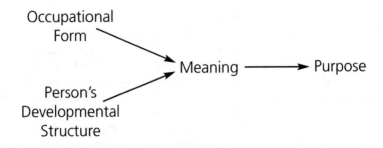

Figure 5-2. Purpose.

future conflict with this student; and fear that a teacher might wonder if the cheating is a conspiracy. Given these meanings, her purposes might include wanting to prevent cheating if possible, wanting to avoid difficulty or trouble with classmates or teachers, wanting to block her classmate's view of her test form, wanting to move her back and shoulder so as to prevent direct visual access by the other student, wanting to succeed on the test without further delay, and in general wanting "to do the right thing." In our example, the student has quite a high level of purpose in this situation, and the associated meanings are stressful.

Through this example we can see that purpose is possible only after meaning is established, yet purpose is identifiably separate from meaning. Unlike meaning, which is a reflection on the past, purpose has a future orientation toward an outcome that is sought. Meaning has to do with figuring out the situation. Once the situation is figured out, different kinds of purposes can be constructed, depending on the person. For example, after the student guessed that cheating might be taking place, she could have developed other purposes. She might have wanted the cheater to be punished, or she might have wanted to please the person cheating by doing nothing and pretending not to notice what was happening.

Multidimensionality of Purpose

Generally, purpose follows directly from what is most meaningful. However, the meanings that an occupational form holds for a person can be complex and contradictory. We get "mixed messages." Sometimes the purposes of the person cannot be made to fit all the contradictory meanings. For example, the meanings associated with knowing the rules about cheating are in conflict with the meanings associated with maintenance of a good relationship with classmates. Purpose and subsequent occupational performance might be in response to some meanings but not to others. Sometimes when a complex situation is figured out, there is no perfect solution. Indeed, occupational forms perceived as no-win situations can lead to a purpose to bypass the situation altogether and to pursue other goals. Purpose can be an internal compromise.

The multidimensionality of purpose can also be viewed in terms of the person's period. Some purposes are short-term (e.g., the young woman taking the quiz has the desire to get the next question correct). Other purposes are long-term (e.g., the act of answering the next question is motivated by the desire to succeed in the curriculum, or even an ultimate desire to be successful in life). At the same time in the same occupation, a person might be experiencing short-term and long-term purposes. In healthy adults, short-term purposes (e.g., wanting to get to work on a particular day) are linked to long-term purposes (e.g., wanting to have financial security). The desire to get to work must be understood in terms of this person's long-term goals.

Many human purposes have very brief periods. When someone is answering questions on an examination, the person experiences an immediate purpose to move one's hand so that the tip of the pen rolls legibly over the paper. If the person did not want to move the hand, the hand would not move. So it is with all voluntary behavior. The smallest movements and maintenance of posture reflect immediate purposes. These purposes are related to longer-term purposes, and these are related in turn to yet longer-term purposes, and so on in a series of relationships leading to the person's ultimate purposes. Characteristic of human experience is a connectedness between the person's goals in the immediate occupational form and the person's ultimate purposes, whatever they might be (e.g., religious, family-oriented). Characteristic of an occupational approach to understanding a person is a concern for the interconnectedness of multiple, inter-related levels of purpose.

Motivational Structure

The purposes of an individual also depend on the individual's developmental structure. Some people tend to have one kind of motivational structure, and some people tend to have another. For example, some people enjoy exploring new territory and others seek the familiar. Some people are oriented to seeking sensory pleasure, whereas others find greater enjoyment in accomplishing things with mastery. Some people tend to do things to get rewards from others, and other people tend to avoid the reward structures set up in occupational forms. These proclivities for specific types of purposes in the person's developmental structure depend on past experiences and on physiologic maturation. Personality theories deal with the analysis of these kinds of proclivities or traits within the developmental structure.

In Figure 5-3, the new arrow from developmental structure to purpose depicts the effect of motivational structure on purpose. Purpose, then, can be thought of as an interaction between meanings experienced in the here-and-now and long-term, well-established personality, or motivational structure. Just as the developmental structure makes it likely that a particular person will find certain kinds of meanings in an occupational form, so the developmental structure makes it likely that the person will develop certain kinds of purposes in the occupational form. In future diagrams, this arrow from Developmental Structure to Purpose will not be drawn so that the picture is less cluttered. Nevertheless, we must acknowledge the effects of motivational structure on purpose even though the diagram does not always include this arrow.

Types of Purpose

There are many kinds of human purpose and many ways of classifying types of purpose. One important kind of purpose is *intrinsic purpose or intrinsic motivation*. Intrinsic purpose involves doing something for its own sake, as in wanting to explore and/or master the occupational form. Here, a person engages in the occupation simply for the sake of engaging in the occupation, with no ulterior motive. For example, a toddler might want to knock over stacked blocks just to see what will happen next, or a scholar might want to wander through the stacks of a library for the pure pleasure of seeing if any interesting reading

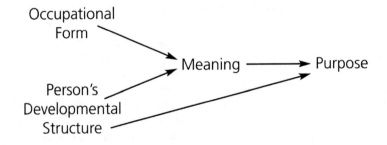

Figure 5-3. Effects of the person's motivational structure on purpose.

material pops out into his or her perceptual field. These are exploratory purposes. Mastery-oriented purposes include the toddler's desire to build a tower of blocks as high as possible or the scholar's desire to write a publishable scholarly article.

In contrast are *extrinsic purposes* or *extrinsic motivators*. Extrinsic purpose involves doing something for some reason that is external to the occupation at hand. An extrinsic purpose is an attempt to qualify for some subsequent occupation, as opposed to doing something for its own sake. For example, a person might dislike the experience of preparing a report at work but might seek the praise that will come later from the supervisor. Another example of an extrinsic purpose is a girl cleaning her room to avoid being grounded. Wanting pay for work, wanting credit in the minds of authority figures, and wanting to avoid punishments are examples of extrinsic purposes.

Extrinsic purposes are felt and experienced within the person, as are intrinsic purposes. An extrinsic purpose has to do with an intention that is extrinsic or external to the occupation at hand — it is not really extrinsic or external to the person. For example, the child cleaning her room feels a personal desire to go out with friends after finishing the unpleasant job of cleaning the room. When the occupational form involves coercion, extrinsic purposes can be felt intensely within the person. For example, when a mugger threatens the life of a person in the demand for money, the person experiences an intense desire to live and therefore wants to comply with the demands of the mugger to escape the danger. In everyday language, we say that the person had "no choice" because of the coercion. This is not really true, however; voluntary occupation always involves an active construction of meaning and purpose (choice). Indeed, in the same mugging situation, a different person might try to fight the mugger, and yet another person might attempt to run away.

Another kind of purpose involves the pursuit of sensory pleasures. For example, tasty food provides the opportunity for gustatory, olfactory, tactile, and visual pleasures. Saunas and spas provide sensory pleasure, as does the "runner's high" experienced after aerobic exercise. The desire for sensory pleasure often occurs simultaneously with other purposes. For example, a person taking a shower might be seeking tactile pleasure from the warm water while simultaneously seeking to conform to social norms regarding cleanliness. A corollary of the seeking of sensory pleasure as a purpose is the avoidance of sensory discomfort and pain. Avoidance of pain can be a powerful purpose (e.g., a woman with arthritis might be highly motivated to learn work simplification techniques to avoid pain).

Other kinds of purpose involve values and/or morality. For example, an elderly man might want to make a toy for the sake of a disadvantaged child, or a middle-aged woman might want to participate in a religious society. As stated earlier, purposes are frequently related to the person's deeply held spiritual convictions. A kind of purpose that is often tied to ultimate values is the desire for long-term health and well-being. Indeed, the range of possible human purposes is as varied as humanity itself. Unfortunately, there are those who want to destroy or control others. Others are motivated mainly by altruism. There are many kinds of purpose, at many levels, and a single occupation can be motivated by several purposes. On the other hand, a person might experience conflicts between different kinds of purpose.

Conscious and Unconscious Purposes

An individual is often highly aware of his or her purposes, but sometimes a person has purposes that escape conscious awareness. Unconscious purposes, just like unconscious meanings, frequently occur in occupations that are habitual. For example, let us consider the occupation of driving a car. In routine driving, the individual moves the steering wheel back and forth without conscious awareness of purpose. Yet purpose is present. The purpose has to be there; otherwise, the person would not engage in the voluntary occupational performance of moving the steering wheel back and forth. Habits with unconscious purposes contribute to the overall efficiency of a person; unconscious purposes allow the person to attend to other meanings and purposes. Thus, instead of devoting conscious attention to the movements of driving, the person can think about work later in the day, listen to the radio, or engage in a conversation. The same principles apply to other routine occupations of daily life. Toothbrushing is done without reviewing all one's immediate and long-term purposes for doing so. A parent cares for a child without questioning why on a daily basis.

A habit occupation is learned over time. In the early stages of learning, purposes are conscious. The beginning driver must focus carefully on his or her purposes in the small movements of operating the steering wheel or the brakes. Only when the habit becomes overlearned does the purpose become unconscious. Nevertheless, even unconscious, overlearned purposes can sometimes rush into consciousness when surprises occur in the occupational form. For example, if a small animal runs out suddenly in front of the car, the driver becomes acutely aware of motives. Or, if a person's regular toothpaste is unavailable and if only toothpowder is available, the person becomes aware of new immediate purposes in the regulation of effective movement.

Purpose Versus the Goals and Expectations of Others

Purpose is always a personal, felt experience of a real person at a particular time. The goal that someone else has for the person is entirely different from the purpose of the person. For example, a mother might want her daughter to be a virtuoso on the piano. This is the mother's purpose, but the purpose of the daughter is to have fun with friends. In occupational therapy, we have a responsibility to be especially careful to differentiate the purposes of one person, the client or patient, from the purposes of the other person, the therapist. The purposes of the therapist include goals that the therapist hopes to see the patient accomplish. However, the client or patient might or might not have the same goals as the therapist. Indeed, it is quite possible that the patient has entirely different purposes in the situation. For example, a patient might engage in an occupation only for the extrinsic purpose of wanting to comply with the requests of an authority figure ("I'll do anything to please these people so I can go home"). Sometimes the patient might engage in an occupation for its intrinsic pleasure, as opposed to having the kind of therapy goal that might appear in the medical chart.

Purpose: A Matter of Degree

From the Conceptual Framework for Therapeutic Occupation point of view, it is an error to say that some kinds of human doing are purposeful and some are not. Given the Conceptual Framework for Therapeutic Occupation definition of purpose, a person cannot engage in any occupation unless there is some minimal level of purpose. For example, even when bored while watching a poor television program, a person must have some level of purpose; otherwise, the watching would not take place. The very idea of a *non-purposeful, voluntary* performance does not make sense.

Purpose is a continuum that can range in intensity from maximal to minimal. Sometimes a person is doing something with minimal interest, and if an alternative arises in the occupational form, attention and purpose are quickly redirected. At other times, as in trying to survive an accident or trying to protect one's child, purpose can become extremely powerful. The overall level of purpose can be thought of as a final common pathway of multiple purposes of different types, different time frames, and different levels of intensities.

OCCUPATIONAL PERFORMANCE

A Definition of Occupational Performance: *Occupational performance is the active doing of the person in the context of the occupational form.*

Occupational performance is the active doing of the individual. After the person interprets the occupational form and wants to do something about it, the person's voluntary doing is the occupational performance (Fig. 5-4).

Overt Versus Covert Occupational Performance

Overt means that the occupational performance is potentially observable. Others need not be present, but if they were present, they could come independently to an agreement about the nature of the movement. Overt occupational performance involves the voluntary neuromuscular system. For example, let us imagine a person throwing a baseball with skill. Here, the occupational performance consists of a complex, coordinated series of movements and restrictions of movement involving most of the major muscles of the body. These movements could be analyzed in great detail in biomechanical and kinesiological terms (e.g., flexion, extension, abduction, adduction, rotation, and forces exerted in terms of the center of gravity). All that we know about voluntary human motor performance can be relevant in the analysis of overt occupational performance. This includes the voluntary maintenance of posture and the maintenance of active co-contraction, even in the absence of movement.

Overt occupational performance includes speaking, facial expressions, and the direction of gaze because they are under the voluntary control of muscles. We must be careful in our analyses of these movements, however, because they are often confused with other things. For example, speaking is an occupational performance, but technically the words produced in speech consist of sound waves that are external to the person (part of the speaker's occupational form). Indeed, the feedback people get from hearing (making

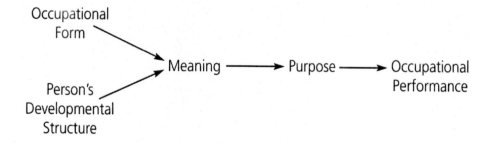

Figure 5-4. The basics of an occupation.

meaning of) their own words (occupational form) is important in regulating future speech (we will discuss this as an "adaptation" later in the chapter). Facial expressions are often confused with meanings. While a facial expression, such as smiling, might indicate pleasure (a meaning), the pleasure itself is not directly observable and objective, whereas the smiling is an objective fact. Later we will discuss how to draw reasonable inferences about meaning from the observation of occupational performance. As for the direction of gaze, this is classified as occupational performance because it involves voluntary movements of the extraocular muscles, the neck, and postural adjustments. However, the experience of seeing something is meaning (perceptual meaning), not occupational performance. The subjective experience of sight is not the same thing as directing one's gaze, even if some words in the English language ambiguously imply both things (e.g., "look at").

In contrast, *covert* occupational performances are not observable and reflect a series of mental images whereby the person imagines that his or her actions (performances) are causing step-by-step changes in the imagined environment. For example, a person could play an entire game of chess mentally. The only overt occupational performances for the person covertly playing chess might be voluntary maintenance of sitting posture, occasional postural adjustments, and voluntary eye movements. The covert occupational performances would be the imagined movements causing step-by-step changes in the imagined locations of the chess pieces (although there is no actual change in the locations).

A common error is to confuse meaning or purpose with covert occupational performance. Meaning, purpose, and covert occupational performance are, by definition, similar in that they reflect mental processes and images that are not observable directly and objectively by others. From the Conceptual Framework for Therapeutic Occupation perspective, however, they are different in that covert occupational performance always involves a multi-step series of mental transformations, each step of which leads to a newly imagined situation requiring a new covert occupational performance. For example, after the first covert occupational performance of moving the queen to a new square, and after the imagined response of the opponent, there is a new covert occupational performance of moving the rook to a new square, and so forth. The imagined chess pieces keep changing locations and keep creating new problems to which the player must respond in an ordered sequence. In contrast, we need not rely on the concept of covert occupational performance to describe the occupation of a beginner playing chess with actual chess pieces and an actual opponent in the occupational form. Here, an objectively observable occupational form (the relative locations of the chess pieces on the board and the rules of the game) take on meanings and purposes to the player, leading to an *overt* occupational performance and an objective change in the occupational form. Although the meanings and purposes of the player might have involved the covert consideration of alternative moves, the concept of covert occupational performance is not needed. The concept of covert occupational performance is needed only if the player moves beyond the level of beginner's play and starts to imagine a multi-step series of performances, effected changes in the situation, and new problems to face.

Covert occupational performances are important in advanced-level chess-playing and are sometimes important in other multi-step occupations involving strategy. However, if materials are available to be transformed, most people will choose overt occupational performance even when devising strategy. For example, the writer continuously responds overtly to the changing words on the computer screen and to previously devised outlines. The changing words are temporal aspects of an actual occupational form external to the writer, not vividly imagined changing situations as in our imagined chess game example.

In like manner, the military student typically studies multi-step battles by analyzing them one step at a time, through changing simulated materials. In these examples, the idea of covert occupational performance is unnecessary, because at each step in the process there are actual changes in an occupational form that can be perceived (meaning) and that can be responded to (overt occupational performance). Indeed, the argument can be made that covert occupational performance is quite rare. Covert occupational performance is definitely restricted to those with strong cognitive skills of imagery and sequencing, such that a series of changing situations and reactions can be imagined. Most of us spend most of our time focusing on actual occupational forms, the changes in those forms, the meanings and purposes they hold for us, and the voluntary responses of our neuromuscular systems. Most of us are very much tied to the physical world around us, and if we lose contact with the actual world of occupational forms (as in sensory deprivation), we begin to engage in hallucinations and we feel confusion, as opposed to engaging in covert occupational performances. In conclusion, the student of the Conceptual Framework for Therapeutic Occupation and occupation is urged to restrict the use of the concept of covert occupational performance to multi-step sequences that involve no changes in the actual occupational form but that are reported later by those who engaged in the covert occupational performances. Please keep in mind that this does not apply to other multi-step occupations in which there is ongoing transformation of materials and the opportunity for feedback. In the remaining sections of this chapter, the term occupational performance will refer to overt performances unless otherwise specified.

Form and Performance

The definitions of occupational form and occupational performance are complementary to each other: one term cannot be understood without understanding the other. For example, let us consider the occupation of a child donning her shoe. The occupational form includes the shoe and sociocultural norms for dressing. If there is a match between the child's meanings and the physical and sociocultural aspects of the occupational form, and if the child has a minimal level of purpose, she will engage in the occupational performance of putting the shoe on her foot. The occupational form is a situation calling for a specific occupational performance. The occupational form involves *something to be done*, and the occupational performance involves the *doing*. These two things are different yet complementary. Both are necessary in occupation: Occupation involves the doing (performance) of something (the form). Another way of saying it is that occupation involves a form, or format, that is performed.

Box 5-2 provides further examples of the relationships between occupational forms and occupational performances and begins to suggest the many varieties of human occupation. It must be kept in mind that the occupations listed in Box 5-2 are oversimplifications. An adequate description of a complete occupational form or occupational performance would take many pages, and subjective elements of meaning and purpose are always involved in occupation.

As can be seen in Box 5-2, some occupational forms are quite structured in calling for a specific performance, whereas others are unstructured or ambiguous. Some occupations involve short-term performances, whereas others involve many years. Some are relatively trivial in the grand scheme of things (many people will find only minimal meaning and purpose in certain occupational forms), whereas others tend to involve high levels of meaning and purpose. Some are highly complex and require great skill in the develop-

Box 5 -2 **VARIETIES OF OCCUPATIONS**	
Part of an Occupational Form	*Part of an Occupational Performance*
A game of football	is played
A religious ritual	is carried out
A banana split	is eaten
A garden	is harvested
A door	is opened
An ambiguous situation	is improvised upon
A circle	is drawn
A messy room	is cleaned
A barbell	is pressed
A symphony	is conducted
A penny	is discarded
A profession	is practiced
A child	is raised

mental structure, whereas others are quite simple. One factor that all the examples in Box 5-2 have in common is that the format in the occupational form suggests a somewhat predictable occupational performance. While keeping in mind that it is always possible for a particular person to find a unique meaning in an occupational form and to respond in a highly unpredictable way, the fact is that much of human behavior is quite predictable in given situations. The concepts of occupational form and occupational performance reflect that general predictability while recognizing the importance of unique responses.

Non-Occupational Motility

One problem in defining occupation is to deal with the relationship between reflexes and occupational performances. Reflexes, by definition, are not under the voluntary control of the individual. Therefore, from a Conceptual Framework for Therapeutic Occupation perspective, reflexive responses are *not* occupational. They are automatic responses to stimuli; they are not voluntary responses to an occupational form. On a neurologic level, reflexes can be simple or rather complex, but the term hard-wired has often been used to describe their automaticity. Examples of reflexes include cardiovascular and digestive activities, stretch reflexes that occur when a muscle is elongated suddenly, nystagmus (the back-and-forth movement of the eyes following certain vestibular and/or visual stimuli), the tonic neck reflexes exhibited in the normal development of infants, and protective equilibrium reactions exhibited when falling. One of the difficulties in distinguishing between reflexes and occupational performances is that many reflexes involve the same muscles and movement patterns used in voluntary occupational performance. For example, nystagmus involves the same extraocular muscles used in voluntary direction of gaze, and a healthy adult can easily mimic the asymmetrical tonic neck reflex. The distinction always comes down to answering the question: Was the movement the result of an involuntary response to a stimulus, or was it the result of voluntarily finding meaning and purpose in an occupational form?

Reflexes must be distinguished from habits, which are occupational in nature. In some ways, habits appear similar to reflexes, because they seem to have an automatic, unconscious quality. Indeed, in everyday language, people sometimes call it "good reflexes" when describing highly skilled habits, such as catching a baseball or reacting quickly in a dangerous driving situation. Neurologically, there are no baseball-catching or driving reflexes. A critical difference between skilled habit occupations and reflexes is that habits were learned over long periods. In the early stages of habit learning, conscious attention to details of the occupational form is necessary. Only after much success and overlearning do meaning and purpose become unconscious. In contrast, reflexes are not learned. Another difference is that the unconscious quality of habit occupations disappears quickly when something surprising occurs in the occupational form. For example, if the baseball player loses sight of the ball in bright lights, the player tends to abandon the "automatic pilot" of habit quickly and becomes acutely conscious of small details. This adaptability is not characteristic of reflex activity.

Another example of non-occupational human motility is passive movement of the body as a result of external physical forces. Movement of a person or a body part from one place to another as the result of being pushed or pulled by others, by machines, or by gravity (as in falling) is not occupational performance. Such movement is not voluntary and therefore does not fit the definition of occupational performance.

We are not saying that reflexes and passive movement are unimportant in human development. On the contrary, reflexes are often necessary for survival, and passive movement is an important fact of life. We are simply saying that these phenomena are not occupational. Another point that must be made is that non-occupational motility frequently interacts with occupational performance. There are many reflexes that operate in close coordination with occupational performance. For example, the first part of swallowing is voluntary, but when the food reaches a point in the throat, the swallowing reflex takes over. Another example is breathing. Under some conditions we can take over voluntary control of breathing (or not breathing); however, if we lose consciousness the breathing reflex begins again. Indeed, there are verifiable reports that some people, through intensive training, can exert conscious control over cardiovascular activities. When they do so, they are engaged in occupational performance. In like manner, there are many complex interactions between passive movement and occupation. A fall involves passive movement, but the person's voluntary movements leading to the fall and the person's voluntary movements to protect the self while falling are occupational performances. For another example, if a person asks another person to move one's arm, the asking is occupational; the voluntary placing of the arm in position so that the other person can move it is occupational; the voluntary relaxation of co-contractors so that the arm can be moved is occupational; the maintenance of sitting posture is occupational; and the engaging in conversation during the passive movement of the arm is occupational. However, the passive movement caused by another person is not occupational. In the Conceptual Framework for Therapeutic Occupation, the distinction between occupational and non-occupational movement depends on the concepts of meaning and purpose, which imply that the movement is voluntary.

Occupational Performance and Inferences about Meaning and Purpose

Meaning and purpose are subjectively experienced by a person and are not directly observable by any other person. So, how does one person learn about the meanings and purposes of another? The answer is that one person can make reasonable inferences about the meanings and purposes of another person by observing occupational performance in the context of an occupational form.

Usually, the best way to learn about the meanings and purposes of another person is to listen to what the person has to say or report. One of the great benefits of language is its use in describing subjective internal states, including perceptions, feelings, and motives. These self-reports involve observable occupational performance (speech, writing, or signing), and in the legal system they can be used as evidence. However, an observer can take other reasonable approaches to the empathetic and accurate understanding of a person's meanings and purposes. A great deal about meanings and purposes can be communicated non-verbally, that is, by how the person directs gaze, by facial expressions, by tone of voice, and by posture. In addition, the person's occupational performance and choices among occupational forms will indicate much about the person's meanings and purposes. For example, sustained effort in occupational performance is often interpreted as suggesting a high level of purpose. The observer expects a degree of consistency between verbal occupational performance and non-verbal occupational performance as a deepening picture of the person's meanings and purposes unfolds.

For most healthy adults, self-reports concerning meanings and purposes are by far the most important indicators of internal states. However, self-reports have limits. Sometimes a person tries to hide his or her feelings from others. There are many possible purposes for misreporting one's meanings and purposes. In addition to wanting to avoid negative sanctions, the person might not want to burden another person or might believe that thoughts and feelings are no one else's concern. Sometimes a person (e.g., a young child) is unable to find the right words to describe motives. Sometimes a person does not know, or does not yet know, how he or she feels. We all have had the experience of gaining new insights about our past feelings and reinterpreting how we felt at earlier times. Sometimes a person forgets how something felt. The occupational performance of talking about feelings takes place after the feelings per se; the longer this interval, the more likely that the self-report is incomplete.

Developing an empathetic understanding of the meanings of purposes of another person is a special achievement. It requires sensitivity, careful observation, and humility. One has to attend very carefully to what the person says and does, and one has to seek ongoing feedback from the person about the accuracy of these observations. One must be willing to admit that one's hunches about the meanings and purposes of another person might be wrong if the situation demands it; the fact is that no person has direct and absolute knowledge of the thoughts and feelings of another. Each person has privacy in one's inner life. Indeed, accurate empathy usually takes place over extended periods. One definition of intimacy is the reciprocal experience of accurate empathy.

In the Conceptual Framework for Therapeutic Occupation, occupation has subjective and objective features. Therefore, to understand an occupation, it is essential to try to understand the meanings and purposes of the person as well as the objective facts (performance in the context of form). This attempt to understand and empathize must always be conducted with humility and an appreciation of the private inner life of the other. Later in the chapter we will see that some models of practice in occupational therapy emphasize subjective factors and others emphasize objective factors. Although emphasis can be given to one or another, depending on the types of recipients of services, it would be an error to focus only on objective factors without considering meaning and purpose, and it would be an error to focus only on subjective factors without paying attention to what the person actually does. An occupational approach to understanding a person requires consideration of the whole person, including the person's experience and performance.

IMPACT

We have described how occupation involves meaningful, purposeful doing by a unique person in relation to an occupational form. Earlier we defined occupation (see page 90) as a dynamic relationship among an occupational form, a person with a unique developmental structure, subjective meanings and purposes, and a resulting occupational performance. Thus, we have defined all the main concepts in the definition of occupation except for the term "dynamic relationship." Now we begin to discuss the dynamics of occupation. We have seen how an occupational form can lead to an occupational performance. Now we will see how occupational performance, in turn, affects other parts of the system. Any definition of occupation must account for the effects of a person's occupational performance on the world around the person. The person is not just a respondent to stimuli; the person has a major impact on the physical and sociocultural world.

> **A Definition of Impact:** *Impact is the effect of occupational performance on the person's subsequent occupational form and on the occupational forms of others.*

The impact of one occupation often serves to set up the next occupation. For example, let us consider a newly admitted college student in his dormitory room who has the opportunity to set up his living space however he likes. His work of setting up the room is an occupational performance that results in an impact (the new layout, with loft beds and extra space for entertaining) that in the future will elicit and support the kinds of occupations he finds meaningful and purposeful.

Figure 5-5 depicts the role of impact in the Conceptual Framework for Therapeutic Occupation's definition of occupation. Note that Figure 5-5 uses abbreviations for the terms we have already defined. One of the ideas depicted in the figure is that the first occupation in a series (occupation$_1$) sets up the second occupation (occupation$_2$). The first occupational performance (OP$_1$) results in an impact (impact$_1$) which affects the next occupational form (OF$_2$). The second occupational performance then has an impact on OF$_3$.

Figure 5-5 also shows that one person's occupational performance can impact the occupational forms of other people. For example, the new college student's roommate has a somewhat changed occupational form because of the young man's efforts. An important point in the Conceptual Framework for Therapeutic Occupation is that the occupational performance of one person never directly affects the meanings and purposes of another person. The occupational performance of another can have dramatic effects on one's occupational form, but this occupational form must be meaningful and purposeful to the individual for an effect on occupational performance to occur. Indeed, the person

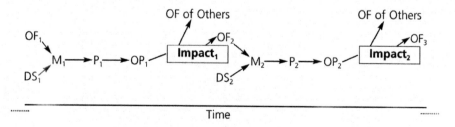

Figure 5-5. Impact. DS, developmental structure; I, impact; M, mental interpretation; OF, occupational form; OP, occupational performance; P, purpose.

could ignore the other person's effects on the environment or could react to it in an unanticipated way.

Occasionally one person has a direct impact on another's developmental structure (but not on the person's meanings and purposes, which are active in nature, not passive). For example, one person could hurt another person or could provide a medical intervention. We will see that this kind of impact of one person on another may be occupational from the point of the doer but non-occupational from the point of view of the person affected.

In Figure 5-5, the line between OP and Impact is not an arrow. Please picture an arrow going all the way from OP to the new OF, with Impact is in the middle of that arrow. The idea is that impact is not really a separate thing from the newly emerging occupational form. Impact is the part of the new occupational form that is caused by the person's own occupational performance.

Types of Impact

Some occupations have obvious impacts, whereas other occupations have subtle impacts. For example, the child building a snowman and the architect designing an office building have definite products reflecting their efforts. In contrast, the solo dancer's only impact consists of her new surroundings (the changing spatial relationships of the occupational form in relationship to her body) and the fairly trivial changes in the surfaces of the floor and her shoes.

In some cases, impact is mainly temporary, as can be seen in the playing of a board game that is put away at the end of the game without any lasting impact on the materials. However, the temporary impacts that occur in the middle of the game, such as the changing locations of board pieces and the exchange of play money, can be important. These temporary impacts (person-caused changes in the occupational form from moment to moment) provide needed structure for the ongoing unfolding of the game, even though the only lasting impacts from the start of the game to the end are fairly trivial (e.g., minimal wear and tear of the game materials). The use of exercise equipment is another example of a type of occupation in which most of the impacts are only temporary (the machine parts or the weights go back and forth but remain untransformed from the start of the game to the end). Each repetition in an exercise can be thought of as a brief occupation, and the changing location of the exercise equipment provides feedback (new meanings regarding personal performance).

Other (Non-Impact) Influences on Occupational Forms

We have described the importance of a person's having an impact on his or her future world (occupational form). However, we have to be cautious to avoid the idea that people can or should be totally in control of their occupational forms. The fact is that the occupational forms of an individual are influenced not only by one's own occupational performance but also by the occupational performances of others and by nature. For example, a man playing golf engages in many occupational performances (including swinging his clubs) and has many impacts (e.g., propulsion of the ball). However, natural forces such as the wind interact with his impacts and influence the locations of the ball. Furthermore, others can influence the form. For example, the groundskeeper might have placed the pin in an awkward part of the green. The talking of his golf partner in the middle of his backswing can further influence his occupational form and distract him, so that he swings badly. Occupational forms are continuously influenced by others and by nature as well as by one's own actions (performances). Sometimes we are relatively in control of the occupational form, but at other times people provide new opportunities or problems. Figure 5-6 depicts this idea graphically.

ADAPTATION

Occupation not only has an impact on the person's external world, but also has a dynamic effect on the person's own developmental structure. In other words, by doing something the person actually changes the self. Please see the definition of adaptation (below). Adaptation can take place in any of the main areas of the developmental structure (the sensorimotor area, cognitive area, or psychosocial area). For example, routine walking in golf (not using carts) results in adaptations in the area of endurance. Solving problems in algebra and geometry enhances one's abilities in deductive logic. Participating in a successful group task such as volunteering to build a house can result in new perspectives on interpersonal relations. The person's ability to adapt reflects the plasticity of the human nervous system.

> **A Definition of Adaptation:** *Adaptation is the effect of occupational performance on the person's developmental structure.*

Adaptations can be small or large. Here are examples of relatively small but still important adaptations. In the cognitive area, each time a person engages in an occupation, there is the opportunity for a memory of the event, and this memory is an adaptation. In the sensorimotor area, the walking that a person does naturally every day changes the developmental structure from what it would be if the person was confined to bed. In the psychosocial area, one's mood is often affected by occupation. Large adaptations also occur. The development of a personal identity is in large part the result of participation in a series of occupations, particularly in childhood. One's interests, values, sense of justice, morality, and ability to love are shaped by occupation. Indeed, much of human development is the result of what is defined here as occupational adaptation.

Figure 5-7 depicts the relationships between adaptation and other Conceptual Framework for Therapeutic Occupation concepts that have already been defined. First, a unique person with a complex developmental structure (DS_1) encounters an occupational form

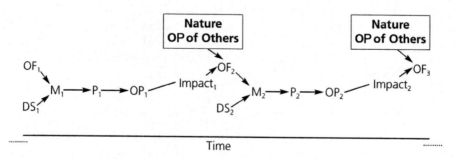

Figure 5-6. Other effects on the emerging occupational form. DS, developmental structure; I, impact; M, mental interpretation; OF, occupational form; OP, occupational performance; P, purpose.

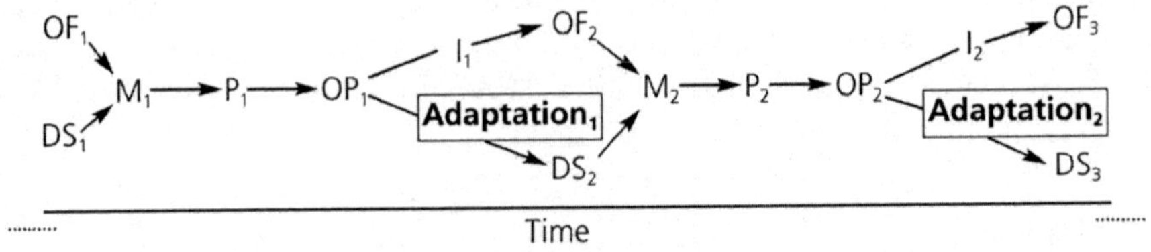

Figure 5-7. Occupational adaptation. A, adaptation; DS, developmental structure; I, impact; M, mental interpretation; OF, occupational form; OP, occupational performance; P, purpose.

(OF_1). From this encounter springs the experience of meaning (M_1): an active mental interpretation with perceptual, symbolic, and affective content. Once some sort of meaning is established, the person develops a sense of purpose (P_1) and voluntarily engages in an occupational performance (OP_1). The person has an impact (I_1) on the world around him and often creates new opportunities in the new occupational form (OF_2). The person's occupational performance also results in a change in oneself ($Adaptation_1$). A somewhat changed person (DS_2) then encounters OF_2 and constructs new meanings (M_2), new purposes (P_2), and new occupational performances (OP_2), causing new impacts (I_2) and new adaptations ($Adaptation_2$) in the ongoing development of the person (DS_3).

For example, let us say that the first occupation (going for a walk in the park) resulted in a new mood (an adaptation in the psychosocial area of the developmental structure). Now that the person is in a better mood, the meaning found in a difficult work task (the new occupational form) is positive and different from what it would have been without the prior occupation of taking the walk. For another example, let us consider the child who, through play, develops conservation abilities (she does not get confused by how tightly or loosely objects are arranged spatially when she is judging quantity). This adaptation in one occupation makes it more likely that she will develop other conservation skills in future occupations, such as the ability to conserve volume when confronted with various containers to measure liquids. One beneficial occupational adaptation leads to the next.

A common error is to confuse impacts and adaptations. In everyday language, one can say that an experience had an "impact" on a person, and one can say that a person "adapted" the environment. However, a rule of thumb in the Conceptual the Framework for Therapeutic Occupation is that there can be no overlap among Conceptual Framework for Therapeutic Occupation terms. Certainly, a change in the person because of occupation is one thing, and a change in the environment (occupational form) because of occupation is a different thing. If they are different things, they should be labeled differently. If in doubt, the student is urged to return to the definitions when using the Conceptual Framework for Therapeutic Occupation terms impact and adaptation.

Adaptation, Purpose, and Occupational Performance

Figure 5-7 shows that adaptation occurs because of occupational performance. However, sometimes adaptation can start to occur even before occupational performance. An example of an adaptation beginning to occur as the result of a purpose just before the occupational performance can be seen in a child's developing a new motor plan when confronted with a plastic tunnel in an obstacle course (the occupational form). Even before the child actually gets into the tunnel (even before the occupational performance), the child's purpose involves the development of a plan for how to creep through the tunnel (with elbows a bit flexed so as to avoid hitting one's head on the top of the tunnel). This new plan is the beginning of a new motor ability. The new motor schema is reinforced when the child successfully gets through the tunnel (after occupational performance). Figure 5-7 shows this relationship between performance and adaptation, but does not show how the adaptation of the developmental structure begins to take place even before the occupational performance.

Learning and Other Types of Adaptation

All learning involves adaptation, whether or not the adaptation begins before the occupational performance. Learning is always the result of active occupation, whether this takes place in formal settings, such as a classroom, or in informal settings, such as a playroom or work environment. Learning can involve the acquisition of motor skills, cognitive skills, or psychosocial skills. Learning always results in some sort of new capacity in the developmental structure, so that the same old occupational form that previously confused the person now makes sense to the person. This is not to say that learning is always permanent. Forgetting is also an adaptation; forgetting tends to occur when a person's occupational performance has nothing to do with what has been learned.

Although all learning is adaptation, not all adaptation is learning. An example of an adaptation that we would not call learning is the development of physical strength after repetitive occupational performance against resistance in the occupational form. Other examples include changes in mood or in level of arousal because of engagement in an occupation.

Maladaptation

Adaptation is not always a beneficial thing. Unfortunately, occupational performance can result in a weakened or less competent developmental structure. For example, an elderly man leaves a store in a humiliated state when he cannot hear what the checkout girl has said to him. He adapts (maladapts) by engaging in avoidance-type occupations in the future (e.g., he avoids going to the store and avoids participation in other occupational forms that might prove humiliating). Here, one problem in the developmental structure (hearing loss) led to another. For another example, a series of failures through occupational performance can result in a learned sense of helplessness, such that the person expects failure (meaning) whenever he or she encounters a new occupational form. A third example is that an inactive lifestyle can lead to decreased physiologic endurance. Just as any of the three main areas of the developmental structure can be strengthened through occupational performance, any can be weakened also. This kind of adaptation can be called *maladaptation.*

Adaptability, Plasticity, and Their Limits

Biologically, the human being is highly structured for occupational adaptation. Adaptability is built into our nervous system. However, there are limits on the plasticity of body systems, particularly in some areas. Some body systems are relatively plastic (for most of us, the strength of a muscle can be increased at any age). Others are relatively stable (e.g., fundamental temperament). Even in areas considered relatively adaptable and plastic, each of us has limits in terms of our ability to change. The person with a spinal cord transection cannot regain lower extremity motor control through occupation no matter how hard she or he tries (here we leave open the possibility for a future medical intervention). There are substantial individual differences from person to person in terms of the ability to learn abstractions, the ability to improve reaction time, and the ability to learn how to gain accurate empathy with another. Therefore, although the human being is structured for adaptability, there are definite limits on occupational adaptation by body system and by individual developmental structure.

Maturation, Disease, and Medical Interventions

Occupational adaptation is a powerful force in human development, but there are other factors that influence the developmental structure of a person (Fig. 5-8).

Maturation is the endogenous physiologic change in the developmental structure resulting from the unfolding of genetic potential. All the body systems change throughout the life span as a result of biological forces. For example, the nervous system supporting cognition is characterized by radical growth in infancy and early childhood. After a period of stability, maturation-based changes occur again in later life. Maturation also accounts for much of sensory development, motor development, and perceptual development. Maturation frequently interacts with occupational adaptation in promoting human development. An infant's occupational performance in a deprived occupational form will inhibit brain maturation. The musculoskeletal system provides another example of the interaction between maturation and occupational adaptation: bone and muscle develop partly as a result of the child's active occupation and partly as a result of maturation.

Nutrition is another factor that interacts with active occupation in human development. Preparing food and eating food are occupational, but the digestive and metabolic processes underlying nutrition are non-occupational. A lack of proper nutrients at the biochemical level can inhibit human development in multiple ways.

Disease processes, including trauma, constitute another important category of non-occupational forces acting on the developmental structure. For example, a traumatic brain injury can result in major sensorimotor, cognitive, and psychosocial changes in the individual. A viral infection of the ear can affect a person's perceptual abilities and endurance. Psychosomatic disease provides an example of an interaction between occupational and non-occupational forces acting on the developmental structure. For example, repeated overchallenges in the occupational forms of a person can result in stomach ulcers, which in turn can result in pain and avoidance-type occupations.

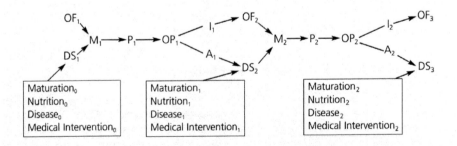

Figure 5-8. Non-occupational effects on the developmental structure. A, adaptation; DS, developmental structure; I, impact; M, mental interpretation; OF, occupational form; OP, occupational performance; P, purpose.

A fourth category of non-occupational effects on the developmental structure involves those medical interventions whereby the patient is the passive recipient of treatment. The distinguishing feature of this type of medical care is the intention to produce a direct effect on the patient's body tissue. For example, the orthopedic surgeon can have a direct effect on range of motion, strength, muscle tone, or somatosensory perception. The internist's prescribed medication might have a specific effect on visual perception, and the psychiatrist's prescription might have an effect on anxiety. In addition to physicians, other health professionals often intervene directly on the developmental structure. For example, the physical therapist might help clear the lungs of a child with cystic fibrosis through postural drainage techniques. Although the patient frequently must engage in occupation to receive the medical treatment (e.g., must drive to the hospital), the treatment itself is non-occupational in nature (e.g., the patient passively receives therapy).

Figure 5-8 shows that all four of these factors can have an effect on the developmental structure in ways that cannot be accounted for by occupational adaptation through active occupational performance. Once the developmental structure is influenced by these factors, future occupations can be affected in major ways. In Figure 5-8 at DS_2, let us assume that maturation has resulted in longer, more powerful limbs. Given this change in the developmental structure, the child finds new meanings in the same old occupational forms that formerly appeared out of reach, and the child is able to engage in a series of occupational performances leading to new perceptual, cognitive, and interpersonal adaptations. Hence, maturation can lead ultimately, but not directly, to occupational adaptations. In parallel fashion, maturation in older persons can include declines in short-term memory, which lead ultimately to occupational maladaptations. The same line of logic applies to changes in the developmental structure because of nutrition, disease, and medical interventions. In all cases, these changes are non-occupational at DS_2, but they can cause major changes at later points in the dynamic unfolding of future occupations and occupational adaptation.

SUCCESS, FAILURE, FUNCTION, AND DYSFUNCTION

Success or failure involves a judgment concerning the quality of occupational performance and/or its impact. The question is: Who makes the judgment? In the Conceptual Framework for Therapeutic Occupation, there are two kinds of success or failure, each of which can be important factors in understanding an occupation. The first kind involves the personal judgment of the individual; the second treats success or failure as a sociocultural matter.

Personal Success or Failure

Definitions of Personal Success and Personal Failure: *Personal success or failure is a judgment about the degree to which one's own occupational performance and/or impact matches one's purposes.*

Personal success involves a judgment by oneself, not a judgment by society. An example of *personal success* is the painter's appreciation of her own work when looking at it. The woman perceives the painting as beautiful and judges that she has accomplished what she set out to do when she started the painting. In personal success, the judgments of others (e.g., the "art world") are irrelevant. What matters is whether the individual accomplishes one's own goal. An example of a personal failure can be seen in a boy's self-disgust after striking out in baseball. The fact that even great baseball players sometimes strike out can be irrelevant in a judgment of personal failure.

It is often the impact of the occupational performance that provides concrete evidence, or feedback, of success or failure. For example, a healthy adult can readily evaluate whether a paper written for a night class matches his or her intentions. When judging success or failure, individuals are often sensitive to the actual materials and products of occupational performance. In judgments of personal success or failure, only the individual's opinion about quality matters.

Personal success or failure is often not an all-or-nothing categorical judgment. An occupational performance can be judged as a partial success or as a mixed success. Depending on the person's values in the developmental structure, the paper written for a night class might be judged successful in originality but rather unsuccessful in terms of scholarly documentation. One person might have very high standards and therefore be reluctant to designate anything as a total success, whereas another person might be the opposite. Indeed, an individual might forget or deny what his or her purposes were in the occupation and therefore see something as a success even though it did not match up to the prior purposes. The individual also might change the criteria for judgment after the fact. For example, an adolescent could judge his first date as a total failure but in later adulthood appreciate the memory of his first date, especially the early naiveté that was impossible to accept as an adolescent. The main point here is that personal success or failure depends on the individual's complex and changing developmental structure.

Sociocultural Success or Failure

Definitions of Sociocultural Success (Function) or Failure (Dysfunction): *Sociocultural success or failure (function or dysfunction) is the degree to which a person's occupational performance and/or impact matches sociocultural norms.*

An example of sociocultural success is the building of a home that is recognized as ideal in community newspapers. An example of sociocultural failure is building a home that does not meet the local government's building codes. Laws define some sociocultural failures (crimes), but there are many less dramatic examples of sociocultural success and failure. A decent paycheck is a mark of sociocultural success for an adult, and failure to wear a shirt and shoes into a restaurant is frequently judged a violation of social norms. As with personal success or failure, sociocultural success or failure is often a matter of degree. For example, a graduate student's "C" work is technically a passing grade in many universities, but there is often a limit on how many "C"s can be received before the student is dismissed from the program.

Sociocultural norms are sometimes clear, but sometimes they are vague or in transition. For example, assassination of a politician is condemned in our society, and the sanctions for such an occupation are severe. However, the assassination of a politician collaborating with an oppressive power might be considered a success in society (consider occupied Europe in World War II). A less extreme example is that norms regarding cellular phone use when driving and when dining are currently in transition. At this time in our culture norms are rapidly changing on many issues, from drinking alcohol to television content, from transnational corporations to child care. Frequently, one level of society considers an occupational performance to be normative whereas another level of society finds it unacceptable. For example, at the level of city government, driving one's wheelchair on the side of the street might be contrary to traffic codes, but at the level of organizations for persons with disabilities, driving one's wheelchair on the side of the street might be sanctioned positively as the only way to get out and do things in the community. This is not to say that everything is relative. A nation or a community could not exist for long if there was not some level of agreement about what constitutes success in living up to social expectations and what constitutes social failure.

Let us consider dressing and hygiene. Each culture and subculture has definite rules about covering parts of the body, and usually there are gender differences. Even within a culture, the rules vary from occupational form to occupational form (e.g., from the beach to the office). Expectations change even within the same setting (e.g., dress-down days at the office). Soiled clothes might be appropriate at the end of a laborer's day or at the end of an infant's meal but would be indicative of failure in most other social situations. Fashion varies from social class to social class and from generation to generation, but certain types of clothing are quickly perceived as indicative of social failure. An oddly dressed person is almost immediately noticeable in a public place. For this kind of occupational performance and impact, there is no formal punishment (there is no law against having poor taste). Yet, there is likely to be informal yet substantial negative sanctions (e.g., avoidance, refusal to help, or laughter). In summary, culture is powerful concerning everyday occupations such as dressing and hygiene, and an understanding of culture is necessary to make judgments concerning sociocultural success or failure.

Function or Dysfunction

In the Conceptual Framework for Therapeutic Occupation, sociocultural success is a synonym for function, and sociocultural failure is a synonym for dysfunction. In other words, when a person's occupational performance or impact is consistent with sociocultural expectations, we say that the occupational performance is functional. We also say that the person has function or that the person is functional. In parallel fashion, when a person's occupational performance or impact does not match up to social expectations, we say that the person has a dysfunction.

The problem with the terms function and dysfunction is that they can apply to so many different things — from human performance to automobile performance, and from physiologic processes (e.g., cardiovascular function or endocrinal function) to physical events that have nothing to do with persons or society (e.g., the functions of mathematics and physics). Because the term function can so readily apply to non-voluntary and even non-human phenomena, it has a mechanistic connotation.

On the other hand, our health care system has become committed to the term function and to related terms such as functional outcome. It is important to be able to translate occupational terms specific to the profession of occupational therapy into terms used in the larger health care system. Therefore, we suggest that function is equivalent to socioculturally successful occupational performance. The positive side of the health care system's focus on function is its emphasis on what we in occupational therapy call occupation. Another benefit is that the concept of functional outcome supports the development of sensitive, reliable, and valid measurements of occupation.

Relationships among the Two Types of Failure and Success

Personal success often occurs simultaneously with sociocultural success (function); sometimes they do not. An example of simultaneous personal and sociocultural success is a work product completed by a person who believes that all her objectives have been realized and who also receives formal recognition for the job by her peers. Another example is the elderly woman's flower garden that is self-pleasing while also standing up well to published criteria for a model garden. On the other hand, it is often happens that an occupational performance meets all one's personal criteria while falling short of social standards. For example, an individual might judge that his personal hygiene is adequate, although others he encounters might disagree. It is also possible for an occupation to be judged a failure personally while it is judged a success socially. A person with low self-esteem can seldom see the quality of his or her own efforts, although they might be universally admired within society.

Challenges: Underchallenges, Overchallenges, and Just-Right Challenges

In the Conceptual Framework for Therapeutic Occupation, the idea of a challenge has to do with the balance between the level of difficulty in the occupational form and the level of competencies in the developmental structure. An occupational form with the appropriate level of difficulty provides a just-right challenge to the developmental structure. Success is the result (this success can be personal success and/or sociocultural success). For example, a covered cup with a straw (occupational form) provides the just-right challenge to a toddler, whose motor control (in the developmental structure) is competent enough for bilateral lifting but not competent enough to prevent tips and spills.

An overchallenge involves an imbalance, such that the level of difficulty in the occupational form exceeds the competencies in the developmental structure. Personal and/or sociocultural failure are the result. For example, a new kitchen with modern devices in an assisted living facility might be an overchallenge to an older woman accustomed to the layout and devices in her old home.

An underchallenge also reflects an imbalance. Here the occupational form is too easy for a person. Failure often occurs, if not at first, then over time. For example, low expectations for school success on behalf of parents and teachers can result in underachievement by a talented adolescent.

In the Conceptual Framework for Therapeutic Occupation, a challenge always originates in the occupational form, not in the person. For example, in the Conceptual Framework for Therapeutic Occupation it would be incorrect to say that the cerebral palsy of a child challenged her. Cerebral palsy is part of the girl's developmental structure. Her challenges are not her sensorimotor problems in isolation but the obstacles she encounters in her everyday occupational forms. The high steps onto a school bus or the insensitive comments of her classmates might be an overchallenge to her, but we should not assume that the overchallenge lies in her developmental structure without due consideration of the difficulties in her occupational forms.

Sociocultural Success/Failure and Therapy

This discussion of success and failure anticipates our discussion of therapeutic occupation. Generally, it is the person experiencing sociocultural failure or the person at risk for sociocultural failure who is a candidate for therapy in our society. In other words, it is the person with dysfunction or the person at risk for dysfunction who is referred to therapy. Objectively measured increases in sociocultural success are often thought to justify the social resources devoted to therapy.

The occupational therapist should often be concerned with whether patients or clients can live up to community and family standards for occupations of daily living and for work. However, many occupational therapy models of practice also emphasize the importance of personally defined success in occupation. Few of us would argue that the goal of therapy and rehabilitation should be concerned exclusively with meeting sociocultural expectations. We must also learn about and respect the personal criteria for success that our patients have when conducting their occupations.

RECIPROCAL OCCUPATIONS AMONG OTHERS

Dyadic Interaction

A principle of the Conceptual Framework for Therapeutic Occupation is that each occupation reflects the effort of a particular person at a particular time. There is no such thing as a group occupation or a shared occupation. For each person involved, there is a different occupation. Two or more people can have reciprocal occupations in relation to each other.

Figure 5-9 depicts an interaction between two persons, each of whom is engaged in a series of occupations. Please note that the relative positions of the developmental structure (DS) and the occupational form (OF) are reversed for Person A, for the sake of graphic convenience. The central idea of Figure 5-9 is that two persons can influence each other's occupational form by engaging in occupational performance and by having impact. Hence, the first occupational performance and resulting impact by Person B (OP_{b1} and I_{b1}) influence the second occupational form of Person A (OF_{a2}). Reciprocity occurs when the occupational performance and impact of Person A (OP_{a2} and I_{a2}) have an impact on the next occupational form of Person B (OF_{b3}).

An example of a simple interaction as depicted in Figure 5-9 can be seen in a card game of rummy between two people. Person B lays down three queens face up and discards a card to the pile (OP_{b1} and I_{b1}). The discarded card presents an opportunity (OF_{a2}) to Person A, who picks up the discarded card, lays down all the cards face up, and says, "Rummy" (OP_{a2} and I_{a2}). The game is over (OF_{b3}). Although this is a simple interaction, several important points can be made about this card game with implications for much more important interactions between people. First, each person's occupational form depends partly on one's own performance and partly on the performance of the other person. The game would have worked out differently if Person B had discarded a different card. A second point is that successful reciprocity depends on the meanings and purposes that each person assigns to the occupational form. If either person did not understand the rules of the game (problems of meaning) or if either person did not want to continue to play the game (a lack of purpose), the game could not have been successfully concluded. Of course, interpersonal life is often much more complex that a card game, but successful interaction of all types depends on each person's meanings and purposes. A third point is that neither Person A nor Person B had a *direct* effect on the meanings, purposes, occupational performances, or adaptations of each other. However, each person did influence the other's occupational form in such a way that was meaningful and purposeful to the individual. Through occupation, we can influence each other in profound ways, even though the effect is indirect.

When we interact in an occupational way, each person has his or her own stream of occupations, with his or her own personally constructed meanings and purposes. It is worth noting that there are other ways to have effects on others in addition to reciprocal occupations. If one person physically moves a second person, the second person's developmental structure can be affected in a passive, non-occupational way. Hence, one person can hurt the other's developmental structure through trauma, or one person can help the other's developmental structure through medical intervention. This point is consistent with our earlier discussion of the effects of disease and medical intervention on the developmental structure.

Groups and Culture

A final point is that group situations are logical extensions of Figure 5-9. It would not be easy to draw, but let us imagine that the occupational performances of each person in the group become components of the new occupational forms of every other person in the group. A coherent, successful group will tend to consist of individuals who find similar meanings in their overlapping occupational forms. Over time, each individual contributes through occupational performance to the formation of a group culture, with its own symbols, norms, and sanctions. This culture in turn becomes part of the occupational forms of

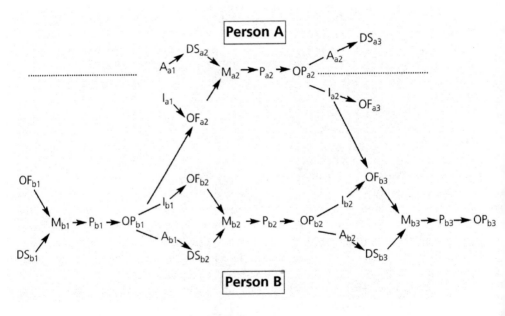

Figure 5-9. Reciprocal occupations. A, adaptation; DS, developmental structure; I, impact; M, mental interpretation; OF, occupational form; OP, occupational performance; P, purpose.

all those in the group. The formation of culture at higher levels of society, such as in organizations, nations, and subcultures, reflects the same basic processes of the formation of culture in a small group, but over longer chunks of occupations and across more participants. In summary, through occupation, each person contributes to cultural stability or change.

SUB-OCCUPATIONS

Levels of Occupation

Occupations taking place over extended periods tend to consist of sub-occupations, each one of which is an occupation in its own right. For example, let us consider the occupation of a person doing laundry. Within that occupation are several identifiable sub-occupations such as gathering the clothes together, operating the washing machine, operating the dryer, folding the clean clothes, and putting them away in drawers and closets. Each of the sub-occupations is also made up of sub-occupations (we can call them sub-sub-occupations). For example, for this occupation, operating the washer consists of putting the clothes in the machine, applying the appropriate cleaning materials, selecting the appropriate controls, and emptying the machine. Each of the sub-sub-occupations, in turn, are made up of sub-sub-sub-occupations. For example, each armful of wet laundry is an occupation in its own right as the person empties the machine. Each time the person reaches down to get more clothes from the washer, there is an occupational form, there is meaning and purpose, and there is occupational performance. Therefore, getting an armful of laundry has all the necessary components of being an occupation.

Just as doing the laundry in an afternoon consists of sub-occupations, doing the laundry can also be a sub-occupation of some higher-level occupation. For example, from this person's point of view, this laundry doing might be an inherent part of "doing Saturday chores." Other sub-occupations in this higher-level occupation might be grocery shopping, house cleaning, and pet grooming.

What are the rules for determining when an occupation starts and stops, and for determining whether a particular occupation is a sub-occupation of another? Just as there are two sets of rules for determining success and failure, there are two sets of rules for determining the relationships among sub-occupations. First, one can use the perspective of the individual engaged in the occupation. Does he or she see the occupation as starting at the point of gathering the clothes, or does she or he see it starting with the loading of the washer? Does he or she see doing the laundry as part of something called "doing Saturday chores?" Second, one can use sociocultural norms in judging the relationships among sub-occupations. How would most people in a culture, or at a particular social level, judge these matters? In this kind of objective determination, the rule of interrater agreement between independent raters would once again be the practical way to judge these matters.

Discontinuous Occupations

Occupations are not always continuous. In our laundry example above, there is a break in time between starting the machine and emptying it. Let us assume that this person engaged in unrelated occupations during this interval (e.g., talking on the telephone with one's sister and checking e-mail). The longer the occupation, the more likely that discontinuities will exist. For example, a person's pursuit of a graduate degree is a clearly identifiable occupation taking place over a period of years. Sub-occupations making up the overall graduate school occupation are marked by many intervals during which family life, leisure, paid employment, maintenance, and other occupations engage the person.

Chains of Sub-Occupations

Sub-occupations can be thought of as links in a chain, with the impact of a prior occupation helping to set up the next occupational form of the next sub-occupation. For example, let us consider a man preparing lunch for his children (Box 5-3). Please keep in mind that we are not fully describing the occupation of the man — we are only highlighting some of his occupational forms and occupational performances in a simplified way.

Please note that the occupational performances involve many different kinds of movement. Indeed, in this brief part of an occupation, most of the muscles of the body are used in one way or another. Analysis of increasingly small units of sub-occupations is especially useful when the focus is on movement quality and motor control. Opening the refrigerator door is only one of seven occupations in Box 5-3. Let us begin to consider the complexity of brief units of occupation by analyzing the opening of the refrigerator door in a little more detail.

Although the man appears to open the refrigerator door in one smooth pattern, careful analysis suggests that even the pulling motion has four important phases, as listed in Box 5-4. These movements are often subtle. For example, he must "ease up" on his pulling once the door begins to open; otherwise, the door on its low-friction hinges would crash to the side. The man must make careful adjustments in response to the moment-by-moment changes in the occupational form from something involving considerable resistance to something involving little resistance. This involves dynamic co-contraction of the agonists and antagonists of his upper extremity and requires careful timing in relation to the temporal aspects of the occupational form.

Analysis of Sub-occupations and a Holistic Approach to Occupation

Some approaches to occupational therapy tend to focus on rather brief units of occupation. For example, analysis of small units of movement might be important to understand the everyday problems of a person with arthritis. Other approaches recommended

Box 5-3	**SUB-OCCUPATIONS WITHIN THE OCCUPATION OF LUNCH PREPARATION**
Occupational Performance	*Aspects of the Occupational Form*
Walks to	the refrigerator
Opens	the refrigerator door
Looks for	leftovers and orange juice
Picks up	leftovers and orange juice
Pushes shut	refrigerator door
Walks to	microwave
Asks	daughter to pour juice

Box 5 -4 **SUB-SUB-OCCUPATIONS WITHIN THE SUB-OCCUPATION OF OPENING THE REFRIGERATOR DOOR.**

Occupational Performance	Aspects of the Occupational Form
Reaches out to	the handle
Grasps (cylindrical pattern)	the handle
Firmly yanks	the handle (rigidly attached to the door with rubber surfaces that adhere tightly to the frame)
Continues to pull while "easing up"	the handle
Stops pulling	the handle on the open door

in occupational therapy focus on long-term occupations, such as carrying out one's roles in raising a family, working, and participating in the community. Approaches with either kind of focus can be analyzed by using Conceptual Framework for Therapeutic Occupation terms, because brief occupations and long-term occupations are made up of occupational forms, meaning, purpose, occupational performance, adaptation, and impact.

Regardless of whether the main focus is on the short-term or the long-term, a holistic approach to understanding the occupations of a person requires at least some appreciation of the links between the short-term and the long-term. It certainly can be reductionistic and short-sighted to focus on how the finger moves in a little task without finding out how the person has used that finger in the past and how the person plans to use that finger in the future. The finger movement seen in the evaluation should be seen as a sub-occupation within the person's larger occupational configuration. In like manner, it is naive to analyze the long-term role occupations of the person without attending to the day-to-day and moment-to-moment realities that make up the long-term role performance. A holistic occupational approach involves the actual doing of things in the here and now, as opposed to an exclusive dependence on talking about how things get done. The brief sub-occupations provide invaluable information about the overall configuration of occupations in the person's life.

Brief units of occupation cannot be understood fully without reference to higher-level occupations, and higher-level occupations cannot be understood fully without reference to brief units of occupation. The purposes of persons engaged in brief occupations usually include future goals that go far beyond the immediate occupation. In other words, the person is not just moving the finger to move the finger. The person is probably moving the finger because the immediate occupation of moving the finger will lead to an impact that relates to short-term goals, while the short-term goals relate to long-term goals. For example, the student taking notes in a class has a purpose to move that finger but the person also has the purpose of wanting to pass the course, which relates to purposes of wanting to graduate, go on to work, raise a family, etc., all of which relate to that student's ultimate purposes in life. To understand the finger movement holistically, one must understand the long-term purposes of the person and how the person sees the links among the sub-occupations. To understand the long-term roles well, we must holistically understand the brief units of occupation (like taking good notes) on which success in the long-term roles depends.

THERAPEUTIC OCCUPATION

To this point, the focus has been on the study of occupation as it occurs in everyday life. This chapter has stressed that a thorough understanding of naturalistic occupation is a prerequisite to an understanding of occupation used as therapy. Therapeutic occupation has special features, but it is first and foremost an occupation, with meaning, purpose, occupational performance, and impact.

Therapeutic Occupational Synthesis

A Definition of Therapeutic Occupational Synthesis: *Occupational synthesis is the design of the therapeutic occupational form by the occupational therapist in collaboration with the recipient of occupational therapy services. Occupational synthesis involves clinical reasoning as guided by an occupational therapy model of practice. Occupational synthesis requires the analysis of the physical and sociocultural aspects of the occupational form in terms of the recipient's developmental structure. The occupational therapist makes predictions as to the meanings, purposes, and occupational performances that the person will experience and display in the context of the occupational form.*

In therapeutic occupation, the occupational therapist synthesizes (i.e., designs or puts together) the occupational form in collaboration with the recipient of occupational therapy services. The person receiving occupational therapy services might be called a patient, a client, a resident, a consumer, or a student depending on the setting and the model of practice. For example, in a nursing home the resident and the occupational therapist might synthesize a self-care situation to work toward a therapeutic goal. As in all occupation, the form must have meaning and must elicit purpose in the resident for there to be a therapeutic occupation.

Occupational synthesis is what each occupational therapist "does for a living." It is the essential occupation of the occupational therapist. The term synthesis is used because many factors must be considered simultaneously when putting together an occupational form that provides a person with the just-right challenge to the developmental structure.

Figure 5-10 depicts occupational synthesis as a collaboration between the occupational therapist and the recipient of services. The recipient's own occupational performance has a collaborative impact on the synthesis. For example, the patient's statement of wishes is an occupational performance that has an influence on the design of the next occupational form. In addition, the patient's nonverbal occupational performance can also have an influence on the synthesis or the next occupational form. For example, if a client performs the prior occupation with ease, the occupational therapist "grades up" the next occupational form by making it somewhat more challenging.

A critical feature of therapeutic occupation is that the person receiving occupational therapy is an active interpreter of the therapeutic situation, as opposed to a passive recipient of care. In other words, the person must find personal meaning in the occupational form if therapeutic occupation is going to occur. This makes therapeutic occupation different from most medical treatments. Please recall the prior figure in which medical intervention was pictured as having a non-occupational, direct effect on the developmental structure of the person. For example, an orthopedic surgeon can have a powerful effect on the developmental structure of a person by installing an artificial shoulder joint. After this medical intervention, the occupational therapist can synthesize therapeutic occupational forms collaboratively with the patient (e.g., safe methods of upper-body dressing). For

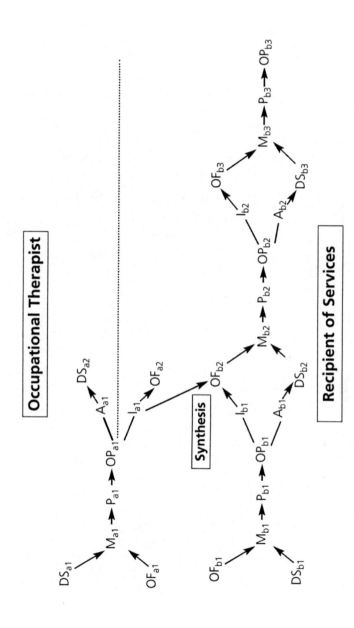

Figure 5-10. Collaborative therapeutic occupational synthesis. A, adaptation; DS, developmental structure; I, impact; M, mental interpretation; OF, occupational form; OP, occupational performance; P, purpose.

these proposed methods of self-care to be truly therapeutic, the patient must find meaning and purpose in them. Whereas the orthopedic surgeon directly influences body tissue while the patient remains passive, the occupational therapist's tool of synthesis will affect the patient's occupational performance only if the patient actively finds meaning and purpose in the situation. In therapeutic occupation, the recipient of occupational therapy is truly an active participant, not a passive set of body systems.

The recipients of occupational therapy are each different in their capacities to collaborate in occupational synthesis. Some are able to synthesize their own forms while receiving minimal input from the therapist. Some do not currently have the capacity to collaborate verbally or nonverbally in synthesis, whether because of immaturity or because of disabilities in the cognitive and/or psychosocial areas. Many are somewhere in the middle (i.e., able to have constructive input into the design of the occupational form but in need of professional guidance). Different models of practice put different degrees of emphasis on this collaboration. A universal guideline is for the recipient of occupational therapy to have as much input into the process as possible. Indeed, an increase in self-determination is often one of the most important treatment goals.

Figure 5-10 depicts the occupational therapist as engaged in occupations also, with meanings, purposes, performances, impacts, and adaptations. As part of the occupational form, the therapist has a socially sanctioned role as a professional person with ethical and institutional responsibilities. An essential part of the therapist's occupational form is the socially established knowledge base of the profession, especially the models of practice. The *clinical reasoning* of the therapist reflects both the subjectivity and the objectivity of the therapist's efforts to establish and maintain a therapeutic relationship. In an ongoing stream of occupations and sub-occupations, the occupational therapist both adapts to the needs of the recipient of services and has a collaborative impact on the person's occupational form. Thus, occupational therapy is a special case of reciprocal occupations between two people.

Occupational Assessment

Definition of Occupational Assessment: *Occupational assessment involves (a) the therapist's direct and indirect (reported) observation of a person's occupational performances and impacts in the context of synthesized occupational forms, and (b) the drawing of inferences about the person's developmental structure and/or occupational configurations.*

Assessment involves gaining information about the developmental structure of the recipient of services. One type of occupational performance that is often an essential part of the assessment process is the self-reporting of the person receiving services. The person's descriptions of past patterns of occupation and the person's voicing of hopes and fears for the future help the occupational therapist construct an overall picture of the individual's developmental structure and occupational configuration. Occupational assessment usually involves other kinds of occupational performance in addition to talking. One of the great ideas of occupational therapy (as stated by Meyer, 1922) is the idea that people will often reveal their abilities and disabilities nonverbally when they are actively engaged in an occupation. What is revealed in the voluntary transformation of materials can be quite different from the verbal self-report of the individual who has little insight or self-awareness. For example, it is characteristic of the person with a borderline personality disorder to sound much more occupationally successful than he or she actually is. The person's problems are often revealed in the context of completing a craft or playing a game. In addition, there are many patients or clients referred to occupational therapy who have difficulty with language, whether because of oral-motor disabilities or cognitive disabilities. The context of meaningful, purposeful occupation provides the ideal opportunity for accurate learning about the person's abilities.

The reports of others, such as family members, are indirect observations of the patient or client. For example, the mother of an autistic child can report on the child's occupational performance in a variety of settings to which the occupational therapist might not have immediate access (e.g., the child's interaction with neighbors or the child's reaction to mealtime). For another example, the husband of a woman with Alzheimer's disease can help the occupational therapist understand the woman's changing occupational patterns over time.

Direct assessment is a problem-solving process. When synthesizing the occupational form, the occupational therapist is aware of the challenges generally provided to developmental structures by this particular occupational form. For example, the occupational therapist knows that a particular recipe challenges an individual's ability to sequence instructions. If the patient succeeds in carrying out this recipe without assistance (occupational performance and impact), and if the recipe was not learned by rote in the past, the occupational therapist can reasonably make the *inference* that the patient has a certain level of sequencing ability in the developmental structure. Then the occupational therapist can go on to assessing other areas. However, if the patient fails in the occupation, the occupational therapist begins a problem-solving process. Was a lack of sequencing ability at the root of the problem, or might there have some other problem or problems, such as an inability to read the instructions or a motor problem, which caused the patient to make errors when trying to carry out the recipe? To answer this question, the occupational therapist later synthesizes a second occupational form that requires an equivalent degree of sequencing abilities but that does not involve written instructions or complex movements. Furthermore, the occupational therapist can assess the patient's ability to read instructions and engage in bilateral coordination in other occupational forms. This is the basic pattern of problem-solving, but the occupational therapist is usually observing and making inferences about more than one ability at a time. For example, in the observation of morning self-care, the occupational therapist can observe performances and impacts that lead to inferences about the patient's motor abilities, short-term memory, sensory abilities, values, interests, coping abilities, receptive language, and many other factors.

Formal or standardized tests work much the same way as informal observation: synthesis, observation, and inference. A major difference is that the authors of the test have provided scientific evidence as to the challenges provided by various items. In other words, the authors of a valid test have already engaged in the problem-solving process, so that the instructions provide little challenge or the individuals unable to understand the instructions have already be excluded from taking the test. For example, there are several tests of gross motor abilities standardized for school-aged children. Each item in each test can be thought of as a carefully designed occupational synthesis. For example, the occupational form for a test of running speed consists of explicit verbal instructions, an indoor space with at least 35 feet by 10 feet of surface appropriate for running, a marker placed 25 feet away from the starting point, and a stopwatch. All test items are structured (the occupational forms are synthesized) in such a way that healthy children will have no problems in terms of cognition, language, and basic sensation. In addition, the instructions to the tester warn about the types of children for whom the test is valid. Therefore, the problem-solving process is simplified for the occupational therapist performing the assessment. The main point here is that standardized tests generally follow the same logic as all direct occupational assessment as depicted in Figure 5-11: An occupational form is synthesized (a test item), and the assessor makes inferences about the individual's developmental structure based on the person's occupational performance and impact.

At the present time, many occupational therapists gain most of their information about clients through informal observations of the clients engaged in occupation, not through standardized tests. Currently available tests may not be sensitive enough to all the factors with which an occupational therapist must be concerned. Furthermore, assessment is an ongoing process that does not stop until discharge. The therapist is always observing the client carefully and making inferences about his or her changing abilities and occupational configuration. Assessment does not stop just because therapeutic intervention starts.

Occupational Adaptation as Therapy

A Definition of Occupational Adaptation as Therapy: *Occupational adaptation as therapy involves the synthesis of an occupational form matched carefully to the person's developmental structure, so that positive change in the developmental structure takes place in accordance with a model of practice.*

The possibility of occupational adaptation through a structured therapeutic relationship is probably the reason that the profession of occupational therapy exists. Although they did not use the same terms, the founders of our profession believed that one person (the therapist) could help synthesize the occupational form of another person (the patient) in such a way as to help the patient make a change for the better in his or her own being (Fig. 5-12).

As with all therapeutic occupation, collaborative occupational synthesis leads to an occupational form for the patient. The therapist hopes and predicts that the occupational form will provide the just-right challenge to the developmental structure and that it will elicit positive meanings and purposes, leading to active occupational performance and positive adaptation. An example of occupational adaptation is the increase in coordination skill of the upper extremities in an elderly woman with mild left hemiplegia. In accordance with a motor learning model of practice, the occupational therapist synthesizes an occupational form in the simulated kitchen of a rehabilitation facility. The occupational form involves a variety of flatware and a sponge in the sink filled with soapy water in addition to instructions to wash the utensils and place them in the adjacent pan of rinse water. Let us assume that the patient found these instructions and the rest of the occupational form to be meaningful, and she went about her occupational performance in a purposeful way. Her occupational performance involves holding the plates with her left hand using a variety of grasp patterns (varying as the objects vary in shape) while simultaneously rubbing the dishes with the sponge in her right hand. This is the first time that the woman has washed dishes since her stroke, and it is just within her abilities. After the occupation, the woman has made a small but significant therapeutic adaptation toward an enhanced ability to use her two upper extremities in coordination with each other.

Developmental promotion and *remediation* are two forms of therapeutic adaptation. In developmental promotion, an ability is developed that was never present before in the developmental structure. An example of a developmental promotion can be seen in the child with a developmental disorder who learns how to dress herself. In contrast, remediation involves regaining a skill that was present in the person's developmental structure

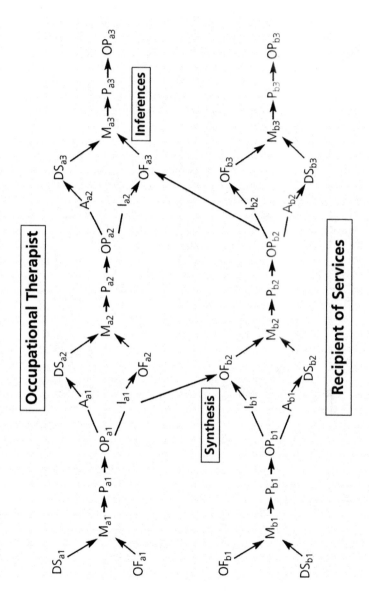

Figure 5-11. Direct occupational assessment. A, adaptation; DS, developmental structure; I, impact; M, mental interpretation; OF, occupational form; OP, occupational performance; P, purpose.

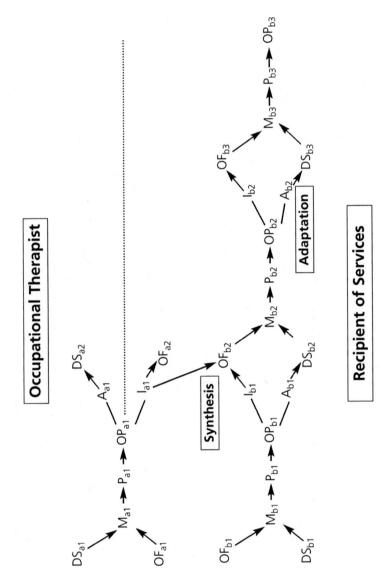

Figure 5-12. Therapeutic adaptation. A, adaptation; DS, developmental structure; I, impact; M, mental interpretation; OF, occupational form; OP, occupational performance; P, purpose.

before the onset of a disease process. Hence, the re-establishment of the ability to feed oneself after a stroke is an example of remediation.

Occupational Compensation as Therapy

A Definition of Occupational Compensation as Therapy: *Occupational compensation as therapy involves four elements: a developmental structure characterized by an intractable problem and latent capacities, synthesis of a somewhat atypical occupational form, substitute occupational performance, and comparable impact.*

Compensation is a way around the problem. In most models of practice, the compensatory approach is used only when some deficit is thought to be unchangeable (intractable). In other words, some part of the developmental structure is incapable of adapting. For example, let us consider a young man with cervical spinal cord injury. The occupational therapist synthesizes a mouth stick in the context of computer word-processing that comes to have meaning and purpose to the young man, even though it is a somewhat atypical occupational form. *Atypical* or *artificial* is the opposite of *natural* or *everyday*; the artificiality or the naturalism of an occupational form is part of its sociocultural aspect. Most people in our society do not use a mouth stick; therefore, it is an atypical occupational form. The mouth stick makes it possible for the young man with a spinal cord injury to engage in a *substitute occupational performance*, to flex and extend his head in substitution for upper extremity movements. His movement pattern has a *comparable impact* in that the letters on a keyboard are depressed and words are thus displayed on a computer screen and stored in computer memory. We call this a *comparable impact* because it is similar to the impact that someone with upper extremity control would have.

As with all therapeutic occupation, successful compensatory occupation depends on an active construction of meaning and purpose on the part of the recipient of services. Although a device might appear to be biomechanically "perfect," the person might see the device (meaning) as insulting, worthless, or too expensive. Therefore, the person might not want to use it (purpose) or might use it only in private situations. A major role for the occupational therapist is to attend to the meanings and purposes of the individual recipient of services.

Another example of occupational compensation (Fig. 5-13) can be seen in occupational therapy for an older woman who has just had hip surgery. The therapist shows the woman how to use a dressing stick to bring clothing up over her feet and legs without flexing more than 90 degrees at the hips. The dressing stick makes the occupational form somewhat atypical. The substitute occupational performance involves hand and shoulder movements instead of flexion beyond 90 degrees at the hips. The comparable impact is that her clothes are on her body.

Sometimes the atypicality of the occupational form is subtle. For example, please consider the bed mobility of a person with spinal cord injury at the lumbar level. The substitute occupational performance involves scooting as a compensation or substitution for lower extremity movements. The comparable impact consists of the new surroundings after the movement. In this example, the somewhat atypical occupational form is the unusual pattern of relationships of the bed to this body as the occupation unfolds. Another example can be seen in the energy conservation movements of a middle-aged woman with rheumatoid arthritis, when she pushes a heavy pot across the counter as a substitution for picking it up. Here the atypicality in the occupational form is the pot's sliding over the counter.

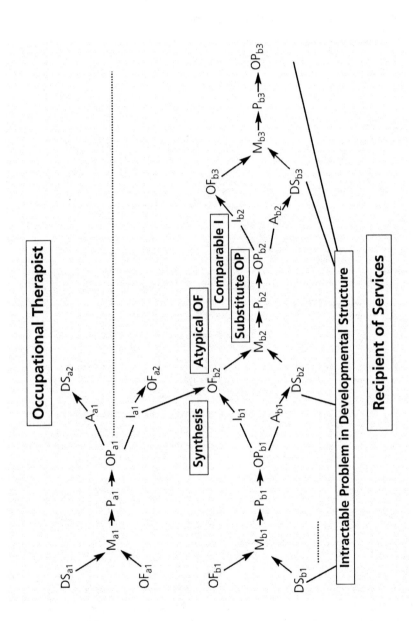

Figure 5-13. Occupational compensation as therapy. A, adaptation; DS, developmental structure; I, impact; M, mental interpretation; OF, occupational form; OP, occupational performance; P, purpose.

Assistive devices, mobility aids including wheelchairs, augmentative communication devices, many prostheses, many positioning systems, and other assistive technology are synthesized to promote compensatory occupation. Whether the assistive device is manufactured or custom-designed, we can still say that it is synthesized by the occupational therapist, because the therapist must introduce each device according to the needs of the individual.

Although therapeutic adaptation is definitely a different process from therapeutic compensation, the two processes can occur in occupational therapy for the same patient. When a patient is first presented with an assistive device that might be helpful, there is usually a period of learning or adaptation that must take place before the person can use the assistive device in an efficient way. For example, the patient with an immobilized arm who is given a buttoning hook has to learn how to insert the hook through the buttonhole before hooking the button. This learning (development of a new memory) is an adaptation to the developmental structure. Once this adaptation is made, the assistive device can serve as a compensation. Sometimes this initial orientation to a compensatory device can be quite complex, as it is for a robotic work station or a myoelectric upper extremity prosthesis. Many sensorimotor, cognitive, and psychosocial adaptations might be necessary before effective use of such devices.

Compensatory occupation can also lead ultimately (in later occupations) to adaptation. For example, the child with cerebral palsy who uses the communication board is compensating for an inability to speak. The impact the child has on the world can be powerful feedback, and this can lead to adaptations in the child's self-concept and sense of personal mastery. This adaptation, in turn, can lead to the child's future willingness to try other devices and to engage in other therapeutic occupations and compensations.

Health Promotion and Therapeutic Prevention through Occupation

Health promotion and prevention are other important goals in occupational therapy. An occupational approach has tremendous potential in promoting high-level wellness. Working collaboratively with the client, the occupational therapist can synthesize occupational forms that elicit deep personal meanings and powerful purposes. Many potential clients could benefit from this sort of consultation with an expert on the nature and uses of occupation.

Prevention of impairment and disability can take place at many levels (Nelson & Stucky, 1992). At the primary level, through occupational assessment the therapist can help identify, through behaviors and physical indicators, medical disorders that others on the health care team might not have noticed. The occupational therapist can then communicate these observations to the medical staff so that preventive action can be taken. Another level of prevention involves various forms of occupational adaptation. Increased range of motion through occupation (an adaptation) can prevent contractures. Increased endurance through participation in a well-planned, long-term exercise group can decrease the likelihood of a cardiovascular disorder. Success as experienced in occupation can prevent some forms of depression. Yet another level of prevention can be seen in much compensatory occupation. Energy conservation techniques and work simplification techniques are compensatory in nature, and they also serve to decrease wear and tear to the musculoskeletal system. In summary, therapeutic prevention through occupation can be accomplished through assessment, adaptation, or compensation.

Models of Practice

A model of practice provides guidelines for occupational synthesis. There are many models of practice in occupational therapy at the present time. Some are relatively well-developed and provide specific guidelines that are consistent with research findings; others are in the early stages of formation. The model of practice and the outline of questions answered by a complete model of practice (Fig. 5-14) draw heavily on the framework provided by Kielhofner (1997). Kielhofner, in turn, was influenced by Mosey (1981), who used the term frame of reference to describe guidelines for practice in occupational therapy.

> **A Definition of Occupational Therapy Model of Practice:** *An occupational therapy model of practice provides theory-based guidelines for occupational therapy practice. A model of practice consists of (a) theory describing relationships between occupation and health, and (b) theory-based guidelines for therapeutic occupation.*

Two models of practice will be used as examples. The reader should keep in mind that all the models of practice in occupational therapy can be analyzed in terms of the ideas presented in Figure 5-14.

Theory describing relationships between occupation and health derives from academic disciplines (such as anthropology, sociology, academic psychology, or biology), from other professions (such as medicine, physical therapy, applied psychology, or education), or from within the profession of occupational therapy. For example, A. Jean Ayres (1972) articulated a model of practice, sensory integration, that draws on the neurosciences, developmental psychology, and prior ideas of physicians, physical therapists, and occupational therapists (e.g., Herman Kabat, Margaret Knott, and Margaret Rood). For another example, Gary Kielhofner (1995) developed his model of human occupation from an interdisciplinary base including humanistic branches of philosophy, psychology (especially social psychology and developmental psychology), sociology, anthropology, early figures in occupational therapy history (especially the physician Adolph Meyer), as well as Mary Reilly, Janice Burke, and other occupational therapists.

A model's domain of concern can be deduced from the interdisciplinary base of theoretical knowledge. For example, the sensory integrative (SI) model of practice focuses especially on the somatosensory systems (the vestibular, proprioceptive, and tactile) as the developmental bases on which visual and auditory systems and higher cognitive functions depend. The SI model also has a focal viewpoint that is developmental in nature, with an emphasis on the plasticity of the person's nervous system. The Model of Human Occupation (MOHO) focuses especially on psychosocial areas, especially what Kielhofner terms "volition" (i.e., personal causation, values, and interests). MOHO also sees the person as capable of adaptation; indeed, the person is conceptualized as an improviser who is continuously updating one's life narrative. Although both models identify a specific domain of concern, this is not to say that they ignore other parts of the person's developmental structure. SI does consider the cognitive and psychosocial areas, and MOHO does consider the sensorimotor and cognitive areas. To have a domain of concern does not mean that the model must be narrow in scope; rather, it provides a focal viewpoint that is a starting point for thinking about the developmental structure of the person.

Each model also defines the *dynamics of healthy occupation* and *threats to healthy occupation*. For example, the SI model of practice emphasizes that somatosensory information must be processed and modulated before efficient learning in school is possible. If somatosensory information is not properly modulated, a learning disability tends to occur (a threat to healthy occupation). In Kielhofner's model of practice, a dynamic of healthy

Models of Practice

I. Theory Describing Relationships Between Occupation and Health

What is the domain of concern?
Which disciplines and professions contribute to the theory?

A. Dynamics of Healthy Occupation (Conceptual Framework for Therapeutic Occupation [CFTO] Terminology)

How is the person's developmental structure conceptualized?
What is successful occupational performance?
What is beneficial adaptation?
What kinds of meanings and purposes are associated with healthy occupation?
How does occupation contribute to health?
How does health contribute to the occupational configuration?
What is the research support for the above?
What further research is needed?

B. Threats to Healthy Occupation (in CFTO Terminology)

What are the relationships between impairments, disabilities, and occupation?
What is dysfunction (unsuccessful occupational performance)?
What is maladaptation?
Does occupation (or its lack) contribute to dysfunction or maladaptation?
How does dysfunction or maladaptation affect subsequent occupation?
What kinds of meanings and purposes are associated with dysfunction and/or maladaptation?
What is the research support for the above?
What further research is needed?

II. Therapeutic Occupation

A. Principles and Technology for Therapeutic Occupational Syntheses

1. Principles and Technology for Occupational Therapy Evaluation

For what types of persons is this model appropriate (i.e., what are the screening or referral criteria and processes)?
Which occupations or components of the developmental structure are evaluated?
How does the therapist decide to evaluate or not to evaluate in a particular area?
What is the sequence used in the initial evaluation? Do parts of the initial evaluation serve as screens for later evaluation?
How is occupational synthesis used in the evaluation?
Are non-occupational techniques used in the evaluation?
How are the person's meanings and purposes considered in the evaluation process?
How does the interdisciplinary team contribute to the process and content of the evaluation?
How do family members/significant others contribute to the process and content of the evaluation?
How does the person contribute to the process and content of the evaluation?
Which assessments are used?
What are the reliability, validity, and sensitivity of these instruments?
What is the research to support the assessments?
When are assessments administered or re-administered?
Does ongoing clinical observation of occupation contribute to the evaluation?
How is the evaluation documented?
How does the occupational therapy evaluation contribute to the interdisciplinary team?
What are the reimbursement issues concerning evaluation?
Overall, how are the principles and technology of assessment consistent with underlying theory (see I above)?

(continued)

Figure 5-14. Outline for occupational therapy models of practice.

Models of Practice *(continued)*

2. Principles and Technology for Occupational Therapy Goal-Setting

   How does the therapist decide to set a goal in a particular area? How does the evaluation contribute to the goal-setting process?

   How are goals prioritized?

   What is the sequence of goal-setting over the course of therapy?

   How does the model involve occupational adaptation, occupational compensation, occupational prevention, occupational maintenance, and/or occupational health promotion? If more than one mode is used, how are goals prioritized among modes?

   Goals are set for which occupations or components of the developmental structure?

   How does a therapist decide on the magnitude of the goal (i.e., the degree of change predicted from the present state)?

   What is the time frame for each goal, and what are the relationships between relatively short-term goals and relatively long-term goals?

   How is occupational analysis used in goal-setting?

   Are goals stated in terms of occupational performance or in terms of components of the developmental structure?

   Are non-occupational goals cited?

   How does the interdisciplinary team contribute to the process and content of goal-setting?

   How do family members/significant others contribute to the process and content of goal-setting?

   How does the person contribute to the process and content of goal-setting?

   How are the person's meanings and purposes considered in the goal-setting process?

   How and why are goals changed?

   Is there research to support the goal-setting process?

   How is goal-setting documented?

   How does occupational therapy goal-setting contribute to the interdisciplinary team?

   Overall, how are the principles and technology of goal-setting consistent with underlying theory (see I above)?

3. Principles and Technology for Occupational Therapy Methods

   What kinds of occupational forms are synthesized in the model of practice?

   Are different types of forms used for different types of goals?

   Are different forms (or variations on forms) used for the same goal?

   Can a single form address multiple goals?

   How are grading and occupational analysis used as a basis for occupational synthesis?

   Are the occupational forms socioculturally typical, simulated, and/or atypical/artificial?

   Are non-occupational techniques used? If so, how are these techniques based in theory?

   How does the therapist decide on a particular occupational synthesis?

   How does the interdisciplinary team contribute to the process and content of occupational synthesis?

   How do family members/significant others contribute to the process and content of occupational synthesis?

   How does the person collaborate with the therapist in the occupational synthesis?

   How are the person's meanings and purposes considered in the synthesis of occupational forms?

   Are materials typically affected?

   How are others part of the synthesized form?

   How is the therapist part of the synthesized form?

Models of Practice *(continued)*

What is the role of the therapist's self-awareness in the clinical reasoning process?

Clinically, how does the occupational therapist decide about the efficacy of occupational synthesis for a particular person?

What is the process of re-synthesis?

Is specific apparatus used? If so, how? Does the model involve protocols to be followed in specific situations?

What is the applied research in support of the efficacy of the methods?

Overall, how are the principles and technology of occupational synthesis methods consistent with underlying theory?

B. General Considerations in Implementation of the Model of Practice

  1. Conceptual Issues

    What is the history of the application of this model of practice (including its components)?

    Does the model have sub-models for different types of persons or different types of settings?

    Can or should the model of practice be used in conjunction with other models of practice, and why? Is the model incompatible with any other model?

    How well-developed is the model, and what are future needed steps in development of the model?

    Does the model involve special ethical problems?

  2. Programming Issues

    In which types of settings is this model appropriate?

    How is the person referred to (e.g., patient, client, consumer, student, resident, etc.)?

    What is the process for initiation of intervention?

    What is the process for termination of intervention?

    What is the occupational therapist's role in assisting the person and the family in transition to other services or to discharge from all services?

    What are the practical aspects of occupational synthesis (e.g., cost, space requirements, non-intervention "down time")?

    What are the issues surrounding funding and reimbursement?

    Does the model involve special problems of management?

    How are evaluation, goal-setting, and methods documented?

    What are the competencies needed for independent practice in this model? Does the model have specific guidelines for training of therapists or for graded levels of supervision? What is the role of the occupational therapy assistant in this model?

---

occupation is a sense of personal causation that promotes successful occupational performance and positive adaptations; on the other hand, a belief that one's destiny is being controlled by others will promote failure in occupational performance. Repeated success or failure can then lead to benign or vicious cycles of healthy adaptation or maladaptation. The person is a dynamic system making volitional use of naturalistic occupational forms.

The second major part of a model of practice involves discussions of *therapeutic occupation*. This is the applied, practical part of a model of practice, and it must be consistent with theory. As posited in the Conceptual Framework for Therapeutic Occupation, *therapeutic occupational syntheses* are at the heart of occupational therapy clinical reasoning. Principles and technology for assessment, goal-setting, and intervention all involve occupational synthesis, the essential occupation of the occupational therapist. An example of therapeutic synthesis in the sensory integrative model of practice is as follows: Self-directed play involving vigorous vestibular, tactile, and proprioceptive stimulation can enhance bilateral motor coordination. In this example, the occupational therapist synthesizes an occupational form that has the sociocultural characteristics of a game while eliciting the desired perceptual meanings. An example from MOHO is as follows: The presence of recognizable options in the occupational form encourages self-directedness and the development of a sense of personal causation. Principles of therapeutic occupation can be deduced from the interdisciplinary base and must be logically consistent with the model's descriptions of success, failure, adaptation, and maladaptation. The emphasis might be on therapeutic adaptation, therapeutic compensation, or therapeutic prevention, depending on the model's focal viewpoint.

The technology used in assessment, goal-setting, and intervention involves practical issues, such as procedures and equipment necessary to carry out the therapeutic occupations. Ayres' model provides the *Sensory Integration and Praxis Tests* (Ayres, 1989), a set of standardized instruments routinely used as part of the assessment process along with a variety of specified observations. Ayres' model also takes advantage of some ingenious equipment (occupational forms) specifically designed to provide somatosensory input in a playful context (e.g., hanging nets, bolsters, and scooter boards). In MOHO, assessment tools include the *Occupational Performance History Interview* and the *Occupational Self Assessment*, to name a few. A prime technique in MOHO is to use naturalistic, everyday settings as contexts for therapy. The many descriptions of MOHO programs with specific populations provide therapists with specific interventions. A model's techniques and tools for assessment and intervention must be consistent with the principles guiding intervention.

In the Conceptual Framework for Therapeutic Occupation format for a model of practice, research is integrated throughout. Research relevant to underlying theory is presented in the first major part of the model, and applied research concerning instrumentation and intervention efficacy is present in the discussions of occupational syntheses. The model of practice should advocate investigating, testing, and expanding on each aspect of the model. An example of applied sensory integrative research would be the testing of the reliability and validity of the *Sensory Integration and Praxis Tests*. An example pertinent to MOHO would be program evaluation research conducted in a particular setting (e.g., a community-based return-to-work program) with a particular population (workers with chronic back pain). The Conceptual Framework for Therapeutic Occupation format also calls for a discussion of conceptual and programming issues. Such a discussion makes the model more practical for therapists.

Differences and Commonalities among Models of Practice

Of the many occupational therapy models of practice, some are oriented to specific populations or settings, and some are general. For example, the occupational therapy version of the psychoanalytical model of practice (Mosey, 1986) is oriented specifically to patients with particular types of psychiatric disorders. In contrast, the developmental model advocated by Llorens (1970) is potentially applicable to all persons at any identifiable chronologic and developmental level. Another difference among models of practice is that some are relatively well-developed, whereas others are in the early stages of development. For example, some models tend to be technique-oriented and seem to be in search of underlying theory, whereas other models are highly principled but rather vague when it comes to reproducible techniques.

In our opinion, the main thing that all occupational therapy models of practice have in common is focus on occupation and occupational synthesis. Regardless of how the developmental structure of the person is conceptualized and regardless of how healthy and unhealthy patterns of occupation are defined, all our models of practice involve a matching up of occupational forms to a person. All involve a prediction of the person's meanings, purposes, and occupational performances. In summary, all involve therapeutic occupation.

SOURCES OF CONCEPTUAL FRAMEWORK FOR THERAPEUTIC OCCUPATION IDEAS

It is often difficult to identify the exact sources of one's thinking. A liberal education, books including novels, good conversation, and a basic education in occupational therapy undoubtedly contributed to many of the ideas in this conceptual framework. Interesting ideas do not always come with a name and a date, and sometimes the sources of the ideas are forgotten. Some ideas, or at least how the ideas are put together, are original. However, there are certain sources that are identifiable. The brief discussion below is not an attempt to discuss the work of scholars in any detail. Its only purpose is to help the reader understand some of the roots of the Conceptual Framework for Therapeutic Occupation.

Certainly John Dewey (1916, 1966), the eminent American philosopher and educator, had a major influence on the development of the ideas in this chapter. His philosophy of pragmatism posited that human development is the result of active occupations, and he even used the term occupation. Reading the early occupational therapists (e.g., Dunton, 1928; Slagle, 1922; Tracy, 1910) and the eminent psychiatrist and proponent of occupational therapy Meyer (1922) confirmed the importance of Dewey's pragmatism on the new profession of occupational therapy. Slagle and Dunton also discussed the ideas of occupational analysis and grading, which involve the match-ups between various occupational possibilities, on the one hand, and the strengths and weaknesses of the patient, on the other hand. Conceptual Framework for Therapeutic Occupation can be thought of as a logical extension of Slagle's system of occupational analysis. The founders of the profession had a powerful belief in the potential of carefully planned (i.e., synthesized) occupations to restore health. Slagle also mentioned the possibility of using occupation as a disease prevention measure.

Meyer (1922) used the word adaptation in the way it is used in the Conceptual Framework for Therapeutic Occupation, but Piaget's idea of adaptation through active doing was more influential in the development of the Conceptual Framework for Therapeutic Occupation's ideas than those of the early occupational therapists. For example, Piaget's two types of adaptation, assimilation and accommodation (Piaget, 1981), are reflected in the Conceptual Framework for Therapeutic Occupation notion that part of adaptation can occur within the process a developing a purpose, even before actual occupational performance.

Colleagues have wondered if the idea of occupational form is indebted to the ecological psychology of J. J. Gibson (1979). Gibson held that perception is direct, that is, that the person looks at the world in terms of what it affords for doing. In some ways, this is similar to the Conceptual Framework for Therapeutic Occupation concept that the world is largely structured into occupational forms and that the person creates meaning by trying to interpret these forms. However, Conceptual Framework for Therapeutic Occupation definitions were influenced more by phenomenology than by ecological psychology. Phenomenologists, such as Husserl (1931) and Ihde (1977), posited that all perception is perception *of something*. The "lived world" is the something to be perceived. The "lived body" is the perceiver. "Intentionality" is the relationship created between the lived body and lived world. These concepts from phenomenology were consciously considered in the writing of the first published paper on the Conceptual Framework for Therapeutic Occupation (Nelson, 1988). In some ways, the lived body is similar to Conceptual Framework for Therapeutic Occupation ideas of meaning and developmental structure. In some ways, lived world is similar to occupational form. Finally, in some ways, intentionality is similar to purpose. However, there are many differences, and most phenomenologists would question the Conceptual Framework for Therapeutic Occupation commitment to the idea of objectivity in the occupational form and occupational performance, and to the idea of an experimental analysis of these objectivities. Readings in anthropology (e.g., Campbell, 1988) also were influential in the Conceptual Framework for Therapeutic Occupation definition of occupational form as consisting of sociocultural norms and symbols embedded in the physical world.

Reilly (1962) was influential in emphasizing a reconsideration of the origins of the profession and in emphasizing occupational terminology. Mosey (1981) provided the idea that the profession involves multiple frames of reference, with practice in each of them guided by underlying theory. Kielhofner (1997) emphasized the need for basic and applied research to refine and test theory and practice and suggested that the profession has a central paradigm that can be applied to all the conceptual models of practice.

Other sources include experimental methodology and behavioral psychology (e.g., the emphasis on inter-rater agreement as a measure of objectivity). It is also important to recognize students as sources of ideas, especially as sources for how to present ideas. The biggest change between this work and that published in 1994 is the use of the new diagrams, and the first discussions of these diagrams took place in occupational therapy classrooms in New York, Michigan, and Ohio. All those students who contributed to the ideas of the Conceptual Framework for Therapeutic Occupation deserve recognition if these ideas become promoters of therapeutic occupations that actually help people. However, they deserve none of the blame if the ideas do not work.

CONTROVERSIES IN OCCUPATIONAL THERAPY TERMINOLOGY

Among theoreticians in occupational therapy, there are many different approaches to occupation. Important terms are used in different ways, and this can be confusing to occupational therapists and to others. In our opinion, past and current attempts sponsored within the American Occupational Therapy Association to eliminate the confusion by providing uniform terms have added to the confusion. Trying to create theory by committee leads to many problems of internal logic in the attempt to make compromises between different points of view. Also, there is a fairness issue whenever there is an attempt to force a consensus in favor of one set of terms at the expense of all the others. In our opinion, our profession is at the stage at which each conceptual framework should strive for internal consistency of logic, completeness, and usability. Over time more of a consensus in the field will develop naturally in the literature, but the consensus cannot be forced by majority vote.

Occupational Form

As the term "occupational form" becomes increasingly used in the profession, it becomes increasingly controversial. The question arises: Why invent a term like "occupational form?" Why not use a label that is used more widely, such as "environment," "stimulus," "context," "situation," or "structure?" This is a valid question. The world does not need more jargon. As a rule in reducing jargon, it is better to use a readily recognized term if the meaning is equivalent. The problem is that none of these other terms is fully equivalent to the use of the term "occupational form" in this chapter. Indeed, the connotations are quite different. These connotations are discussed in Nelson (1997).

There is another reason to commit ourselves to the term occupational form. This reason has to do with the label of our profession: We are *occupational* therapists. That means that *occupation* is our focus. We need to reaffirm that occupation is our method of therapy and our reason for existing. Although occupational therapists are not always clear about what their title means, one term with the word occupation ("occupational performance") has been used for many years — for example, in several of the official documents of the American Occupational Therapy Association (e.g., AOTA, 1995). Given the widespread use of the term occupational performance, what should we call the contextual structure of that performance? Let us analyze the word performance. In Latin, the word *per* means to go "through." In the word performance, "per" is immediately followed by "form." Thus, performance literally means to go "through a form." In other words, for there to be a performance, there has to be a form that is gone through. Therefore, the term occupational form is the perfect term to match up to the term occupational performance.

Another controversy concerning occupational form is that other theorists in the profession have started to use the term but have defined it in different ways. For example, Kielhofner (1997) defines occupational form as just one part of the environment. To Kielhofner, occupational form has to do with sociocultural expectations, not with objects, settings, and social interactions in the environment. The Conceptual Framework for Therapeutic Occupation argument against Kielhofner's definition is the integrated unity of the physical aspects of a situation and the sociocultural expectations. It is recommended that the reader return to this discussion of unity in the section on occupational form. In addition, the Conceptual Framework for Therapeutic Occupation idea of occupational form simplifies the essential role of the occupational therapist: to synthesize occupational forms.

Occupation Versus Activity

Getting comfortable with occupational terminology requires us to consider alternative words for occupations or sub-occupations. The most common alternative term for occupation is *activity*, and activity tends to be used especially in describing brief units of human doing (what are called sub-occupations in the Conceptual Framework for Therapeutic Occupation). Darnell and Heater (1994) gave two reasons for avoiding the term activity in our literature. First, the term activity is overly broad in that it refers to many reflexive and even non-animate events. Consider the terms reflex activity, cardiovascular activity, molecular activity, atomic activity, volcanic activity, and solar activity. Indeed, the term activity can refer to anything that is moving. In contrast, the term *occupation* always refers to the meaningful, purposeful doing of a real human being, even if the person is holding still in a purposeful way. Second, the founders of the profession of occupational therapy chose the name carefully, but over time the meaning of the term *occupational* in our title has gotten lost in the minds of the public, and even in our own minds. This has created a problem of identity. If we begin to use terms like occupation, occupational analysis, and occupational synthesis with confidence, then the public will catch on to the essence of our profession. If we do not use the word occupation with comfort, how can we expect the public to understand our profession?

It would be convenient if new terms could be identified for each level of sub-occupation, and various terms such as activity and action have been proposed. Despite the apparent usefulness of this approach, we believe it is impossible to use the same hierarchical classification scheme for all occupations. Real occupations are too different from each other. One occupation may have seven identifiable levels of sub-occupations, and another may have only five. Some occupations seem to fit nicely into higher-level, long-term roles in life, but others do not. When occupations are defined as being made up of a series of activities, it turns out to be impossible to determine clearly what are the occupations and what are the activities. Where exactly is the line to be drawn? Each occupation has its own configuration of sub-occupations, and the Conceptual Framework for Therapeutic Occupation posits that these sub-occupations can be defined both in terms of sociocultural criteria and personally defined criteria.

Adaptation and Compensation

In the occupational therapy literature, the term *adaptation* and related terms such as adapt, adaptive, and adapted are frequently used in a way that is contrary to the Conceptual Framework for Therapeutic Occupation definition. For example, the term *adaptive device* is commonly used instead of the Conceptual Framework for Therapeutic Occupation-preferred *assistive device*. In addition, therapists talk about adapting the environment. Indeed, some theorists (e.g., Toglia, 1991) have used the term *adaptation* as a synonym for what the Conceptual Framework for Therapeutic Occupation means by the term *compensation*. As stated in a prior section, we choose the word adaptation to label the change in a person because of his or her own active doing, because important historical figures in occupational therapy (e.g., Meyer, 1922) and in other fields (e.g., Piaget, 1981) have used the word in the same way. In biology and psychology, the organism adapts to the environment, as opposed to the organism adapting the environment. In addition, the terms assistive device, assistive technology, and compensation are widely used in rehabilitation and gerontology in the same way as defined in the Conceptual Framework for Therapeutic Occupation. The basic rule of terminology in the Conceptual Framework for Therapeutic Occupation is that a single term should have a single, unique meaning. If the term adaptation refers to a change in the person because of occupational performance, it should not also mean a change in the environment or a mechanical device.

Other Controversies

For some in occupational therapy, *purpose* refers to society's standards for importance, whereas *meaning* reflects subjective experience. For others, meaning is something that is stored within the person. Another controversy is between the term *frame of reference* and *model of practice*. It will be interesting to see how a consensus develops over time in relation to these controversies as well as others. While acknowledging that there are currently many approaches to terminology in occupational therapy, we offer the Conceptual Framework for Therapeutic Occupation as an approach that carefully defines each term and relates that term to every other term in the conceptual framework in a precise way. We think the Conceptual Framework for Therapeutic Occupation is useful in analyzing everyday occupations, in describing and teaching clinical reasoning in occupational therapy, and in analyzing research. That is our opinion, but it is up to people like you, the reader, to decide if this conceptual framework is a valid and useful one for our field.

A FORMAT FOR OCCUPATIONAL ANALYSIS

Figure 5-15 presents a brief format for analyzing therapeutic occupation from a Conceptual Framework for Therapeutic Occupation perspective. The format might look brief, but the carrying out of the format requires astute observation skills, careful clinical reasoning, thorough understanding of all Conceptual Framework for Therapeutic Occupation terms, understanding of an occupational therapy model of practice, and excellent writing skills. Carrying out this format is the best way to take the next step in mastering the Conceptual Framework for Therapeutic Occupation. When used as a teaching technique, this format can be introduced by a series of brief videotaped occupations. The instructor is urged to review the Conceptual Framework for Therapeutic Occupation terms as the class discusses each part of the format.

CONCLUSION

Occupation is the core of our profession; hence, our title as *occupational* therapists. We are the experts in the use of occupation as a therapeutic method. That is what makes us unique. That is what makes our identity potentially much clearer than the identities of other professions.

It is hoped that this chapter helps in defining and thinking about some of our most basic concepts and principles. This chapter grounds the reader in *occupation* and suggests a way that all of our models of practice (past, present, and future) can be described in occu-

---

Analyzing a Therapeutic Occupation

(a) name (only) of the model of practice used, with primary (not secondary) reference;

(b) brief summary of evaluation (parts relevant to the planned occupations);

(c) short-term therapeutic goals;

(d) the planned occupational form, including planned instructions and temporal aspects (be very specific and detailed about <u>relevant</u> details only) and the predicted meanings, purposes, performances, impacts, and adaptations/compensations;

(e) the actual occupational form at the beginning of the occupation (note: a description is necessary only if circumstances required a change from the plan);

(f) the actual occupational performances observed and temporal changes in the occupational form over the course of the occupation (underline those words in this section that refer to the occupational form);

(g) the inferred meanings and purposes (these should be related to observable performances and impacts);

(h) adaptations and/or compensations made by the patient or client and any assessment information gained through observation of occupational performance (note: one-session adaptations are usually small and can be described by phrases such as "began to learn ..." or "took an initial step toward ....");

(i) how and why you would re-synthesize the occupational form in the future.

Note: When describing the occupational form, describe the most relevant aspects first. First name the form by putting it into quotations (e.g., "shaving"). When describing the <u>most</u> relevant features, do not only name the dimension (e.g., length) but give specifics (e.g., "approximately 12 inches"). The use of body-scaled information is often appropriate (e.g., "about the length of the patient's forearm"). Let the reader assume certain factors without need of mention (e.g., appropriate lighting) unless this factor is particularly relevant in this occupation (e.g., "the midday sun created a glare").

Figure 5-15. Format for analyzing a therapeutic occupation.

pational terms. Perhaps this chapter has assisted the reader in meeting the goal of our founders as stated in Article 1, Section 3 of the Constitution of the National Society for the Promotion of Occupational Therapy (1917):

> *"The object of the society shall be the advancement of occupation as a therapeutic measure; the study of the effects of occupation upon the human being; and the dissemination of scientific knowledge of this subject."*

LEARNING ACTIVITY — BEGINNER

5.1. Nelson and Jepson-Thomas refer to occupation as a construct. What does this mean?

5.2. Define each of the following and give an example:
- Developmental structure
- Occupational performance
- Occupational form

5.3. A very important point is made in this chapter — each occupation is unique and actual. What does this mean to you?

5.4. Compare objective and subjective and relate them to the terms developmental structure, occupational performance, and occupational form.

5.5A. Identify an occupational form that you encountered this week. Regarding that occupational form, delineate each of the following:

Physical dimension including the:
- Objects present
- Presence of others
- Temporal aspect

Sociocultural dimension including the:
- Ethnicity
- Financial considerations
- Role expectations
- Signs and symbols and their meaning
- Norms
- Typical uses and variations
- Language

5.5B. Take the occupational form you identified in 5.5A and describe the cultural bias or setting of the form. Hypothesize how the occupational form would be different if set within a different culture.

5.5C. Elaborate on the following statement: A social norm is an expectation for future occupation.

5.6 Within your own life, what cultural changes have you observed? You might want to start with a simple example like the Internet. How has it changed during your experience with it? How can such cultural change influence occupational performance and occupational form?

5.7 There are sociocultural dimensions to occupational forms. For the occupational form you identified in 5.5A, further analyze it in terms of each of the following social levels:
- Subcultural
- National
- Institutional

- Organizational
- Neighborhood
- Subgroups

5.8. How does law or legal considerations play a role in occupational forms?

5.9. Explain how an occupational form can be ambiguous or contradictory.

5.10. Mentally walk through where you live. For each room or distinct space, list the occupational forms associated with it. Compare your listing with a classmate. What is similar? What is different?

5.11. Mentally walk through the places where you have been today. For each space, list the occupational forms associated with it. Compare your listing with a classmate. What is similar? What is different?

5.12. Consider and identify at least three occupational forms you would like to encounter. Label each occupational form as scenarios as the authors did in this chapter. Explain your rationale for selecting each occupational form.

5.13. How does an occupational performance complete or integrate with an occupational form?

5.14. Explain why the occupational performance is different for two people participating in or completing approximately the same occupational form. According to Nelson and Jepson-Thomas, could they ever experience the same occupational performance? Explain the rationale for your answer.

5.15. Of what does developmental structure consist? Speculate how development structure changes over the lifespan.

5.16. Define each of the following types of meaning related to a particular occupational form:
- Affective
- Symbolic
- Perceptual

5.17. Meaning of an occupational form and purpose of an occupational performance are invisible. How can one infer meaning and purpose? How can one validate a hypothesis about persons' meaning and purpose?

5.18. Another very important point made in this chapter is that a characteristic of an occupational approach to understanding a person is a concern for the interconnectedness of multiple, inter-related levels of purpose. What does this mean to you? How could such an approach be manifest?

5.19. Differentiate intrinsic purpose and motivation from extrinsic purpose and motivation.

5.20. Why is it important to differentiate the purpose of the client from the purpose of the occupational therapist?

5.21. Differentiate between overt and covert occupational performance. Give an example of each.

5.22. According to the authors, occupation involves the doing (performance) of something (the form). If this is the case, speculate about the following: If one is doing something that is novel or not labeled, is it an occupational form?

5.23. Why are reflexes not occupational?

5.24. Why are habits occupational?

5.25. Why and how do occupational performance and choices among occupational forms inform us about a person's meanings and purposes?

5.26. What is humility?

5.27. What is an occupational approach?

5.28. How do the authors define function and dysfunction?

5.29. The authors do not believe in shared occupations. Explain their rationale.

5.30. Explain how a focus on occupation and occupational synthesis is common across models of practice in occupational therapy.

LEARNING ACTIVITY — ADVANCED

5.31. In what ways do concepts in this chapter overlap with anthropology? In what ways are concepts in this chapter distinct or unique from anthropology?

5.32. Uniform Terminology is referred to in this chapter. Currently, an updated alternative called the "Practice Framework" has been adpoted by the Representative Assembly. Obtain a copy of the "Practice Framework" and analyze it in terms of occupational form and occupational performance.

5.33. Argue the pro and the con viewpoints related to the following statement: A person's tendency toward certain occupational forms is inherited.

5.34. How could the Human Genome Project be related to occupational performance?

5.35. Can affective, symbolic, and perceptual meaning be ascribed to occupational performance? Explain.

5.36. The authors identified persons with immaturities, persons who are not acculturated, and persons with disabilities as three groups of people who tend to misinterpret common occupational forms. What other groups of people may deliberately choose to misinterpret occupational forms and why?

5.37. Compare to the voluntary doing of something (occupational performance), speculate what the compulsory doing of something might be termed.

5.38. Why is the concept of a non-purposeful, voluntary performance not sensible?

5.39. The authors speculate about occupations, sub-occupations, and sub-sub-occupations. Do you agree with these concepts? Why or why not?

5.40. The authors do not believe in shared occupations. Argue why this is a false assumption. Argue why it is a true assumption.

5.41. What is therapeutic occupation?

5.42. Explain occupational synthesis.

Acknowledgments

Special thanks are due to our Medical College of Ohio colleagues and students, who are implementing this chapter's ideas and terminology within our curriculum. Thanks are due also to colleagues and students around the world who are investing their occupational resources in trying to understand and apply the ideas of the Conceptual Framework for Therapeutic Occupation. We are interested in your comments and applications.

References

American Occupational Therapy Association. (1994). Uniform terminology for occupational therapy — third edition. *American Journal of Occupational Therapy, 48*, 1047–1054.

American Occupational Therapy Association. (1995). Position paper: Occupational performance: Occupational therapy's definition of function. *American Journal of Occupational Therapy, 49*, 1019–1020.

Ayres, A. J. (1972). *Sensory integration and learning disorders.* Los Angeles: Western Psychological Services.

Ayres, A. J. (1989). *Sensory integration and praxis tests.* Los Angeles: Western Psychological Services.

Campbell, B. G. (1988). *Humankind emerging* (5th ed.). New York: Harper Collins.

Christiansen, C. (1990). The perils of plurality. *Occupational Therapy Journal of Research, 10*, 259–265.

Darnell, J. L., & Heater, S. L. (1994). Occupational therapist or activity therapist — Which do you choose to be? *American Journal of Occupational Therapy, 48*, 467–468.

Dewey, J. (1916, 1966). *Democracy and education (1966 Free Press ed.).* New York: Macmillan.

Dunton, W. R., Jr. (1928). *Prescribing occupational therapy.* Springfield, IL: Charles C. Thomas.

Gibson, J. J. (1979). The theory of affordances. In R. Shaw and J. Bransford (Eds.), *Perceiving, acting, and knowing: Toward an ecological psychology* (pp. 67–82). Hillsdale, NJ: Lawrence Erlbaum.

Husserl, E. (1931) [Ideas]. (W. R. B. Gibson, trans.). New York: MacMillan.

Ihde, D. (1977). *Experimental phenomenology: An introduction.* New York: Putnam.

Kielhofner, G. (Ed.). (1995). *A model of human occupation: Theory and application* (2nd ed). Baltimore, MD: Williams & Wilkins.

Kielhofner, G. (1997). *Conceptual foundations of occupational therapy* (2nd ed.). Philadelphia, PA: F.A. Davis.

Llorens, L. A. (1970). Facilitating growth and development: The promise of occupational therapy. *American Journal of Occupational Therapy, 24*, 93–101.

Meyer, A. (1922). The philosophy of occupational therapy. *Archives of Occupational Therapy, 1*, 1–10.

Mosey, A. C. (1981). *Occupational therapy: Configuration of a profession.* New York: Raven.

Mosey, A. C. (1986). *Psychosocial components of occupational therapy.* New York: Raven.

National Society for the Promotion of Occupational Therapy. (1917). *Constitution.* Baltimore, MD: Sheppard Hospital. (Box 1, File 2 of the American Occupational Therapy Association Archives, Rockville, MD).

Nelson, D. L. (1988). Occupation: Form and performance. *American Journal of Occupational Therapy, 42*, 633–641.

Nelson, D. L. (1994). Occupational form, occupational performance, and therapeutic occupation. In C. B. Royeen (Ed.), *AOTA self study series: The practice of the future: Putting occupation back into therapy,* Lesson 2 (pp. 9–48). Rockville, MD: American Occupational Therapy Association.

Nelson, D. L. (1996). Therapeutic occupation: A definition. *American Journal of Occupational Therapy, 50*, 775–782.

Nelson, D. L. (1997). The 1996 Eleanor Clarke Slagle Lecture. Why the profession of occupational therapy will continue to flourish in the twenty-first century. *American Journal of Occupational Therapy, 51*, 11–24.

Nelson, D. L., & Stucky, C. (1992). The roles of occupational therapy in preventing further disability of elderly persons in long-term care facilities. In J. Rothman and R. Levine (Eds.), *Prevention practice: Strategies for physical and occupational therapy* (pp. 19–35). Philadelphia, PA: W.B. Saunders.

Piaget, J. (1981). *The psychology of intelligence.* Totowa, NJ: Littlefield, Adams & Co.

Reilly, M. (1962). Occupational therapy can be one of the great ideas of 20th century medicine. *American Journal of Occupational Therapy, 16*, 1–9.

Slagle, E. C. (1922). Training aides for mental patients. *Archives of Occupational Therapy, 1*, 11–17.

Toglia, J. P. (1991). Generalization of treatment: A multicontext approach to cognitive perceptual impairment in adults with brain injury. *American Journal of Occupational Therapy, 45*, 505–516.

Tracy, S. E. (1910). *Studies in invalid occupation: A manual for nurses and attendants.* Boston, MA: Whitcomb & Barrows.

6

Occupational Science: The Study of Humans as Occupational Beings

Ann A. Wilcock

OBJECTIVES

This chapter will help you to:

- Describe the nature and purpose of occupation according to occupational science.
- Discover the historical basis of occupational science.
- Characterize the philosophical underpinnings of occupational science.
- Discuss research related to occupation according to occupational science.
- Apply occupational science, an interdisciplinary theoretical approach, to occupational therapy practice situations.

⌐ABOUT THE AUTHOR

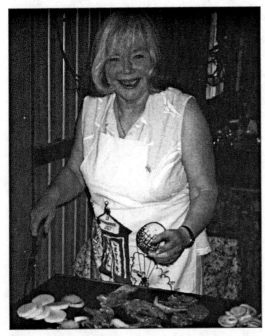

Ann cooking dinner on the barbeque.

Ann Wilcock is surprised at the amount of attention that her work has generated. She has always perceived herself as a rather simple soul who finds that to comprehend complex ideas she has "to write in a way that I understand." She works slowly and laboriously to set down her research findings, thoughts, and views in a clear straightforward manner, attributing much of her writing ability to her doctoral supervisor, Dr. Neville Hicks, whom she found to be an important mentor. Dr. Hicks is a historian of social and public health, and Ann recognizes his influence in her current thoughts and writings.

Ann has also been influenced by noted leaders in the United Kingdom, where she undertook her basic occupational therapy education. In particular, she cites Mary S. Jones, an occupational therapist who was a leader in establishing rehabilitation in the United Kingdom. In the 1940s, Jones coined the term "reablement" for a dynamic approach that was both holistic and specific. Her practice and the term were close to the enabling concept of the 1990s. Another mentor was Grisel McCaul, one of the pioneers of the activities of daily living (ADL) and independence movement in the United Kingdom. Ms McCaul's energy and commitment inspired Ann.

Her most recent work focuses on the history of occupational therapy from the beginning of time to the present day. She has just completed two volumes, commissioned by the British College of Occupational Therapists (COT). The first volume tells the story of how occupation was used for health purposes through to the end of the 19th century. The second volume takes up the tale of the establishment of occupational therapy in the United Kingdom in the 20th century. In both, the importance of the social context is made clear. This work is available through the COT website.

Ann is also committed to promoting the work of occupational therapists within public (population) health. In the future, she would like occupational therapists to become known for what they can contribute to the quality of people's lives overall. They have the potential to inform people about the importance of occupation as an agent for health, but this means that they take an active role in influencing public and social policy. She sees the educational system as critical, in that there is a need to educate and socialize students to become more politically aware and to take an active role in the process. She fears that dire consequences may result if occupational therapists do not begin to be active in the broader institutional/political arena. Further, the concept of occupational justice adds to her commitment in that direction because it suggests consideration of the need for all people to experience meaning and well-being through what they do.

Personally, the recent past has been difficult for Ann, filled with the loss of her husband and other people and pets that were very dear to her. She states that she "has been trapped by circumstances into spending too much time writing" and looks forward to balancing her life as an occupational being. Although she talks of retirement, she remains excited by thoughts and ideas yet to be developed.

INTRODUCTION

The subject of this chapter is occupational science as a potential knowledge base for occupational therapy. Occupational science is a discipline, which now has a following around the world. It was formally created in the last decades of the 20th century to study humans as occupational beings. Research into the purpose, meaning, and complexities of the interaction between people and what they do is of primary importance to inform, not only occupational therapy practice, but also almost all disciplines, professions, and agencies responsible for sociocultural, political, and health planning. Because occupation is so all-embracing, and apparently, so mundane, its significance has failed to be appreciated sufficiently. That is so despite parts of what "human occupation" embraces being studied by many diverse disciplines apart from occupational therapists. The diversity of the topic and of such study has made it difficult to gain a holistic perspective of occupation's overall purposes and importance, particularly within the field of health. This is responsible, in part, for some of the difficulties occupational therapists have experienced in having their services appreciated. An increased understanding by others of the importance and meaning of occupation in human existence will assist appreciation and development of occupational therapy philosophies, beliefs, and practices.

In the process of helping readers to understand the potential breadth of occupational science and its place within occupational therapy, a historical approach dating to before the 20th century will be taken to set the development of occupational science in context and to suggest its potential. The formal origins of occupational science are traced from occupational therapy pioneers in North America in the first decades of this century, through the work of Mary Reilly and Elizabeth Yerxa, to its establishment as a separate discipline at the University of Southern California. The idea of occupational science was taken up by occupational therapists in other countries and by some people in other disciplines. The consequences and potential benefits of an occupational knowledge base to underpin the practice of occupational therapy will underlie this chapter's discussion of many of the papers published in the *Journal of Occupational Science*. The place to start, however, is with defining and explaining the nature and purpose of occupational science.

NATURE AND PURPOSE OF OCCUPATIONAL SCIENCE

The need for occupation is an inbuilt physiologic mechanism that motivates, energizes, and enables people to meet and obtain the requirements for living, survival, health, and well-being (Wilcock, 1998). Like most needs it has been acted on, in most part, unconsciously, which accounts for its multi-various expressions as socio-politico-cultural beliefs, environment, and knowledge change. Occupational therapists are most interested in the relationship between occupation and health, although it is almost impossible to separate one purpose from another because they are so closely linked. Health, in a holistic sense, has been defined by Kass (1981) as the well working of the organism as a whole and as a state of being revealed in activity relative to each species as a standard of bodily exercise or fitness. Although Kass is not a professed occupational scientist, his definition of health lays the foundation for the idea of "people as occupational beings."

The simplest definition of occupational science is that it is the study of humans as occupational beings. What does that mean? It is easy to say "humans are occupational beings" but it is, in fact, a remarkably complex concept. At the very least it suggests that engagement in occupation is an innate behavior that is an integral aspect of humanness; that occupation (doing) and humanness (being) have an intimate relationship; and that occupation has evolutionary and biological as well as social and economic functions — factors which all need to be taken into account in occupational therapy when practicing holistically.

Indeed, the simple definition of occupational science previously stated touches on some of the most fundamental ideas about the nature of humans and the meaning of life which have been considered throughout recorded history by philosophers and scholars. Plato, for example, recognized that individuals have a unique collection of physical, mental, and spiritual capacities and, like Aristotle, his pupil, discoursed on the nature of praxis (action). Defining praxis as creative labor, Hegel, Marx, and Engels based their revolutionary philosophies on the nature and purpose of praxis as the nature of our species; while existential theorists hold that meaning, purpose, and choice in the lives of each unique individual are as important as scientific truths.

While occupational therapists have long espoused similar ideas, the importance of occupation to humans, to me it is surprising that so little research has been based on something apparently so important. Occupational therapists have, in the main, chosen to explore medical aspects and outcomes of treatment and have not studied humans, sick or well, as occupational beings. Perhaps because of this they find it difficult to explain effectively what the occupation part of the title has to do with therapy in a way acceptable to modern society. Indeed, many appear to welcome being called something different, such as hand therapists.

One reason for the scarcity of research on humans as occupational beings may be that there is little agreement about what the central issue of concern — "occupation" — encompasses. Whereas this lack of agreement could produce a position of strength from ongoing debate and research, few occupational therapists have engaged in this type of inquiry. Although this situation is changing, acceptance of conflicting ideas sits uneasily with many occupational therapists' frame of mind, which is based on a strong foundation of the need to be adaptable and to create a warm, friendly environment. Prevailing models or health policy, the strongest or most persistent voices, with or without research to back them up, still tend to set the agenda for practice in many countries. Even so, many different ideas about the nature of occupation have been proposed, despite it being a natural human phenomenon that is taken for granted because, as Cynkin and Robinson (1990) said, it forms the fabric of everyday lives.

A few examples of the range of views about occupation held by occupational therapists suggest the potential extent of the science, along with potential debate about whether or not all should be included or are relevant. McColl, Law, and Stewarts' (1993) annotated bibliography of the theoretical basis of occupational therapy provides a starting place for the debate. In their database (drawn from North American Occupational Therapy Journals), 211 entries beginning from the first decade of the 20th century addressed the concept of occupation. The subject dramatically tailed off in the 1950s and 1960s, beginning to appear again in the 1970s and 1980s following work by Reilly, Kielhofner, and others. A similar pattern was found to be the case in the United Kingdom, although that tended to be some 10 years later (Wilcock, 2001b).

Most commonly, occupational therapists advance the notion that occupation includes work (productivity), play (leisure), and self-maintenance (self-care, activities of daily living) (AOTA, 1989; CAOT, 1986). Despite that obviously simplified version of the subject, many have also attempted to capture or at least explain occupation's complexity. Carroll (1910), in the *Journal of the American Medical Association,* provides an early insight which viewed "work" as life and discussed the action-orientation of the human body as part of discussion of the "Law of Work." Meyer, in his 1922 seminal philosophical paper, advanced the idea that it includes rest and sleep as well as work and play. Both Carroll's and Meyer's views anticipate later propositions that occupation is a biological need. Licht's book (1950) provides a mid-20th century view in *Occupational Therapy: Principles and Practice.* Theorists argued that the "occupation" in occupational therapy refers to occupation of mind and body rather than the type of work performed. All those notions suggest that occupation can be defined in other than component parts, and especially that occupation is more than paid employment despite current usage of the word. It has been described as purposeful use of time, energy, interest, and attention (AOTA, 1972), including activities that are playful, restful, serious, and productive (Kielhofner,1985). Nelson (1988) discussed it in terms of a relationship between occupational performance and the environmental context in which it takes place, which he called occupational form. Yerxa (1993), referring to occupation's Latin root, *occupacio,* meaning to seize, take possession, or control, described it as "units of activity classified and named by the culture according to the purposes they serve in enabling people to meet environmental challenges successfully" (p. 3). Culturally sanctioned, occupation is a primary organizer of time and resources, enabling humans to survive, control, and adapt to their world as well as to be economically self-sufficient (Yerxa et al., 1989). Even those few examples provide an idea of the wide-ranging debate which surrounds the basic idea of occupation and which makes the science so necessary. The range of concepts also make the topic interesting, if only to study all the practical concerns such ideas raise, not least in a therapy which purports to use occupation as its mode and its media.

Bearing that debate in mind, it is useful to consider the beliefs, vision, mission, and aims of the International Society of Occupational Scientists (ISOS), which was formed in 1999. The Society was established on four main beliefs, namely that:

1. Occupation encompasses all human pursuits (mental, physical, social, and spiritual; restful, reflective, and active; obligatory and self-chosen; paid and unpaid).
2. Occupation is fundamental to autonomy, health, well-being, and justice.
3. Occupational science generates knowledge about the rich diversity of human occupation (and the sociocultural, political, financial, and other conditions needed to support healthy, satisfying, and meaningful occupation for individuals and communities in diverse world contexts).
4. Occupational science embraces a multidisciplinary, multiperspective approach to research, debate, and activism.

It holds as its vision that:

By 2005, there will be a worldwide network of occupational scientists across diverse disciplines and interested groups and organizations advocating occupational justice for world health and well-being. (ISOS, 2000)

The beliefs and vision provide some key pointers to the discipline. Firstly, that it is generalizable and applicable to people of different cultures across the world. Secondly, that interest is not restricted to occupational therapists, and that its findings will meet needs across a broad spectrum of concern. Thirdly, that it is a topic of such importance that equity of access to occupations which meet individually different needs can be considered a matter of justice, especially in terms of the health and well-being of all. The mission of ISOS, which follows those beliefs and vision, is:

To advance world health, well-being and justice by energising a worldwide network of individuals, groups and organizations to research, debate and activate towards equity of opportunity for all people, in accordance with their occupational nature. (ISOS, 2000)

The aims of the International Society of Occupational Scientists are:

To promote study and research of humans as occupational beings within the context of their communities and the organization of occupation in society.

To disseminate information to increase a general understanding of peoples' occupational needs and the contribution of occupation to the health and well-being of communities.

To advocate for occupational justice internationally.

To encourage a range of disciplines to consider and frame their own research from an occupational perspective (so they may expand their influence on sociocultural, political, medical, environmental, and occupational processes.)

Those extracts from the Constitution of the International Society of Occupational Scientists include not only mention of its interdisciplinary nature, but also the understanding that the human need to do crosses many socially determined boundaries such as those which address cultural, economic, political, medical, and environmental issues. It is anticipated that the study of humans as occupational beings will generate knowledge about the rich diversity of the subject and the sociocultural, political, financial, and other conditions needed to support healthy, satisfying, and meaningful occupation for individuals and communities in diverse world contexts.

HISTORICAL FOUNDATION FOR A SCIENCE OF OCCUPATION

From either an evolutionary or a Biblical perspective of the origins of human life, occupation played an important role in individuals maintaining their own health. It is known that early humans lived in small communities which provided protection and succor to them, and in which the health of the "group" was deemed to be at least as important as individual survival. It was through their social organization as well as their physical toil and rest, mental planning, creativity, and spiritual fulfillment that they maintained or enhanced the well-working of the organism as a whole (Wilcock, 2001a). Looking at such lifestyles and comparing them with the present, with a view to understanding the critical relationship between what and how people carry out their lives in ways which maintain health naturally, could be one direction for occupational science investigation in the future.

During the classical period of Greece and Rome, a concept existed which was remarkably similar to that of humans as occupational beings. Then, as noted earlier, the idea of humans as "praxic beings" was studied and articulated by prominent philosophers. Aristotle sometimes used praxis to describe all human activity. Mostly he regarded it along with *theoria* (truth) and *poiesis* (the production of something). Aristotle's School, which largely followed his teachings, divided all human activity between the theoretical and the practical; the latter including both poiesis and praxis. Accepted in medieval scholastic philosophy, that dichotomy was integral to later philosophies and remains part of modern thinking (Petrovic, 1983). Indeed, debate still continues about whether praxis is characterized by human activity in all its forms or whether it is only one aspect of human nature or action. There is even current disagreement about the extent to which the concept of praxis can be defined or clarified:

> The definitions range from that which treats it simply as the human activity through which man changes the world and himself, to more elaborate ones which introduce the notions of freedom, creativity, universality, history, the future, revolution, etc. (Petrovic, 1983, p. 435-440)

It is instructive that in classical times when the study of "praxis" was a central factor, the use of occupation as part of health regimens was commonplace (although frequently translated or understood as exercise of capacities). It was advocated by well-respected physicians such as Hippocrates and Galen at that point in history when modern medicine is said to have had its origins. The "great Galen," Burton explained, in *Anatomy of Melancholy* (1651, p. 266–267), preferred "Exercise before all Physicke, Rectification of diet, or any regiment in what kinde soever; 'tis Natures Physician."

However, it was not only in medicine that the importance of occupation was recognized during classical times. Indeed, in some places, it warranted state intervention. Across much of Greece, the education of children of both sexes was carried on at public expense in gymnasia (educational complexes), where the officials were responsible for the development and maintenance of their pupils' health, exercise, intellect, and morals. The overlap between these was a part of a holistic view which recognized the interaction between mental and bodily occupation, education, and health status. It appears that the system, as well as being aimed at the safety of the State, was more focused toward the promotion of health and the development of pupils' inherent strengths than their economic futures.

In line with the objective of healthy, strong, sound, beautiful, and balanced citizens, the leaders of ancient Greece deemed physical training to be of the utmost importance. Because of the demotion of everyday physiologically based occupation into the hands of slaves and conquered peoples, it was necessary, though probably unconscious, to invent occupations to take their place (Wilcock, 2001a). So little was this understood at the conscious level that we see the resurgence of gymnasia today without also realizing they are made necessary by the loss of the physiological requirements of mundane occupations because of technology. A science of occupation could help clarify the occupational requirements for health as long as it is sufficiently broadminded and honest. If it restricts exploration according to particular doctrine or ethnic beliefs, it could be as short-sighted as the classical science of praxis which put one set of people's requirements above another's, that is, according to whether they were citizens or slaves. This appears to suggest that study of humans as occupational beings should not divide any groups, including those with handicap or illness, from other and all people, but rather consider any special or different factors from those held generally, including differences according to individual rights and needs as well as cultural beliefs.

The notion of "physical" perfection and mind/body balance as it was sought in the gymnasia gave way to notions of spiritual perfection as monastic power and life-after-death rationales gained ground during the Middle Ages. Because disease was often attributed to sin, people needed to engage in "morally right" occupations according to the Christian creed (Porter, 1997/1999). Health of a spiritual kind embraced notions of labor being necessary for a healthy soul. Likewise, such was the case with pilgrimages, crusades, and charitable "good works," along with prayer. The physical nature of those occupations, and labor such as agricultural and household occupations, also fulfilled physical and mental health requirements. Because spirit, mind, and body influence each other, such regimens may have appeared effective, in comparison to other medical interventions of the time, in maintaining physical and mental health (Wilcock, 2001a). Without a science of occupation, or of praxis, to study, explain, and enable their benefits as time went on, occupation became viewed as a largely economic phenomenon.

Driven by materialism and sophisticated political agendas, social status and class distinctions began to divide, arbitrarily, types of occupation available to individuals. This led, in many instances, to occupationally unjust situations in which people were occupationally deprived, exploited, or alienated. Many sought solace in occupations thought to be of a depraved nature. During the reign of England's King Edward VI (1547–1553), calls from the public demanded action to reduce the numbers of occupationally deprived and depraved in London. Hence, a "Royal" hospital, Bridewell, aimed solely at the remediation of occupational illness, was established along with four others that offered care to unwanted children and the physically and mentally sick. In Bridewell, "Art-Masters" were employed to develop and to restore skills. Although the term hospital was used in a broader sense than currently is the case, that early recognition of the need to remediate "occupational sickness" is a significant milestone worthy of further study (Wilcock, 2001a). The significance of that establishment was partly due to the belief that industriousness was morally, mentally, socially, and physically valuable. Indeed, for centuries it appears to have been valued for its own sake.

John Locke (1632-1704) was an English philosopher probably influenced, to some extent, by those values. In his greatest work, *Essay concerning Humane Understanding* (1690), he advised:

> . . . it will become us, as rational Creatures, to employ our Faculties about what they are most adapted to, and follow the direction of Nature, where it seems to point us out the way. For 'tis rational to conclude, that our proper Imployment

lies in those Enquiries, and in that sort of Knowledge, which is most suited to our natural Capacities, and carries in it our greatest interest . . . (Locke, 1690, p. 327)

Locke made a plea for what he considered to be the right approach for the acquisition of knowledge and "scientific" understanding which would eventually benefit humankind. He argued that science, which he recognized as the means to explore, discover, and understand the whys and wherefores of the world as far as it was possible, could be divided in three distinct fields (in closest to modern day terms): biological science, communication science, and occupational science — "Actions as they depend on us, in order to Happiness" (p. 362). He called the latter ethics. He described as the "three great Provinces of the intellectual World, wholly separate and distinct one from another":

All things that can fall within the compass of humane Understanding, being either, First, The Nature of Things, as they are in themselves, their Relations, and their manner of Operation: Or, Secondly, that which Man himself ought to do, as a rational and voluntary Agent, for the Attainment of any Ends, especially Happiness: Or, Thirdly, The ways and means, whereby the Knowledge of both the one and the other of these, are attained and communicated. (Locke, 1690, p. 361)

Two centuries later Thomas Carlyle's (1843, p. 220) conjecture that "even in the meanest sorts of Labour, the whole soul of a man is composed into a kind of real harmony, the instant he sets himself to work!" provides some indication of the almost religious fervor that continued to be given to industriousness. Despite that, or Locke's proposals for scientific endeavors, little formal research was carried out to determine how much or how little "industriousness" is valuable to health and well-being, so that social planning could occur on a sound basis in the future. This has led to the current situation in which many people recognize that stress and illness are caused by too much work as well as by too little, yet economic policies that accentuate an obviously unhealthy dichotomy continue.

Also growing from the idea that "industriousness" was of value in itself was "Moral Treatment." Based on the success of Phillipe Pinel's experiments at the Bicetre in Paris (Pinel, 1806), and William and Samuel Tuke's (Tuke, 1813) at the Retreat in York, that approach to insanity used occupations as the major element of treatment. The benefit of specially chosen occupation was its capacity to divert patients from the "mad" thoughts which held them captive. To use it effectively was seen as a difficult but essential task. There were many reasons for moral treatment's demise despite occupation having been used as a treatment media to a far greater extent than was ever the case in the 20th century (Wilcock, 2001a). Peloquin (1989), reports that because moral treatment was touted as successful in America, with some superintendents recording up to 90% cure, asylums became overcrowded to a point at which treatment deteriorated into custodial care. At the same time, medicine was reconsidering the causes of insanity in the light of new physiologic knowledge in which ideas about occupation did not seem of importance, and the reported success of moral treatment was challenged as exaggeration. Moral treatment disappeared from psychiatric practice across the Atlantic. Peloquin concluded:

Moral treatment's decline relates closely to a lack of inspired and committed leadership willing to articulate and redefine the efficacy of occupation in the face of medical and societal challenges. The desire to embrace the most current trend of scientific thought led to the abandonment of moral treatment in spite of its established efficacy. The failure to identify and address the social and institutional changes that had gradually made the practice and success of moral treatment virtually impossible led to the erroneous conclusion that occupation was not an effective intervention. (Peloquin, 1989, p. 544).

As a counter to the industriousness demanded by the dominant manufacturing industry, also in the 19th century, there was a resurgence of interest in many things medieval. That interest was led by people such as John Ruskin and William Morris, leaders of the Arts and Crafts Movement (Yates, 1987). They recognized the well-being potential of the creative occupational milieu of the Middle Ages. In trying to encourage understanding of people's physical, mental, and spiritual occupational nature and needs, they used their own "creative natures" to combat urban industrialization, capitalism, and economic expansion. Whereas both argued for social reform, Ruskin sought to spread enthusiasm for manual labor and Morris for a return to earlier craft ideals. The latter articulated an occupational theory of social health which holds value today and it too is worthy of further study. He said:

> It is assumed by most people nowadays that all work is useful, and by most well-to-do people that all work is desirable.... (They) cheer on the happy worker with congratulations and praises, if he is only "industrious" enough and deprives himself of all pleasure and holidays in the sacred cause of labour.... it is of the nature of man, when he is not diseased, to take pleasure in his work under certain conditions. And, yet, we must say in the teeth of the hypocritical praise of all labour, whatsoever it may be, ...that there is some labour which is so far from being a blessing that it is a curse; that it would be better for the community and for the worker if the latter were to fold his hands and refuse to work, and either die or let us pack him off to the work-house or prison — which you will. (Morris, 1884, p. 603-604)

Morris's argument preempts the need for occupational therapists and scientists to be aware of the negative as well as the positive effects of occupation, just as drug trials are undertaken to find out the benefits and the damaging effects of pills and potions.

That brief journey into the past reveals that, from time to time, some occupationally based ideologies or philosophies were obviously germinating. It is also fascinating that when they were at their zenith, however insignificant that may have been in the great scheme of things, that some form of occupational treatment to improve health and well-being was also formulated or established. Science and practice have influenced each other over time. Occupational scientists studying humans as occupational beings have to take ideas seriously which were raised at earlier times, even though the ideas might take occupational therapists well and truly into a political arena in which they have little experience. The founders in the United States must have recognized that when they set out their objectives in 1917.

FORMATION OF THE DISCIPLINE

Objectives

The initial objectives of the National Society for the Promotion of Occupational Therapy, which was formed in the United States of America in 1917, point to the need for a science of occupation. The objectives read:

> *The advancement of occupation as a therapeutic measure, the study of the effects of occupation upon the human being, and the dissemination of scientific knowledge of this subject.* (Dunton et al, National Society for the Promotion of Occupational Therapy, 1917)

Although the first of these three objectives has been pursued with some vigor, the second and third have been largely overlooked. Occupation, in some form or other, has been used throughout the 20th century by occupational therapists for therapeutic purposes, but the study of the relationship between occupation, health, and humans has not been rigorous or systematic. In part, that can be seen to have led to a profession which has difficulty explaining its own philosophy, or of confidently describing to others how it is different or special. Most disciplines of applied sciences have a particular basic science which provides ongoing sustenance and nurture for clinical work. They share their particular science with others, which in itself adds to understanding of their potential contribution and to the prestige in which the profession is held. Without a basic and particular knowledge base, the applied discipline of occupational therapy has had ongoing difficulties in nurturing itself and has succumbed to trends, fads, and fashions of health care throughout its existence. Whilst the ability to be adaptable to changing contexts is also a necessity, without adequate or specific sustenance a profession can fade away. Successful health initiatives based on occupation have been discontinued before. As noted above, such was the fate of occupation as part of moral treatment.

It might be said that the objectives of the American founders were only applicable to the time of origin. Indeed, in some measure, they do reflect the complex interaction of the mental hygiene movement, social activism, pragmatism, and the arts and crafts movement, within the context of a rapidly developing industrial culture, along with other ideas and values which were prevalent in the United States at that time. However, throughout occupational therapy's 20th century journey, the notion of the need to understand better the nature of occupation has waxed and waned. The latest resurgence of interest across many academic occupational therapy establishments in the United States has lasted for more than 30 years. It has been manifest by numerous occupation-based frames of reference or models of practice, as well as calls for practice to be based on the relationship between occupation and health. Indeed, from the 1960s on, a group of leaders in the field were encouraging the profession to aim, through occupation, at "maintaining optimum health rather than...intermittent treatment of acute disease and disability" (West, 1967, p. 312). Wilma West, for example, proposed it was time to change occupational therapy's long-held focus on activities of daily living (ADL) for the disabled toward advocating balanced regimens of age-appropriate occupations before disease or disability occur (West, 1970). Along the same lines, Geraldine Finn (1977) proposed that, as primary prevention is aimed at the relationship between the basic structural elements of society and health and of what keeps people in a state of health, occupational therapists should make their contribution with a greater understanding of the effects of occupation on health. Laukaran (1977), who held similar views, suggested occupational therapists found it difficult to make a shift in that direction because of long-held values associated with clinically based medicine. This had led to the idea that occupational therapy is concerned only with ill or disabled people, rather than having potential benefit for all people, an idea which was reinforced by many occupational therapy models developed according to medical model values. With views such as those being expressed by such eminent therapists, it would seem that the establishment of a basic science of occupation was an idea in a chrysalis.

Such was the flavor of the times, it could have been at any number of American universities that a science of occupation was suggested as a new discipline. However, it was at the University of Southern California (USC) that it was envisaged. There Mary Reilly had acted as the catalyst. As Director of Graduate Programs, she had begun emphasizing the importance of occupation and the need for occupational therapists to value their unique base of practice during the 1970s. Advocating that people have a vital need to produce, to create, to master, and to improve their environment through occupation, which she claimed was "wired" into them through the process of evolution, she developed an occupational therapy frame of reference known as "Occupational Behavior" (Reilly, 1962, 1969, 1974). This frame of reference proposed the use of occupation to promote life satisfaction for people thwarted in the attainment of competence by disease or injury (Reilly, 1974). It recognized that humans acquire interests, abilities, skills, and habits of cooperation or competition through the process of meeting their need for achievement, which, incidentally, also support their various occupational roles throughout life (Van Deusen, 1988). Reilly's frame of reference introduced some new directions for theory development based on concepts about occupation, especially among graduate students such as Gary Kielhofner and fellow workers such as Elizabeth Yerxa.

Kielhofner went on to develop the Model of Human Occupation (1985), which reached a wide audience across the world and successfully influenced many to return to the basic promise of health through occupation. Yerxa, over a number of years, became an advocate for the development of a science of occupation which, as early as 1983, she identified as a basic science as distinct from the applied science of occupational therapy. Six years later in *Occupational Therapy in Health Care,* a special issue about occupational science, Yerxa and her colleagues explained that:

> *By identifying and articulating a scientific foundation for practice, occupational science could provide practitioners with support for what they do, justify the significance of occupational therapy to health, and differentiate occupational therapy from other disciplines.* (Yerxa et al., 1989, p.3)

They also suggested that the science could help occupational therapy to "contribute new knowledge and skills to the eradication of complex problems affecting everyone in society."

Yerxa (1993), in the first issue of the *Journal of Occupational Science: Australia,* explained how the foundation for the science grew from past traditions of occupational therapy as well as from Reilly's vision. Despite her earlier writing, she extended the credit for the naming of the science at USC to anthropologist Paul Bohannan, the Dean of Social Science and Communication, as well as faculty members and graduate students of the Department of Occupational Therapy, along with herself. Occupational science was accepted as the basis of a new PhD program offered at USC which came under the directorship of Florence Clark in 1989. Specifications and criteria established for the emerging science outlined that the study would center on individuals in interaction with their environment, "not on a cell or reflex," would be developmental in nature, and address the complexities of occupation (Yerxa et al., 1989).

Going on to talk about the new science, Yerxa explained that as all "sciences are embedded in assumptions and values, even though the scientists may be unaware of them," making them explicit could determine which other disciplines may be relevant participants within occupational science. She identified several which would fit with occupational therapist-scientists' "optimistic view" of human nature, such as evolutionary biology, anthropology, and social and developmental psychology. Articulating an exciting vision, she proposed that:

> *As a basic science it (occupational science) is free to pursue the widest and deepest questions concerning human beings as actors who adapt to the challenges of their environments via the use of skills and capacities organized or categorized as occupation. Thus the science is not constrained in its development by preconceptions of how its knowledge will be applied in occupational*

*therapy clinical practice. This sort of freedom is essential in enabling the sci-
ence to explore potentially fruitful lines of inquiry and to assure its perspectives
will contribute not only to occupational therapy but to the mainstream of
thought in society.* (Yerxa, 1993, p. 5)

She added that society would be served "by new knowledge of how human beings
become competent and how people with disabilities discover and use their adaptive
resources" (p. 5).

In 1991, Florence Clark, the present Professor and Chair of the Department of Occupational Science and Occupational Therapy at USC, and her colleagues wrote that because
of its focus on occupation, the knowledge gained by studies carried out by this new academic discipline is bound to nurture occupational therapy. As findings from this science
are brought to public attention, our profession will be better understood because the heart
of its practice — occupation — will cease being an enigma. At that time they put forward
the view that:

*Occupation cannot be explained through the focus on a single level of the human
system; occupation must be studied within the context of both the immediate
environment and the person's history; occupation is fired by the person's drive
for efficacy and competency; although it may be observed as behavior, occupation cannot be fully understood without consideration of it's significance to the
individual; the most productive study of occupation requires a synthesis of
knowledge from the biological and social sciences.* (Clark et al., 1991, p. 303).

In the 1996 publication, *Occupational Science: The Evolving Discipline*, edited by
Zemke and Clark, suggestions of how the basic science could inform the applied science
of occupational therapy were made. They described how although originally occupational
science was conceived as a basic science, the first two major publications about it contained "applied content." Indeed, the second paper was titled *Occupational Science: Academic Innovation in the Service of Occupational Therapy.* "One of the most thrilling
aspects inherent in the development of the academic discipline," they wrote, was untan-
gling the complexities of occupation and coming to recognize its centrality in human lives
(Zemke & Clark, 1996, pp. x–xi). Because it is embedded in the lives of people taking on
different nuances dependent on context and culture, sociologically based studies, for
example, could assist therapists to apply practice concepts according to broad social needs
rather than verbatim from literature related to the culture of origin, as has so often been the
case. On such grounds they rejected Mosey's (1992) call for the complete partitioning of
occupational science from occupational therapy (Clarke et al., 1993).

In their publication, Zemke and Clark included the contributions of eminent scholars
from many disciplines whose work was seen as tangential and who had participated in the
USC Occupational Science Annual Symposiums. Taking the proactive stance of inviting
and including such scholars as Mary Catherine Bateson, Jane Goodall, and Stephen Hawk-
ing to consider their work in relation to the concept of "occupational beings" provides an
ever growing pool of thought to draw on in considering what is proving to be a science of
enormous complexity and excitement.

Occupational science was taken up by Wilcock in Australia, in 1988, after chance reference to its genesis at a meeting with another member of the profession from a different
part of the globe. In a sense, the establishment of the science in Australia began separately
from what occurred in the United States, simply because at that time nothing had been
published which reached Australia before early 1990. So important did the need for such

a science appear to be, that action was taken to establish a multidisciplinary, international journal to facilitate its growth. The *Journal of Occupational Science: Australia* (JOS:A) started at the University of South Australia (UofSA) in Adelaide in 1993. Some 9 years later, it is now known simply as the *Journal of Occupational Science* (JOS). This receives support from USC, the Auckland University of Technology in New Zealand, and the UofSA. Established as a specialist journal dedicated to publishing articles about the study of humans as occupational beings, it holds as a policy that it does not compete with designated journals of occupational therapy and so does not publish articles about therapy per se. Instead, it concentrates on explorations which have the potential to inform practice in many diverse ways, and to increase general understanding in the academic community about the importance of taking an occupational perspective of people's lives, not least, in health care. Whilst this approach is sometimes criticized as one which is of little use to therapists, that is only really the case in terms of immediate practice issues. JOS is a far-sighted rather than a short-sighted publication. It is aimed at building up a foundation of future resources for the profession and society in general.

Overview

An overview of some of the studies and the issues reported in JOS since its beginnings is appropriate at this point to demonstrate the present trends of research and findings to date. The articles are diverse, as might be expected with a subject which is able to be defined in many ways. However, it is salutary that there are very few which do not have significance or relevance to the practice of occupational therapy.

Occupational therapists' interest in defining and describing what they mean by occupation has already been noted, and it is not surprising that several occupational science studies sought to address that issue. Some, like the one by Wu and Lin (1999), revisited and discussed earlier definitions, whereas Gray (1997) sought to discover the essence of occupation, drawing from the work of the founders of phenomenology. She argues that such study is prerequisite to exploration of "the relationships between occupations, between occupations and people, or between occupations and adaptation or health" (p. 15) as well as to the experience of meaningful or productive occupation as a vital component of people's daily lives. Her investigation found that, in essence, occupation was perceived as "doing" by individuals and carried meaning for them, was goal directed, and was repeatable. Christiansen (1993) took a different approach, setting about identifying taxonomies for "describing and differentiating between phenomena of relevance to occupational science" (p. 3). He recognized that many already existed in fields such as ergonomics, sociology, and psychology. Recommending familiarity with existing taxonomies, he predicted that occupational scientists would develop additional classifications of relevance to occupation, health, and well-being which should advance both theory and practical applications.

Other researchers have studied the basis of occupational behavior. Wilcock (1993) found substantial support from evolutionary science and anthropology of a biological basis. Using history of ideas methodology, she found that occupation is the mechanism by which people fulfill basic needs, closely linked with survival, health, and their ability to flourish in environments which allow them to grow toward their potential. Because of the brains' integrative and adaptive capacity, she also found that the innate need for occupation is influenced by sociocultural forces and values (Wilcock, 1995). A slightly different view of some primatologists, put by Fortune (1996), highlights one possible explanation of how the symbolically limited occupation of proto-humans developed into symbolically meaningful occupation which is a distinguishing feature of humans. That view suggests that collective rituals associated with blood taboos related to menstruation were significant in the transition. Wood (1998), coming from another perspective, proposed that humans' biological requirement for occupations is an aspect of phylogenetic continuity. Based on a detailed examination of the occupational patterns of a group of chimpanzees living in captivity, her findings suggest that human occupations have grown from earlier ones such as foraging, nest-building, play, grooming, and object manipulation. A further naturalistic study of prosimians (*Coquerel sifakas*) led to the idea that occupational behavior engages living beings as both agent and environment, is "intentional" and purposive toward some objective or goal, and can be discriminated from non-occupational behavior on that basis. Such studies can inform potentially valuable applied research with "human new-borns, people awakening from coma or suffering from profoundly paralyzing conditions" (Wood, Towers & Malchow, 2000, p. 16).

Occupation has also been looked at from the point of view of particular types or aspects. Hocking (2000a) considered it in relation to object acquisition, creation, and use in everyday life. Taking a history of ideas approach and drawing on literature from psychology, consumer research, sociology, anthropology, disability studies, and popular literature, she suggests that people in Western cultures take for granted that the objects they have and use reflect their individuality. She goes further, proposing that the way people use objects in constructing identity and notions of self are informed by a strange mix of Stoicism and Romanticism, and have the potential to be the "stuff of transformation, of transcending the mundane everyday world to experience and portray ourselves as the best that we can be" (p. 154). However, the making of objects also has the potential to create change of a cultural nature. With that perspective, Gilbert (1996) examined an attempt by the Quichua people of Ecuador to strengthen their traditional culture through the development of a market for their ceramics. In the same journal, artisan occupations and craft production in terms of their economic and social significance were the topics of exploration by Dickie and Frank (1996). They found occupation can be used to challenge ideology. Frank (1996a), for example, cites traditional crafts being used to mobilize resistance to political and economic domination in Chile and in Israel on the Occupied West Bank. Traditional crafts are but one aspect of occupation still being seen as useful in multiple ways. Feasting, too, can be considered as part of traditional occupations which play an important role within cultural mores. Moore (1996) explored feasting as ritual among the Yanomami people of South America, recording how changing circumstances and procedures can transform ordinary mundane acts, such as food preparation and eating, into a ritual for orchestrating political and economic events.

In addition to considering different aspects of occupational engagement, and biological and healthy survival explanations of occupation, the notion of enhancing and promoting health has been a subject of a large number of articles. Successful aging has been addressed by several. Hugman (1999) discussed how the dominant popular image of old age as a time of steady decline and withdrawal from ordinary life is a product of urbanized industrial society. Suggesting the possibility of an "age irrelevant society, in which... who you are and how you are occupied all displace age defined roles as the fabric of social identity," (p. 65) he argued that "the challenge is to develop policies and practices that enable all, rather than just some, older people to look towards a lively later life..." Part of the challenge for older women, Gattuso (1996) suggests in her research about the body, self, and aging using personal narrative, is to the integrity of self, particularly as contemporary stereotypes depict them as "ugly, asexual, and dependent." She proposed the use of narrative assists the process of self preservation and provided fascinating stories told by three women of how they meet the challenges of aging "passionately, with meaning" (p. 108). Pentland, Tremblay, Spring, and Rosenthal (1999) also considered engagement in occupations for women as part of the aging process, but for those facing the additional complication of disability. Using focus groups and key informant interviews with 41 Canadians, they too found story-telling was useful in the process of adapting to and coping with change associated with aging. Of concern was the informants' view that the opportunity for sharing narratives with others was generally unavailable, particularly as they reported that "their problems and concerns are frequently not anticipated, understood or responded to by service providers or health care personnel" (p. 121). One possible clue to some of the lack of understanding comes from an investigation of older men's occupational role performance following stroke. Hillman and Chapparo (1995) found that when they invited participants to classify their occupations according to the main reason they engaged in them, their classification seldom coincided with those of the interviewer in terms of meaning, value, and satisfaction of their post-stroke roles. That suggests that the individual variation of the meaning which different occupations hold for people is as unique as their various talents, interests, and physiology.

Retirement as an occupational transition was the focus of research undertaken by Jonsson, Borell, and Sadlo (2000). Interviews of 29 participants 66 years of age or older revealed several themes. Retirees developed new occupational structures, and many described how the meaning of what they did appeared to have changed. There were temporal changes also, experienced as a slowing down in the execution of occupations. That was perceived as less stressful than pre-retirement, and provided a sense of "being master of one's own time" (p. 32), but without more time for other occupations. Participants explained that although retirement was positive, it felt as though something was missing, and that plans for the future did not extend beyond the coming year. With views that decline was inevitable, keeping things basically the same was found to be a positive view of the future. Baum (1995), in her consideration of dementia of the Alzheimer type (DAT), a condition usually associated with aging, studied 72 couples (one spouse, one DAT). She found that individuals who remain actively engaged in occupation demonstrated fewer disturbing behaviors and required less help with basic self-care. Their care-givers also experienced less stress.

Noting the urgent challenge to promote successful aging in the light of increasing longevity in modern society were articles by do Rozario (1998) and Carlson, Clark, and Young (1998). The first articulates a social, transpersonal vision in which the occupation of elders could provide them with the opportunities to "heal, share, celebrate, mentor, and give service toward the growth and development of the future generations" (p. 124). The second describes the USC Occupational Science Based Well-elderly Program Model. In that, coaching by an occupational therapist enabled elders to "consciously articulate and gain appreciation of the importance of occupations in affecting health" and "successfully employ occupationally based principles of healthy living" (p. 111). Didactic presentation, peer exchange, direct experience, and personal exploration were utilized as enabling strategies. The program resulted in "strong positive benefits in multiple outcome areas reflective of successful aging" (p.114). Without programs such as that, it might be that many people find it difficult to understand the value of meaningful occupations. In some ways that was supported by the findings of a study by Stanley (1995) conducted in South Australia, in which sampling followed random door knocking. Using time-budget methodology with 58 subjects whose ages ranged between 70 and 89 years, she found they had difficulty grasping the notion of "valued" occupation to the extent that some participants refused to answer.

In considering the restorative dimensions of occupation, Howell and Pierce (2000) refer to the almost forgotten Meyer insight about the part of sleep and rest in the occupation cycle. They blame the advent of electricity, which freed people and productivity ideals from the age-old tempo of light and dark, plunging them into "chronic and culture wide sleep disturbance." They discuss the issue using quilting as an example of restorative occupation because of its "quiet focus" and associations with rest. Also challenging industrial societies' preoccupation with productivity above human costs (which have not truly been explored), do Rozario (1994) discussed the meaning-making rituals of traditional cultures. She argued that greater consideration of the significance and power of subjective experiences would be of value in the use of therapeutic procedures to address the art of living in a way restorative to chronic disabilities and illness.

Particular Disabilities

Other authors have considered how the notion of humans as occupational beings relates to some particular disabilities. For example, building on Moore's (1996) explanation of the importance of the visual system in making sense of all other sensorimotor systems and how it is integral to the occupations of daily life, Pearson's (1994) exploration considers the effect of homonymous hemianopia on occupational engagement. She found in a phenomenological study with three people that right homonymous hemianopia resulted in a decline in skills resulting in familiar occupations becoming more demanding and less satisfying. Particularly affected were the occupations of driving, personal mobility, literacy, and locating objects. In a study by MacKinnon, Avison, and McCain (1996) which addressed rheumatoid arthritis (RA), occupation, and psychological adjustment, interviews with approximately 140 subjects with RA were compared with about the same number without the disease. They found a significant association between depression and ADL for individuals with RA. In a follow-up study to find whether occupation could be a mediator of depression in people with RA, MacKinnon (1998), this time with Noh and Miller, found that whilst occupational competence in work, self-care, leisure, and sleep (as opposed to rest) was a strong mediator of depression, time spent in occupations of perceived value was not a mediator. Law and her colleagues (1999) chose to explore environmental constraints which children with physical disability encounter within their environment. This Canadian study with 22 families used focus groups and individual interviews as the method for gathering data. They found that physical accessibility did not emerge as the most important factor, with parents perceiving that the "major barriers to occupation are in the social and institutional environment" and that removal of such barriers will "enhance their children's ability to participate in occupations of their choice" (p. 108).

Apart from particular disabilities, the issue of caregiving emerged as one of interest to occupational scientists. Scoggin (1999), using the ethnographic methodology of participant observation over a 3-month period with a group of hospitalized children in Peru, tells how caregiving occupations were central to the children's progress. Of particular importance in the children's cognitive and psychological development were when caregiving occupations, such as singing to the child or playing with them, were "enfolded" with other aspects of a nurse's work. In a very different study of caregiving, Segal (1999) studied families with children who have special needs and discussed the reasons for their engagement in family occupations. These were being together, sharing the children's life experiences, and providing learning opportunities for them. Citing the work of Bellah et al. (1985), Segal suggests that the sharing activities can be understood in terms of "the principle of commitment" or "an obligation to sacrifice one's needs for the well-being of another." Although those researchers chose qualitative research to explore caregiving occupations, Ujimoto (1998) makes a strong case for using time budget methodology to capture the range of caregiving occupations which individuals carry out on a daily basis.

Time Use Studies

"Time use methodologies" are, arguably, the most established research techniques which explore important aspects of human occupation. Occupation within occupational science is perceived as having a temporal nature which unfolds over time and may even be broken down into stages or phases. People may experience temporality differently from each other and even during the course of a single occupation. Clark (1997), in her article about the tempo and temporality of human occupation, explains temporal character as occupations being "imbued with meaning in relation to one's past, present and the future" (p. 89). That perception of temporality changes with occupational experience is suggested in Farnworth's (1998) exploration of boredom as lack of challenge and as information overload. Her work with young offenders led to her proposition that boredom is alive and well for the employed as well as the underemployed, and that it is a little understood but critical concept.

Time use studies have been used to investigate different aspects of people's health, satisfaction, and quality of life. Using experience sampling method in a study of 182 Canadian adults, Zuzanek and Mannell (1993) found, for example, not only gender differences in distribution of daily and leisure activities, in behavioral motivations, and in mood states, but also differences according to the day of the week. Zuzanek (1998) also considered mental health, personal stress, and life satisfaction along with time use and time pressure using data collected as part of the 1986 and 1992 Canadian General Social Surveys and the 1994 National Population Health Surveys. He found that low as well as excessive levels of time pressure seemed to correlate negatively with mental health, and the lowest levels of life satisfaction were reported by the unemployed, students, and divorcees. Harvey (1993), with a view that the potential of occupational science is its application to improve quality of life and well-being, examined the role of time use studies in relation to those factors. He concluded:

> *Evaluation of quality of life is closely connected with how one lives out one's daily life — the degree of congruence between one's environment, one's preference structure and one's behaviour. Time use studies capturing the living of one's life as it is lived in terms of what is being done, with whom, where and in what frame of mind make an ideal contribution to the evaluation of the quality of life.*
> (Harvey, 1993, p. 29)

With Singleton (1995), Harvey also used the Canadian General Social Survey time budget data to determine if the stage of lifecycle affects a person's activity patterns. They found activity patterns were related to the presence or absence of children or significant others, and all impacted on time allocation and the selection of occupations. Pentland, Harvey, and Walker (1998) used time diaries and interviews to gather information about daily time use of men with spinal cord injuries. That study led to the recommendation that:

Rehabilitation, education, and resources need to go beyond personal care independence such that persons with disabilities can expand their leisure and productivity roles and become better socially and economically integrated into society. (Pentland, Harvey, & Walker, 1998, p. 14)

Not only does such research support the need for resources to develop practice in ways that have a sound backing, but it can also be used to measure impact of disease, as Albert and his colleagues' 1994 study of time allocation and disability in HIV infection concluded.

In a pilot study to test methodologies which would capture the experience of everyday occupations, Persson, Eklund, and Isacsson (1999) used a combination of experience sampling method (ESM), occupational story telling, and the Sense of Coherence Scale. Their findings have led to preparations using the same methodology for a larger study comparing healthy people with those suffering chronic pain. ESM is the chosen time use methodology of Csikszentmihalyi, arguably one of the best known of the time use researchers whose theory of "flow" is based on a comprehensive body of research using it. In the first issue of JOS:A, Csikszentmihalyi (1993), discussed some of the implications of time use methodologies from the point of view of a science of occupation. He deliberated over the constantly changing way that either "viva activa" (immersion in activity) or "viva contemplative" (immersion in mental reflection and analysis) has been valued, noting that at present the latter is prized over action to an unprecedented extent. Yet his research has indicated that occupation which entails challenge and the use of personal skills is more effective in improving quality of life than therapy based on thinking things through. If, he cautioned, only mindless or violent opportunities for action are available, it is unlikely that individuals will recognize challenges of a more subtle nature or develop skills. Such factors provide him with an important rationale for a science such as the one under discussion.

A totally different and challenging look at temporal issues came from Yalmambirra, a Wiradjuri man who presented the views of time held by Australian Aboriginals in a 2000 issue of JOS. Explaining that indigenous time began with creation, in contrast to the invention of the calendar, sundial, and clock of "white time," he discussed how whilst indigenous time was in tune with the environment, white time has resulted in family instability, the decline of resources, and deterioration of the air we breathe. Willis (2000), in the same issue of JOS addressed a not unrelated concept: that of deadlines, rationalization of time, and time anxiety. Relating those to the medieval idea of purgatory, she recognized similarities between that and "each new management strategy for work enhancement" in places such as schools, hospitals, and government offices. Described firstly as a solution to the problem of lack of time, new management strategies then became a place where missed opportunities were raked over in neurotic detail. She concluded that both purgatory and work enhancement strategies are a form of occupational punishment. Those articles, whilst entertaining in the extreme, give pause for thought about the negative health effects of many present day occupational structures. Surely the structures and the lack of occupational understanding which allowed their creation are in need of therapy before they create and continue to create occupational illness for individuals.

Occupation and Work

Another area of interesting research has been that about women as occupational beings. Papers have addressed such issues as the multiple workloads of women, adaptation to socioeconomic change, and impact on their health in Africa (Barrett, 1997; Barrett & Browne, 1993); and the negotiation of adult women in transition to lesbianism and the consequent effects upon occupational behavior. In the latter case it was concluded that sexual identity and occupational behavior are so closely linked that "coming out" seems to be a "state of doing" as well as a "state of being" (Birkholtz & Blair, 1999).

Perhaps not surprisingly in view of the contemporary idea that occupation and work are synonymous, the subcategory of work has been addressed frequently and in many different ways. Jones (1993), an Australian politician and author of some note, discussed the evolution of postindustrialism, describing the enormous changes in work patterns in the Western world. He suggested that changes in the future would be basically conceptual and not enacted through legislation. With the view that work is central to living, "to all economic and social life and probably to the human condition itself," (p. 11) he suggested that all people would need to play active, life-enhancing roles rather than negative, defensive ones in effecting that change. In 1998 he went further, and although basing his concerns on Australia, he suggested that discussion of economic issues occurs in an extraordinary narrow way which ignores historical, social, or human context, with ends being more important than the means. In his opinion a balancing process is required to counteract "bottom line economics." He argues that universities and research communities are two of several groups who need to be proactive in the process. I suggest that his view is applicable to all postindustrial economies, and that both occupational scientists and therapists need to take part in the balancing process to improve the health and well-being of populations as well as individuals.

As occupational therapists during the Second World War and some 20 years after concentrated much of their effort on the "return to work" ethic which pervaded much of the world, it appears that "work" is an interest they hold. With the rise of postindustrial economies and the slump in levels of employment, occupational therapists' professional interest largely swung to the arena of self-care and work in the home. In recent years, in some countries, like the United Kingdom, there is a trend back to practice centered around paid work. Because of the massive changes which have occurred over the years, it will be necessary to approach "return to work" strategies from an entirely different perspective than in the earlier days. The new approach will need to be informed by research which considers the issues from a point of view compatible with therapists and their clients interests. One would hope that this scenario may be facilitated by research into the occupational needs of people in the present and future work situations by occupational scientists.

With some concerns similar to those of Jones, Kenny (1994) discussed how the outbreak of commercial disasters brought home to many how insidiously occupation has been tied to notions of money and power. She put forward the notion that when occupation is directed to attaining kudos or acquiring value in purely monetary terms, that is the moment when self-interest takes over. That essentially stifles the value of occupation which originally created conditions for survival, then conditions for civilization, and then for civic societies. She holds that the large scale of those effects has engendered feelings of helplessness. In spite of that, individuals can be helped by participation in shared meaning.

Hocking (2000b) suggests that the specific cultural meanings of work are a potential rich area for research by occupational scientists, and points to Cox's (1997) findings that household tasks are perceived as "non work" even by paid domestic workers, because they are most commonly undertaken as unpaid labor by the female members of a household. It may also be the case in household work. In a study, by Primeau (2000), she found gender-based divisions of household work persist despite the changes to the work force outside the home. Ten families with preschool-aged children took part in the exploration which used interviews, participant observation, and a questionnaire. She argued that both intensive interviewing and participant observation are required to gain a true picture of how families divided work to sustain themselves.

Not a few studies were interested in the relevance of identity and notions of self to occupation. Some have already been mentioned. Another, by Christiansen (2000), reported a study addressing self-construction and identity in everyday action, personal projects, and happiness or subjective-well being. Using a battery of validated instruments with 120 adults between the ages of 19 and 79 years, the findings supported the view that goal-directed projects provide important opportunities for shaping identity, and that the "expression of self influences satisfaction and well being throughout the lifespan" (p. 105). Whiteford and Wicks (2000) also addressed the issue of self from an occupational perspective in the second of two articles that provided a reflective analysis of the "Occupational Profiles" published in the journal over a period of years. Naming the theme "occupational persona" they described it as:

> That dimension of self shaped by a myriad of factors both biological and socio-cultural, which is predisposed, as well as driven toward, engagement in certain types of occupations. Through the process of such engagement and the outcomes generated, the occupational persona is shaped, and to some extent reinvented, over time. (p. 48)

"Escaping boredom, pursuing vocation" and "Having a passion, needing a challenge" were ideas addressed by interviewees within that theme. The interviewees' unique personal and social environments appeared to have had a significant impact on the development of their occupational persona particularly in their early childhood and adolescence.

The other themes which emerged from Whiteford and Wick's analysis were the occupational environment, engagement, and outcomes. In the first of those, specific people, cultural and socioeconomic milieus were discussed, as influential in terms of their view of themselves as occupational beings. For example, Justice King's description of his early occupational environment was one characterized by "hard times." He explained:

> My boyhood was spent in the depression years and, as my family had fallen on very hard times indeed, there was no prospect my continuing at school beyond the permissible leaving age of fourteen. It was necessary to leave school and help support the family. (Wilcock &White, 1995, p. 30)

Leaving a deep impression on King, that early environment appeared to be influential in shaping his subsequent occupational choices and his orientation toward social justice.

Within a collection of ideas categorized as "occupational engagement" were rich descriptions of how the interviewees went about "the multiple occupations to which they were drawn, in order to bring their ideas, beliefs and visions to fruition" (p. 52). Some set goals, others allocated time, seized opportunities, were flexible, worked hard, or created fun. The apparent relationships that emerged between occupational engagement, personae, and environments prompt ongoing questions for further study to provide insight into the complexities and multidimensional nature of occupational beings.

The fourth theme was described as "occupational outcomes." This referred to the results of occupational engagement at individual or collective levels, "tangible, long-term consequences," and in some cases "ephemeral, spiritual experiences" (p. 54). Important ideas that surfaced were the drive to perform at the highest standards to a point of "being physically and mentally exhausted." David Lange vividly recalled the price he paid when he was Prime Minister of New Zealand:

> *The demands of the work were enormous. I used to get to work at quarter past six on a Monday to be briefed and then have two press conferences and all day Cabinet. I would have to be on top of it for the press and for the Cabinet, and it was just devastatingly hard (p. 54).*

More positive outcomes were classified as "feeling proud, feeling satisfied" and "creating a better world" (p. 55).

Clark's 1997 view of the articles that appeared in JOS:A was that they had greatly enhanced her understanding of the complexities of considering humans as occupational beings in postindustrial societies. She pointed to resounding themes such as concern with the structurally unemployed, worries about the decoupling of biological needs and occupation, attempts to systematically study the time investment in occupation on health and happiness, and the cultural and historical differences in occupational patterns.

Picking up on many of those issues, Townsend (1997) reflects:

> *Since occupation is so basic to life, we need to recapture the pre-industrial understanding that we can occupy life in many ways and for many purposes. Certainly transformation into an egalitarian society seems utopic. Yet we can move towards visions of health and justice by recognising the personal and social as well as the economic value in occupations. Moreover, if people with mental health problems or other difficulties face barriers in living, there is urgency in changing the ways in which education, health, welfare, and other institutions organize opportunities for engagement in occupation. (p. 24)*

SUMMARY

If readers are looking for direction, I suggest that the first task is to try to develop an occupational perspective. This takes time but is very stimulating. I have found it easier to consider issues external to occupational therapy, in the first instance, as these are less colored by intense professional molding and personal experience. Rethinking social structures or political or education policies from an occupational perspective is invigorating, creative, and productive in helping to develop a new mind-set. The next step for an occupational therapists is trying to consider clients' problems from an occupational perspective.

At the 1997 Australian Occupational Science Symposium, Dr. Florence Clark explained that she and Dr. Ruth Zemke had found that the discipline was developing in marvelous ways they could never have imagined or predicted at its beginning. "Its shape, substance, direction and character were being molded by scholars throughout the world" (p. 86). Her statement, I suggest, alludes to the strength which comes from openness to different points of view so that understanding grows, and with it the potential to use the information to benefit occupational beings throughout the world and in the future. Occupational therapists, by the very choice of their title, have to have a large stake in understanding better the occupational needs of people, even if in the future, they chose to restrict their practice to the needs of those with medically defined illness and disability, as they have, on the whole, done in the past. I believe occupational therapy has much more to offer than that in terms of population, community, and individually based health promotion initiatives as well as preventive approaches which serve a holistic vision of well-being.

STUDY QUESTIONS — BEGINNER

6.1. What does it mean to study humans as occupational beings?

6.2. Explain the paradox of occupation being all embracing and yet mundane.

6.3. What is the nature and purpose of occupational science?

6.4. Delineate a holistic definition of health.

6.5. Differentiate occupation (doing) from humanness (being).

6.6. Hypothesize as to why praxis therapy could potentially be another name for occupational therapy.

6.7. Within your country, hypothesize how health policy influences the occupational therapy practice agenda.

6.8. Explain how occupations form the fabric of everyday lives.

6.9. Delineate how occupation is a primary organizer of human beings.

6.10. Relate the American Occupational Therapy Association's Code of Ethics to the call for occupational justice.

6.11. In ancient times, what was nature's physician?

6.12. Explain what an occupational perspective means.

STUDY QUESTIONS — ADVANCED

6.13. Speculate about anticipated differences between occupational patterns in a culture valuing individualism (Western culture) compared with occupational patterns in a culture valuing the group (non-Western culture).

6.14. Review a historical religious book such as the Koran, Bible, or Talmud. Identify the occupations identified in the book.

References

Albert, S., Todak, G., Elkin, E., Marder, K., Dooneief, G., & Stern, Y. (1994). Time allocation and disability in HIV infection: A correlational study. *Journal of Occupational Science: Australia, 1* (4), 21–30.

American Occupational Therapy Association. (1972). Occupation therapy: It's definition and functions. *American Journal of Occupational Therapy, 26*, 204–205.

American Occupational Therapy Association. (1989). Uniform terminology for occupational therapy. *American Journal of Occupational Therapy, 43* (12), 808–815.

Barrett, H. R., & Browne, A. (1993). Workloads of rural African women: The impact of economic adjustment in the Sub-Saharan. *Journal of Occupational Science: Australia, 1* (2), 3–11.

Barrett, H. R. (1997). Women, occupation and health in rural Africa: Adaptation to a changing socioeconomic climate. *Journal of Occupational Science: Australia, 4* (3), 93–105.

Baum, C. M. (1995). The contribution of occupation to function in persons with Alzheimer's disease. *Journal of Occupational Science: Australia, 2* (2), 59–67.

Bellah, R. N., Madsen, R., Sullivan, W. M., Swidler, A., & Tipton, S. M. (1985). *Habits of the heart: Individualism and commitment in American life.* Los Angeles: University of California Press.

Birkholtz, M., & Blair S. E. E. (1999). "Coming out" and its impact on women's occupational behaviour. *Journal of Occupational Science, 6* (2), 68–74.

Burton, R. (1651). *The anatomy of melancholy.* Oxford: Printed for Henry Cripps.

Canadian Association of Occupational Therapists. (1986). *Intervention guidelines for the client-centred practice of occupational therapy.* Ottawa: Ministry of National Health and Welfare.

Carlson, M., Clark, F., & Young, B. (1998). Practical contributions of occupational science to the art of successful ageing: How to sculpt a meaningful life in older adulthood. *Journal of Occupational Science, 5* (3), 107–118.

Carlyle, T. (1843). Past & present: Work. In C. Knight (Ed.), (c 1850) *Half hours with the best authors.* London: Frederick Warne & Co.

Carroll, R. S. (1910). The therapy of work. *Journal of the American Medical Association, 54*, 2032–2035.

Christiansen, C. (1993). Classification and study in occupation: A review and discussion of taxonomies. *Journal of Occupational Science: Australia, 1* (3), 3–17.

Christiansen, C. (2000). Identity, personal projects and happiness: Self-construction in everyday action. *Journal of Occupational Science, 7* (3), 98–107.

Clark, F. (1997). Reflections on the human as an occupational being: Biological need, tempo and temporality. *Journal of Occupational Science: Australia, 4* (3), 86–92.

Clark, F., Parham, D., Carlson, M. E., Frank, G, Jackson, J., Pierce, D., Wolfe, R. J., & Zemke, R. (1991). Occupational science: Academic innovation in the service of occupational therapy's future. *American Journal of Occupational Therapy, 45* (4), 300–310.

Clark, F., Zemke, R., Frank, G., Parham, D., Neville-Jan, A., Hedricks, C., Carlson, M., Fazio, L., & Abreu, B. (1993). The issue is: Dangers inherent in the partition of occupational science and occupational therapy. *American Journal of Occupational Therapy, 47*, 184–186.

Cox, R. (1997). Invisible labour: Perceptions of paid domestic work in London. *Journal of Occupational Science: Australia, 4* (2), 62–68.

Csikszentmihalyi, M. (1993). Activity and happiness: Towards a science of occupation. *Journal of Occupational Science: Australia, 1* (1), 38–42.

Cynkin, S., & Robinson, A. M. (1990). *Occupational therapy and activities health: Towards health through activities.* Boston: Little, Brown & Company.

Dickie, V. A., & Frank, G. (1996). Artisan occupations in the global economy: A conceptual framework. *Journal of Occupational Science: Australia, 3* (2), 45–55.

do Rozario, L. (1994). Ritual, meaning and transcendence: The role of occupation in modern life. *Journal of Occupational Science: Australia, 1* (3), 46–53.

do Rozario, L. (1998). From ageing to saging: Eldering and the art of being as occupation. *Journal of Occupational Science, 5* (3), 119–126.

Dunton, W. R., Johnson, S. C., Slagle, E. C., Barton, G. E., Newton, I. G., & Kidner, T. B. (1917). *Certificate of incorporation of the National Society for the Promotion of Occupational Therapy, Inc.* Clifton Springs, NY: National Society for the Promotion of Occupational Therapy.

Farnworth, L. (1998). Doing, being, and boredom. *Journal of Occupational Science, 5* (3), 140–146.

Finn, G. L. (1977). Update of Eleanor Clarke Slagle Lecture: The occupational therapist in prevention programs. *American Journal of Occupational Therapy, 31* (10), 658–659.

Fortune, T. (1996). The proto-occupation/occupation interface. An exploration of human occupation and its symbolic origins. *Journal of Occupational Science: Australia, 3* (3), 86–92.

Frank, G. (1996). The concept of adaptation as a founda-tion for occupational science research. In R. Zemke & F. Clark (Eds.), *Occupational science: The evolving discipline* (pp. 47–55). Philadelphia, PA: F.A. Davis.

Gattuso, S. (1996). The ageing body and the self-project in women's narratives. *Journal of Occupational Science: Australia, 3* (3), 104–109.

Gilbert, W. (1996). Quichua pottery: Cultural identity and the market. *Journal of Occupational Science: Australia, 3* (2), 72–75.

Gray, J. M. (1997). Application of the phenomenological method to the concept of occupation. *Journal of Occupational Science: Australia, 4* (1), 5–17.

Harvey, A. S. (1993). Quality of life and the use of time theory and measurement. *Journal of Occupational Science: Australia, 1* (2), 27–30.

Hillman, A. M., & Chaparro, C. J. (1995). Occupational role performance in men following a stroke. *Journal of Occupational Science: Australia, 2* (3), 88–99.

Hocking, C. (2000a). Having and using objects in the Western world. *Journal of Occupational Science, 7* (3), 148–157.

Hocking, C. (2000b). Occupational science: A stock take of accumulated insights. *Journal of Occupational Science, 7* (2), 58–67.

Howell, D., & Pierce, D. (2000). Exploring the forgotten restorative dimension of occupation: Quilting and quilt use. *Journal of Occupational Science, 7*, 68–72.

Hugman, R. (1999). Ageing, occupation and social engagement: Towards a lively later life. *Journal of Occupational Science, 6*, 61–67.

International Society of Occupational Scientists. (2000). Constitution. Refer to *Journal of Occupational Science.* Occupational Therapy Dept. University of South Australia, Terrance Adelaide, SA 5000.

Jones, B. (1993). Sleepers, wake! Ten years on. *Journal of Occupational Science: Australia, 1* (1), 11–16.

Jones, B. (1998). Redefining work: Setting directions for the future. *Journal of Occupational Science, 5* (3), 127–132.

Jonsson, H., Borell, L., & Sadlo, G. (2000). Retirement: An occupational transition with consequences for temporality, balance and meaning of occupations. *Journal of Occupational Science, 7* (1), 29–37.

Kass, L. R. (1981). Regarding the end of medicine and the pursuit of health. In A. R. Caplan, H. T. Engelhart, & J. J. McCartney (Eds.), *Concepts of health and disease: Interdisciplinary perspectives.* Reading, MA: Addison Wesley Publishing Co.

Kenny, V. C. (1994). Functional containment and the work complex in mass society. *Journal of Occupational Science: Australia, 1* (3), 22–27.

Kielhofner, G. (Ed.). (1985). *A model of human occupation: Theory and application.* Baltimore, MD: Williams & Wilkins.

Laukaran, V. H. (1977). Toward a model of occupational therapy for community health. *American Journal of Occupational Therapy, 31*, 71–74.

Law, M., Haight, M., Milroy, B., Willms, D., Stewart, D., & Rosembaum, P. (1999). Environmental factors affecting the occupations of children with physical disabilities. *Journal of Occupational Science, 6 (3)*, 102–110.

Licht, S., (Ed.). (1950). *Occupational therapy: Principles and practice.* Springfield, IL: Charles C. Thomas.

Locke, J. (1690). *An Essay Concerning Humane Understanding*. London: T. Bassett.

MacKinnon, J. R., Avison, W. A., & McCain, G. A. (1996). Rheumatoid arthritis, occupation profiles and psychological adjustment. *Journal of Occupational Science: Australia, 3* (1), 16–17.

MacKinnon, J. R., Noh, S., & Miller, W. C. (1998). Occupation as a mediator of depression in people with rheumatoid arthritis. *Journal of Occupational Science, 5* (2), 82–92.

McColl, M. A., Law, M. C., & Stewart, D. (1993). *Theoretical basis of occupational therapy: An annotated bibliography of applied theory in the professional literature*. Thorofare, NJ.: Slack.

Meyer, A. (1922). The philosophy of occupational therapy. *Archives of Occupational Therapy, 1*, 1–10.

Moore, A. (1996). Feasting as occupation: The emergence of ritual from everyday activities. *Journal of Occupational Science: Australia, 3* (1), 5–15.

Moore, J. (1996). The visual system and engagement in occupation. *Journal of Occupational Science: Australia, 3* (1), 16–17.

Morris, W. (1884). Useful work versus useless toil. In G. D. H. Cole (Ed.). (1934). *Centenary edition. William Morris. Stories in prose. Stories in verse. Shorter poems. Lectures and essays*. New York: Random House.

Mosey, A. C. (1992). The issue is: Partition of occupational science and occupational therapy. *American Journal of Occupational Therapy, 46*, 851–853.

Nelson, D. L. (1988) Form and performance. *American Journal of Occupational Therapy, 42*, 633–641.

Pearson, S. (1994). An exploration of the effect of right homonymous hemianopia on engagement in occupation. *Journal of Occupational Science: Australia, 1* (4), 3–10.

Peloquin, S. M. (1989). Moral treatment: Contexts considered. *American Journal of Occupational Therapy, 43* (8), 537–544.

Pentland, W., Harvey, A. S., & Walker, J. (1998). The relationship between time use and health and well-being in men with spinal cord injury. *Journal of Occupational Science, 5* (1), 14–25.

Pentland, W., Tremblay, M., Spring, K., & Rosenthal, C. (1999). Women with physical disabilities: Occupational impacts of ageing. *Journal of Occupational Science, 6* (3), 111–123.

Persson, D., Eklund, M., & Isacsson, A. (1999). The experience of everyday occupations and its relation to sense of coherence — a methodological study. *Journal of Occupational Science, 6* (1), 13–26.

Petrovic, G. (1983). Praxis. In T. Bottomore, ed. *A dictionary of Marxist thought* (2nd ed.). Oxford, UK: Blackwell Publishers.

Pinel, P. (1806). *A treatise on insanity*. Translated from French by D. D. Davis, Sheffield, Strand., London: Printed by W. Todd, for Messrs. Cadell and Davies.

Porter, R. (1997/ 1999). *The greatest benefit to mankind: A medical history of humanity from antiquity to the present*. London: Harper Collins.

Primeau, L. A. (2000). Household work : When gender ideologies and practices interact. *Journal of Occupational Science, 7* (3), 118–127.

Reilly, M. (1962). Occupational therapy can be one of the great ideas of 20th century medicine. *American Journal of Occupational Therapy, 16*, 1–9.

Reilly, M. (1969). The education process. *American Journal of Occupational Therapy, 23*, 299–307.

Reilly, M. (1974). *Play as exploratory learning*. Los Angeles: Sage.

Scoggin, A. E. (1999). Caregiving as an occupation: Developmental intervention for a group of hospitalised Peruvian children. *Journal of Occupational Science, 6* (1), 34–41.

Segal, R. (1999). Doing for others: Occupations within families with children who have special needs. *Journal of Occupational Science, 6* (2), 53–60.

Singleton, J. F., & Harvey, A. S. (1995). Stage of lifecycle and time spent on activities. *Journal of Occupational Science: Australia, 2* (1), 3–12.

Stanley, M. (1995). An investigation into the relationship between engagement in valued occupations and life satisfaction for elderly South Australians. *Journal of Occupational Science: Australia, 2* (3), 100–114.

Townsend, E. (1997). Occupation: Potential for personal and social transformation. *Journal of Occupational Science, 4* (1), 18–26.

Tuke, S. (1813). *Description of the retreat: An institution near York for insane persons of the Society of Friends containing an account of its origin and progress, the modes of treatment, and a statement of cases*. York: Printed by W. Alexander and sold by him.

Ujimoto, K. V. (1998). Frequency, duration, and social context of activities in daily living: Time-budget methodology for caregiving research. *Journal of Occupational Science , 5* (1), 6–13.

Van Deusen, J. (1988). Mary Reilly. In B. R. J. Miller, K. W. Sieg, F. M. Ludwig, S. D. Shortridge, & J. Van Deusen (Eds.), *Six perspectives on theory for the practice of occupational therapy*. Rockville, MD: Aspen.

West, W. (1967). The occupational therapists changing responsibilities to the community. *American Journal of Occupational Therapy, 21*, 312–316.

West, W. (1970). The emerging health model of occupational therapy practice. Proceedings of the 5th International Congress of the WFOT, Zurich.

Whiteford, G., & Wicks, A. (2000). Occupation: Persona, environment, engagement and outcomes. An analytic review of the Journal of Occupational Science Profiles. Part 2. *Journal of Occupational Science, 7* (2), 48–57.

Wilcock, A. A. (1993). A theory of the human need for occupation. *Journal of Occupational Science: Australia, 1* (1), 17–24.

Wilcock, A. A. (1995). The occupational brain: A theory of human nature. *Journal of Occupational Science: Australia, 2* (2), 68–73.

Wilcock, A. A. (1998). *An occupational perspective of health*. Thorofare, NJ: Slack.

Wilcock, A. A. (2001a). *Occupation for health: Volume 1: A journey from self-health to prescription*. London: COT.

Wilcock, A. A. (2001b). *Occupation for health: Volume 2: A journey from prescription to self health*. London: COT.

Wilcock, A. A., & White, J. (1995). Occupational profile:

An interview with South Australia's Chief Justice, Leonard King. *Journal of Occupational Science: Australia , 2* (1), 30–33.

Willis, E. (2000). Deadlines and the purgatorial complex. *Journal of Occupational Science, 7* (3), 128–132.

Wood, W. (1998). Biological requirements for occupational primates: An exploratory study and theoretical analysis. *Journal of Occupational Science, 5* (2), 66–81.

Wood, W., Towers, L., & Malchow, J. (2000). Environment, time-use, and adaptiveness in prosimians: Implications for discerning behavior that is occupational in nature. *Journal of Occupational Science, 7* (1), 5–18.

Wu, C-Y., & Lin, K-C. (1999). Defining occupation: A comparative analysis. *Journal of Occupational Science , 6* (1), 5–12.

Yalmambirra. (2000). Black time...white time: My time...your time. *Journal of Occupational Science, 7* (3), 133–137.

Yates, N. (1987, September). Victorian values: Pugin and the medieval dream. *History Today,* 33–40.

Yerxa, E. J. (1983). Oversimplification: The hobgoblin of occupational therapy. American Occupational Therapy Association Annual Conference. Kansas City, MO.

Yerxa, E. J. (1993). Occupational science: A new source of power for participants in occupational therapy. *Journal of Occupational Science: Australia, 1* (1), 3–10.

Yerxa, E. J., Clark, F., Frank, G., Jackson, J., Parham, D., Pierce, D., Stein, C., & Zemke, R. (1989). Occupational science: The foundations for new models of practice. *Occupational Therapy in Health Care, 6* (4), 1–7.

Zemke, R., & Clark, F., (Eds.) (1996). *Occupational science: The evolving discipline* (pp. x–xi). Philadelphia, PA: F.A. Davis.

Zuzanek, J. (1998). Time use, time pressure, personal stress, mental health, and life satisfaction from a life cycle perspective. *Journal of Occupational Science, 5* (1), 26–39.

Zuzanek, J., & Mannell, R. (1993). Gender variations in the weekly rhythms of daily behaviour and experiences. *Journal of Occupational Science: Australia, 1* (1), 25–37.

7

Occupational Adaptation

Janette K. Schkade and Sally Schultz

OBJECTIVES

This chapter will help you to:

- Define, according to Occupational Adaptation, the following key terms: occupations, adaptive capacity, relative mastery, and Occupational Adaptation process.
- Explain the assumptions underlying Occupational Adaptation.
- Describe the structures and processes of the Occupational Adaptation process.
- Differentiate among the following Occupational Adaptation key phrases: adaptation energy, adaptive response modes, adaptive response behaviors, and adaptation gestalt.
- Discuss the seven principles of Occupational Adaptation intervention.
- Use Occupational Adaptation as an intervention framework for individuals and programs.

ABOUT THE AUTHORS

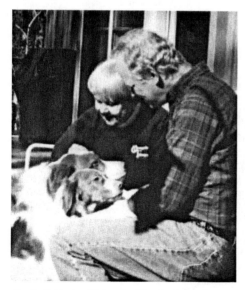

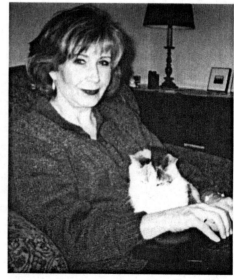

Janette Schkade with her significant other and beloved pets.

Sally Schultz and friend.

"Occupational Adaptation is a phenomenon in which a person engages, rather than does what an occupational therapist says."

> I have tremendous regard for Sally's intellectual acumen . . . her genius.

> As an individual, Janette is a person of great vision, clarity about whom she is and where she wants to go, and a great deal of strength in knowing what she is about.

Two southern accents are heard when they talk, indistinguishable to one not attuned to Southern accents. When one speaks, the other is apt to finish the sentence. Janette brings a background in experimental psychology to occupational therapy. Sally brings a background in counseling and psychosocial occupational therapy. Together they have forged the "grand theory" of Occupational Adaptation — "a tool that guides your thinking process." Genuine respect is shown between them.

Their work epitomizes true collaboration. Sally summarized it as follows:

> I've found people were surprised that there wasn't competition between us. It was questions like, "How do you fight out whose name goes first?" and stuff like that. What I would say to that is there was never an issue of whose name went first. It seemed to occur naturally without any need for discussion.

They both believe that developing theory requires creativity, along with a strong ego, ". . . because you put yourself out on a pretty significant limb, often times without much to hold you up." Who would ever think that developing a theory is "fun?" These two do.

> We had run people out of adjacent offices because we were so noisy, and they couldn't believe we were doing anything serious because we were having so much fun. We would get so excited, and high five each other, and laugh. It was really cool.

Although never explicitly stated, the quality of fun is clearly a part of the adaptive process in which they engage, and for which it is a reward, as they engage in scholarship and theory building. Key concepts emerge from their ongoing conversation. Things like:

Occupational Adaptation is the highest level or form of occupational therapy.

Occupational Adaptation is holistic.

Adaptive process refers to intervening variables between occupation and occupational functioning.

Issues with which they have struggled long and hard during development of Occupational Adaptation theory similarly emerge. Things like:

How can you tell if you have affected someone's internal adaptive capacity?

Can change in internal adaptive capacity be a positive feedback cycle, which engenders more change?

Can change in internal adaptive capacity generate spontaneous generalization?

Does adaptive capacity consist of self-initiated adaptations?

The pair developed Occupational Adaptation to guide practice and to serve as a research tool. Additionally, their view on Occupational Adaptation brings yet another twist in how to think about occupation. "It is not the activity that is therapeutic, and it is not the occupation that is therapeutic, but it is the therapeutic process and its relationship that establishes what the patient will find (or accomplish)." This harkens back to the importance of therapeutic use of self, something in which all three editors of this text were steeped.

Schultz and Schkade believe that a major contribution of Occupational Adaptation to occupational therapy is to facilitate occupational therapy intervention using a theoretical base to drive it. By doing so, their goal is to improve practice in occupational therapy.

INTRODUCTION

Occupational Adaptation, a theoretical frame of reference, emerged from the discussions of a committee of the occupational therapy faculty at Texas Woman's University which was developing a Doctor of Philosophy in Occupational Therapy. This perspective was first published in Schkade and Schultz (1992) and Schultz and Schkade (1992). This committee wanted to develop a focus on which to build a research program. This focus was to be grounded in basic assumptions of the profession of occupational therapy. After much discussion, it was concluded that the focus must include occupation and adaptation. These two concepts are historically important and central to occupational therapy.

These two concepts, occupation and adaptation, were inextricably linked to what has been labeled "Occupational Adaptation." This integrated notion represented a phenomenon that existed and captured the therapeutic uniqueness, thrust, and intent of this program. Thus, Occupational Adaptation as a theoretical frame of reference became the foundation for the doctoral curriculum in occupational therapy. This involved addressing the following four points. First, Occupational Adaptation should be a theoretical umbrella broad enough to cover a wide range of therapeutic and research interests but narrow enough to provide an approach that is distinctive. Second, it should be applicable across the life span. Third, it should represent an approach to intervention that conceptualized the occupational nature of the individual as holistic. Fourth, it should incorporate the occupational performance components and areas into its thought and language under this holistic theme. Schkade and Schultz developed the theoretical notion of Occupational Adaptation described in this chapter. Throughout this chapter, Occupational Adaptation is capitalized to identify our theoretical perspective and its body of knowledge.

Our experiences as occupational therapists and our conclusions regarding the nature of the adaptive process as seen in our clients, as well as our educational backgrounds, guided the development of the constructs. Other Texas Woman's University faculty have approached Occupational Adaptation as a broad rubric, choosing to follow a qualitative, grounded theory approach (e.g., Spencer & Davidson, 1998; Spencer, Daybell, Eschenfelder, Khalaf, Pike & Woods-Petitti, 1998; Spencer, Hersch, Eschenfelder, Fournet, & Murray-Gerzik, 1999; White, 1998). These are viewed as complementary rather than conflicting efforts.

Drs. Anne Henderson, Lela Llorens, and Kathlyn Reed consulted on the development of Occupational Adaptation and involved themselves freely and openly in our discussions, critiqued our ideas, and shared their wisdom and their knowledge. It was Lela Llorens who insisted that a figure was needed to depict this model visually. Following her advice, the figure that represents the Occupational Adaptation process was created (Fig. 7-1). This figure will be referred to frequently throughout this chapter. Relevant portions of the figure will be featured when discussing particular constructs.

Figure 7-1 depicts the components and relationships of the Occupational Adaptation process. The arrows indicate the process flow. This figure represents a cross-section of the process as a freeze-frame sketch. This cross-section slows the process to a halt so that the structures can be examined and analyzed in more depth. It is much like a computerized tomography (CT) scan that shows the shapes and proximity of physiologic structures but does not show the dynamic nature of the interactions of those structures. In real time, the Occupational Adaptation process may be operating at a very rapid speed, as the individual deals with multiple occupational challenges simultaneously. It is also important to note that Figure 7-1 represents one "pass" or cycle through the Occupational Adaptation process. Individuals may require more than one activation of the process "loop" before achieving an adaptive and masterful outcome.

Occupational Adaptation is presented as a comprehensive theoretical model that is based on a defined process that is supported by articulated assumptions and postulates.

PERSON
Element

INTERACTION
Element

OCCUPATIONAL
ENVIRONMENT
Element

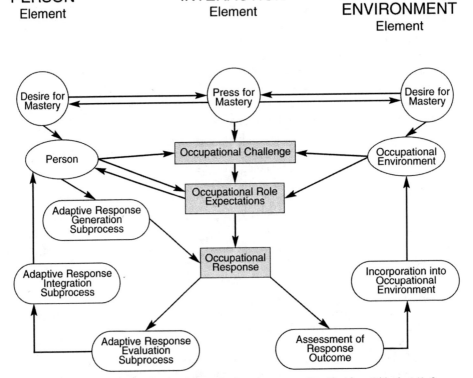

Figure 7-1. Model—schematic of the Occupational Adaptation process. (Modified from Schkade, J. K., & Schultz, S. (1992). Occupational adaptation: Toward a holistic approach to contemporary practice, part 1. *American Journal of Occupational Therapy, 46,* 832.) Reprinted with permission.

This chapter first defines the critical terms that are used in Occupational Adaptation. Following this, some of the assumptions that undergird the theory are discussed. These assumptions fall into two categories: general assumptions and those that are specific to particular constructs. The general assumptions will be presented first. The construct-specific assumptions will be presented as each construct is introduced, followed by a description of the construct and an example. The examples are labeled by occupational role and challenge (e.g. "homemaker: caring for young infant" [occupational role: occupational challenge]). Thus, the "rhythm" of the presentation here will be construct/assumptions/description/example. Finally, the intervention approach of Occupational Adaptation and its distinctive properties will be discussed, along with examples taken from intervention.

Definition of Terms

Occupational Adaptation, a theoretical system, is based on clearly defined concepts and constructs. Definitions can be hard to understand, particularly at first reading. Theorists spend a great deal of time and thought in developing definitions. Definitions are important because they describe exactly what the theorists have in mind, particularly when there may be many definitions for a particular idea. As the reader proceeds through this chapter with its explanations and examples, the definitions, their meanings, and their significance should become clearer.

Occupations

Occupations have three properties: (1) they actively involve the person, (2) they are meaningful to that person, and (3) they involve a process with a product, whether that product is tangible or intangible. To qualify as occupation, the task, activity, or action must demonstrate all three of these properties.

Adaptive Capacity

Adaptive capacity is the capability an individual possesses to perceive the need for change, modification, or refinement (adaptation) of an occupational response in order to respond with positive relative mastery. The strength of this capacity is the cumulative result of experience with responding adaptively and masterfully to occupational challenges over the lifetime of the individual.

Relative Mastery

Relative mastery comes into play as the person evaluates occupational responses. It consists of these properties: (1) efficiency (use of time, energy, and resources), (2) effectiveness (extent to which the desired goal was achieved), and (3) satisfaction to self and society (the extent to which the individual engaging in the occupation finds it personally satisfying and the extent to which it is socially well regarded).

Occupational Adaptation Process

The Occupational Adaptation process consists of a series of actions and events that unfolds as an individual is faced with an occupational challenge that occurs as the result of person/environment interactions within an occupational role. This process exists to enable the individual to respond adaptively and masterfully, that is, to meet both self-produced (internal) role expectations and environmentally produced (external) role expectations. Occupational Adaptation consists of three elements: person, occupational environment, and interaction of person and occupational environment. Each element is built on a constant that is invariably present as the person engages in occupation. These constants are the desire for mastery (person), the demand for mastery (occupational environment), and the press for mastery (interaction of person and occupational environment).

General Assumptions that Undergird the Theory of Occupational Adaptation

Assumption

Occupation is universal. People all over the world engage in actions on a daily basis that are productive, playful, or restorative. They engage in actions designed to maintain their homes, their health, and their well-being. The exact nature of these actions or occupations is the product of individual capacities, histories, and predispositions interacting with environmental influences that are physical, social, and cultural.

Assumption

Occupational therapy has long identified the significance of occupation as a tool for healthy participation in life. This belief goes back as far as the writings of Meyer (1922). Reilly's work on the theoretical notion of occupational behavior was crucial in helping our profession to see the theoretical potential in the therapeutic tool of occupation and its power to influence society (Reilly, 1962, 1969). Trombly (1995), in her Slagle lecture, encapsulated the idea that occupation is both means and end of therapeutic intervention. Competence in occupational functioning is the end therapeutic goal in Occupational Adaptation. However, the means by which one reaches that goal is to improve the client's adaptive capacity through the vehicle of occupation.

Assumption

Occupation is reemerging as our core intervention medium. With movement toward practice within a medical model, occupation became devalued as an articulated force which guided the thinking of therapists in many settings (Kielhofner, 1992). As a cadre of occupational therapists began to develop their theoretical perspectives (e.g., Christiansen & Baum, 1991; Clark et al., 1991; Kielhofner 1985; Law, Cooper, Strong Stewart, Rigby, & Letts, 1996; Nelson, 1988; Schkade & Schultz, 1992), occupation reemerged as the central theoretical construct. Its potential as a powerful therapeutic tool was revisited, reconsidered, and amplified. The Guide to Practice (Moyers, 1999) gives new credence to the prominence of occupation in the thought, language, and intervention application of current practice.

Assumption

Occupation requires adaptation. Competence in occupational functioning develops as the cumulative effect of adaptations that individuals employ to experience some degree of mastery over the challenges that occur during engagement in occupation. Thus, adaptation through and in the service of occupation leads to competence in occupational functioning. The philosophy of the profession, first formally developed in 1979 and reaffirmed in 1995 (AOTA, 1979/1995), acknowledges the central role of adaptation in the occupational process.

Both occupation and adaptation have been accepted as critical constructs within occupational therapy. It is proposed that integrating them into an interactive construct maximizes their power, both as a theoretical perspective and as an approach to intervention.

STRUCTURES OF THE OCCUPATIONAL ADAPTATION PROCESS: THE CONSTANTS (FIG. 7-2)

Constant

The constant in the person element is a desire for mastery. Infants demonstrate this desire as they seek to influence persons and objects in their world. The earliest cry that says, "I'm hungry," expresses a desire for mastery of nutrition-seeking actions. Further, it is contended that the desire for mastery lasts throughout life. Thus, an occupational therapist practicing from this perspective may never conclude that a client is unmotivated. Emotional or physical dysfunction may have devastated the desire. If the client cannot express this desire, the therapist must uncover it through exploratory occupation and input from other sources close to the client.

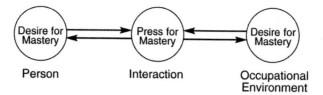

Figure 7-2. Constants in the Occupational Adaptation elements.

Constant

The constant in the occupational environment element is a demand for mastery. The world in which we live expects that we behave with at least a minimal level of mastery. The physical, social, and cultural features of a particular occupational environment specify what constitutes the expected mastery. Failure to respond with sufficient mastery produces lack of reinforcement at best and punishment at worst. An occupational therapist must learn, from the client and/or others, what the demands of a particular occupational environment are and tailor intervention to those demands. Otherwise, the intervention may be directed toward occupational expectations that do not match the client's abilities and needs.

Constant

The constant in the interaction element is a press for mastery. The individual's desire for mastery and the occupational environment's demand for mastery interact to produce this "press." This constant then reflects both the person's expectations and those of the occupational environment. It is this interactive press that spurs the demand for the client to produce an adaptive response.

STRUCTURES OF THE OCCUPATIONAL ADAPTATION PROCESS

Occupational Environment

Environments are described in many ways. The occupational performance areas have been used as the language of the occupational environment. In Occupational Adaptation, the modifier "occupational" is added to identify environments in which an occupational response is required (Fig. 7-3). This designation prompts the therapist to think of the con-

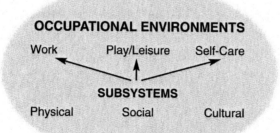

Figure 7-3. Occupational environments — constant press for mastery.

texts in which clients operate. An occupational environment consists of a complex of external stimuli that call for a masterful response. These stimuli affect the individual in a work, play/leisure, or self-maintenance context. The occupational environment is unique to the person. Each occupational environment has expectations for occupational perform-ance that result from physical, social, and cultural influences. The physical, social, and cul-tural influences are the subsystems of the occupational environment. Thus, work environ-ments differ from one another as do leisure and self-maintenance environments because of differences in these influences.

Physical Subsystems

Physical subsystems include factors such as time, space, and materials. Time frequently becomes an important factor in the person's ability to respond masterfully. Properties of space such as lighting, temperature, color, sound, texture, condition (clean or dirty, organ-ized or disorganized), and size affect performance expectations. Materials and supplies that may be required such as equipment, furniture, machinery, and tools all create per-formance demands.

> **Example 7-1:** *Occupational therapist: Effectiveness in a rural community.* An occupa-tional therapist is working in an impoverished rural community. The therapist may be required to improvise equipment if none is available or "make do" with equipment that is less than state-of-the-art.

> **Example 7-2:** *Heavy equipment operator: Returning to work.* An injured heavy equip-ment operator desires to return to work in his previous setting. The equipment moves over uneven terrain with stress to the body. If he wishes to continue in this vocation, the phys-ical subsystem (as seen in the equipment and the terrain) influences significant job per-formance expectations.

Social Subsystems

Social subsystems are made up of the interpersonal interactions among the participants in a particular setting. Social leadership, both formal and informal, can determine perform-ance expectations. In some social subsystems, for example, newcomers are welcomed and included. In others, newcomers are viewed with suspicion and must "pay their dues" before being invited to participate in that social subsystem. These two situations imply very different occupational responses on the part of the newcomer if that person is to expe-rience mastery in that occupational environment.

> **Example 7-3:** *New occupational therapist employee: Fitting into the social structure.* An occupational therapist is on her first day at a new job. The organization has experienced recent downsizing. The remaining "old-timers" resent the new therapist who has taken the place of former co-workers who were "released" during organizational changes. The newcomer must be sensitive to this social influence if she is to respond masterfully in this situation.

> **Example 7-4:** *The social group member: Re-entering the group following hospitaliza-tion.* A client with bipolar disorder wants to re-enter her community of friends at work after hospitalization. This social group highly values consistency on the part of their members. The expectation of this group of friends is that she will behave in the incon-sistent and unpredictable manner she exhibited before hospitalization. They have let her know that if she does so, she will no longer be welcome to participate in the group.

Cultural Subsystem

The cultural subsystem consists of the values, mores, ethics, standards, rules, communication methods, and so on in a particular environment. This subsystem creates the "rules of the road" by which participants are expected to function. In formal organizations, policies and procedures are important facets of the culture. There may be codes of conduct and expectations regarding acceptable behavior that may reflect positively or negatively on the organization. The occupational performance expectations are substantially impacted by the cultural subsystem.

> **Example 7-5:** *The therapist employee: Performing public relations function.* A health care facility depends heavily on outside donor contributions. Therefore, each professional employee is expected to perform a certain number of public relations tasks. A therapist has been asked to speak to a community group outside of work and without additional compensation. He refuses to do so since he will not receive compensation. He believes that he will be exploited by the facility if he agrees to this request and that additional such requests will follow. At his next employee evaluation, he receives an unfavorable performance review based on this refusal. He has violated a norm of the facility culture.

> **Example 7-6:** *The student: Functioning successfully in the school culture.* A child in the school setting is expected to conform to the cultural expectations within the classroom and the larger school. She is expected to know where to hang her coat, recognize which desk is hers, and come to school with homework assignments prepared. She is expected to be familiar with the classroom schedule as defined by the teacher. She is expected to know and follow the routine for negotiating the requirements in the cafeteria at lunch time, to wait in line as necessary, and remove her trash at the end of the lunch period and place it in an appropriate receptacle. In the schoolroom, the culture is defined by the teacher, and the teacher monitors and maintains the culture in that occupational environment. The principal is responsible for monitoring and maintaining the culture in the larger school arena.

There are frequently clearly identifiable individuals who serve as "keepers" of the culture, such as the teacher and the principal in the above example. In other complex adult settings, keepers of the culture may be greater in number, and the cultural features of the setting may be found in documents such as policy manuals. Regardless of who monitors and maintains the culture, masterful, and adaptive functioning in all occupational environments requires knowledge of the particular culture in question.

Occupational roles are carried out in occupational environments or contexts that have occupational performance demands. These demands come from a combination of sources that are physical, social, and cultural. The individual wishing to perform adaptively and masterfully must attend to these demands. The therapist facilitating the occupational performance of a client must learn what the demands are for that particular client, operating within a particular set of demands in his or her chosen occupational environment. To provide effective intervention, the therapist must be keenly aware of these demands, because they are the expectations against which an occupational environment will judge the quality of client performance.

Person Systems

Knowledge of occupational environments is necessary to understand the context in which individuals carry out their various occupations. However, the environment comes into play in Occupational Adaptation only insofar as the person's occupations are performed there. The person is the focus in intervention, and the person is the focus of Occupational Adaptation.

Just as there are multiple ways one might represent the environment, there are many possibilities for how to represent the person. The person is described, once again, in occupational performance terminology. The occupational person is viewed as consisting of sensorimotor, cognitive, and psychosocial systems (Fig. 7-4). The person, like the occupational environment, also has subsystems that contribute to the sensorimotor, cognitive, and psychosocial capabilities in a particular individual. These subsystems consist of genetic, familial, and physiologic influences; personal history and experiences; and phenomenological factors. The person systems contain certain occupational response capabilities that are the result of innate abilities, previous experiences, and current influences. It is recognized that both nature and nurture play a role, but it is not useful to include those in Occupational Adaptation. The person is considered in this parsimonious way, because it allows for both a simplicity and a complexity as one looks at the occupational person with a view toward intervention. Because the person is viewed in the particular manner just described, the term "Person" (with a capital "P") is used to refer to the individual about whom Occupational Adaptation is concerned. Hence, whenever the reader sees "Person," he or she will know that this refers to an individual consisting of sensorimotor, cognitive, and psychosocial systems with genetic, familial, and physiological influences; person history and experiences; and phenomenological factors.

OCCUPATIONAL ADAPTATION PROCESS

The following discussion describes the comprehensive Occupational Adaptation process. Important features of the comprehensive process are the subprocesses that represent the functions of creating an adaptive response, evaluating its outcome, and integrating this occupational experience into the Person for ongoing use. These subprocesses will be discussed as they occur during the comprehensive Occupational Adaptation process.

The Occupational Adaptation process begins with perception of an occupational challenge (Fig. 7-5). As the arrows in Figure 7-1 indicate, both the Person and the Occupational Environment contribute to the nature of this challenge. The challenge always sug-

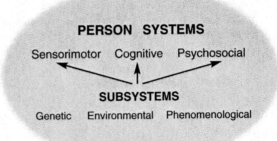

Figure 7-4. Person systems.

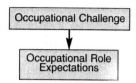

Figure 7-5. Occupational challenge initiates the process.

gests occupational role expectations. The Person brings individual expectations and pre-dispositions as well as sensorimotor, cognitive, and psychosocial capabilities to the occupational role expectations. Likewise, the occupational environment also contributes to those expectations through the physical, social, and cultural subsystems discussed earlier. These contributions to the role expectations are reflected by the arrows leading to the expectations. The arrow returning to the Person indicates that the individual has a perception of the interactive internal and external expectations. This perception may be fairly accurate or it may be faulty. Nevertheless, it is this mix of expectations that prompts the Person to create an occupational response, perform it, assess its efficacy, and integrate the information surrounding this occupational event into the Person for subsequent use. The creation, assessment, and integration occur through subprocesses available to the individual that we referred to earlier. These subprocesses are named the adaptive response generation subprocess, the adaptive response evaluation subprocess, and the adaptive response integration subprocess, respectively. As each subprocess is presented, the representation will be featured in Figure 7-1, and the relevant portion will be enlarged for clarity.

Adaptive Response Subprocesses

The subprocesses described will represent potential points of intervention for the therapist. To practice from an Occupational Adaptation perspective requires an in-depth understanding of these subprocesses. Since it is proposed that Occupational Adaptation is a process that lives in all humans, it will be described it as a "normative" process as well as discussing the kinds of dysfunction seen in clients. Because it is a normal and naturally occurring process, therapists are encouraged first to try the constructs in their own lives of occupational functioning. It has been our experience that therapists who practice from this perspective most competently find that the constructs seem to resonate in their own lives as they deal with the occupational challenges of day-to-day living.

Each of these subprocesses bears the modifier "adaptive response." This label conveys the idea that these subprocesses exist to enable occupational responses that are adaptive. The output of these subprocesses does not always result in a response that turns out to be masterful and adaptive. Nevertheless, to promote adaptation is why the subprocesses exist. They may be dysfunctional at times, but their intended function is still adaptation.

Adaptive Response Generation Subprocess (Fig. 7-6)

This is where the response is created or generated. Upon perception of the occupational role expectations, this subprocess comes into play. It has two major components: (1) the adaptive response mechanism and (2) the adaptation gestalt. This subprocess is the most abstract concept in Occupational Adaptation. It is also the most unique theoretically and is of great significance in the Occupational Adaptation process. This subprocess represents the anticipatory part of the adaptive process. It is very important to understand for

Adaptive Response Mechanism

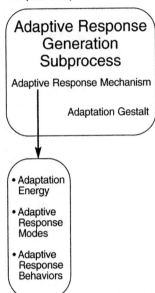

Figure 7-6. Adaptive response generation subprocess — adaptive response mechanism.

intervention. This is the portion of the process where the therapist ultimately hopes to have an impact if the client's adaptive capacity is to be enhanced. In other words, a client whose Occupational Adaptation process is functioning well will be more likely to anticipate the need for adaptation and make those adaptations before the occupational response occurs. Let's consider first the adaptive response mechanism since it is the first to go to work.

Adaptive Response Mechanism

The adaptive response mechanism consists of three constructs: adaptation energy, adaptive response modes, and adaptive response behaviors. They do not occur in the subprocess in any particular order and should not be viewed as hierarchical. Their actions are occurring simultaneously. Once again, the constructs are broken apart artificially to understand their nature and their function. The action of the adaptive response mechanism is a precursor to planning the response.

Adaptation Energy — Assumptions

Assumption. *Adaptation energy is a finite supply present at birth (based on the assumption from Selye, 1956).*

Assumption. *As a protective mechanism, there is some upper limit to the amount of adaptation energy that an individual can use at any discrete point in time.* It can be focused on one activity or divided among activities designed to respond to multiple occupational challenges.

Assumption. *There is a threshold of adaptation energy activation that must be present to potentiate an occupational response.* Failure of the individual to call up that energy in sufficient quantity to activate the Occupational Adaptation process will preclude responding adaptively and masterfully.

Assumption. *Adaptation energy is active at two levels of awareness: a primary level at which creating the response occurs at a high awareness level, with high usage of the finite supply of adaptation energy; and a secondary level at which the response creation is being processed at a sub-awareness level, with a lower energy expenditure* (Table 7-1).

In developing the construct of adaptation energy, this perspective was influenced by the work of Selye (1956) in his work on stress. Although the construct is used quite differently, it is still appropriate to acknowledge Selye's influence. Selye's work was conducted in the laboratory, and his focus was the effect of stress on the adrenal glands in laboratory animals. Nevertheless, he extrapolated his findings to the human situation in a very compelling manner.

In Occupational Adaptation, it is adaptation energy that fuels the adaptive process. This finite supply is enough to last a lifetime. There are other parallels in nature to a finite supply present at birth. For example, it is thought that humans are born with all the neurons we will ever have. (The current focus on stem cell research may produce a way to create new neurons, but as a naturally occurring phenomenon, the finite supply is the norm.) This supply of neurons is enough to last a lifetime barring abuse, trauma, or illness. It is also believed that female infants are born with all the ova they will have. Once again, the finite supply is present at birth. The reason for this theoretical assumption is that the finiteness of the supply provides a compelling reason to manage it wisely. Adaptation energy is a very abstract construct and is not to be confused with an automobile gas tank. Finite does not necessarily mean small just as the number of neurons is not small. Finite just means bounded.

It is assumed that secondary energy is more efficient, more sophisticated, and more creative than the primary level. The individual first works to generate a response at the primary level. Then by choice or as the result of life role tasks, the response generation work is shunted to the secondary level while the individual engages in other tasks. Upon return to the original response generation work, the individual finds progress toward the solution or even a solution not previously considered. When one tries to problem-solve at a primary

---

Table 7-1 **SUMMARY OF ADAPTATION ENERGY**

Adaptation energy operates at two levels
  Primary
  • Focused attention
  • High energy usage at intense activity
  • More structured
  Secondary
  • More creative, sophisticated
  • Lower energy usage
  • Disregards structure in favor of alternative approaches

From Schultz, S., & Schkade, J. (1997). Adaptation. In C. Christiansen & C. Baum (Eds.), *Occupational therapy: Enabling function and well being* (2nd ed.) (p. 476). Thorofare, NJ: Slack.

energy level, the tendency is to put a structure on our possible solutions. Secondary energy is not bound by that structure but goes outside those bounds, thus approaching the problem with more flexibility and more potential for creative approaches. Another advantage of secondary energy use is that the solution is achieved at a lower energy expenditure.

It is believed that this view has significant implications for a balanced life style. In other words, by varying activities among work, leisure, and self-maintenance, this capability for problem solution is maximized at a sub-awareness level while one is engaged in other pursuits at an awareness level. The person, therefore, operates more efficiently with respect to the use of the supply of adaptation energy.

> **Example 7-7:** *The graduate student: Planning and completing a term project.* A graduate student is working on a major term project that represents a significant portion of the course grade. She works on it at a primary energy level until she reaches an impasse in her thinking. She goes with her family to a baseball game after which she tucks the children in bed and does a load of laundry. She then returns to her project and finds that she now knows how she wants to develop her project.

> **Example 7-8:** *Minister: Returning to preaching.* An elderly minister who has sustained a stroke has been in rehabilitation for some time. He desires to learn to walk again. In accordance with his expressed wishes, the intervention team focuses on the occupational performance components of walking: standing tolerance, weight shifting, and crossing midline. However, the team of therapists has recorded that after much therapy, his standing tolerance is extremely low (a maximum of 5 minutes with maximum assistance), his weight shifting is virtually nonexistent, and his ability to cross midline is severely restricted. The team has concluded that this client is not a candidate for ambulation.

The occupational therapist decides to try approaching intervention from an Occupational Adaptation perspective. In addition to the minister's expressed desire to walk, she learns that he wants to return to preaching, despite the concerns of his family. She brings a podium from which he can preach to an informal Bible study group that meets in the facility. The minister stands and preaches for 20 minutes, weight shifting and gesturing cross midline as far as his limitations allow. Three days later he begins to walk again.

The example above is based on a case reported by Jessica Dolecheck, MA LOTR (Schultz & Schkade, 1997). Through the use of occupation, the minister focused on preaching at a primary energy level. The sensorimotor tasks were shunted to secondary energy, and his residual sensorimotor capability emerged naturally without his having to "think" about it.

Adaptive Response Modes

Assumption. When confronted with an occupational challenge, the first strategy is to use an existing mode.

Assumption. The capability to develop adaptive response modes in response to occupational challenges is in place throughout the life span.

Adaptive response modes are another construct in the adaptive response mechanism. Adaptive response modes are the repertoire of Person system response patterns when interacting with the environment in occupational challenges. This repertoire develops as the result of maturation, the challenges presented, and the outcomes experienced. The development begins as innate, reflexive, or random patterns in the young infant. As the engagement in these patterns produces adaptive outcomes (i.e., outcomes that result in a positive relative mastery experience), the response modes become part of the collection of approaches available for use. These same modes are reinforced as they generalize successfully to meet a variety of challenges. What may be "successful" at an early age may be unsuccessful at a later age but still perpetuates in the individual as a mode. These modes are referred to as existing adaptive response modes (Table 7-2).

Example 7-9: *The toy seeker: Retrieving a toy (1).* A toddler has learned to pull to stand and reach to retrieve an object. He sees a toy placed near the edge of the kitchen table. He pulls to stand and reaches for the toy. As the use of this approach in acquiring objects results in successful outcomes, the strength of this mode increases and he will use it frequently.

When the individual encounters new challenges, the immediate response is to use an adaptive response mode from the existing repertoire. This approach can be very efficient. However, if the response fails to produce the desired outcome, a different way of approaching the task becomes necessary. A slight modification to the mode may be all that is necessary.

Example 7-10: *The toy seeker: Retrieving a toy (2).* The toddler mentioned above now wishes to reach an object that is placed just out of reach on the kitchen table. This time there is a cloth on the table. As he reaches for the toy, he inadvertently grasps the cloth and pulls it. The result is that he retrieves the toy with a variation on the pull to stand and reach mode. This is known as a *modified* adaptive response mode (i.e., it is a variation on the existing mode of pulling to stand and reaching).

There are occasions when neither existing nor modified modes succeed. A new mode is required.

Example 7-11: *The toy seeker: Retrieving a toy (3).* Our same toddler now confronts an object at the center of the table. This time there is no cloth. His previous adaptive response modes will not allow him to reach the object. He moves a chair to the table, climbs onto the chair, and successfully retrieves the desired object. He has now created a new adaptive response mode, that of climbing. The pulling to stand and reaching as well as the pulling to stand and pulling the cloth do not succeed. He now adds the new mode of climbing to his adaptive response repertoire.

The repertoire of adaptive response modes expands when the individual is confronted with occupational challenges that are different from those previously experi-

---

Table 7-2 **SUMMARY OF ADAPTIVE RESPONSE MODES**

Existing adaptive response modes
  • Response patterns in adaptive repertoire from previous successful uses
Modified adaptive response modes
  • Changes in existing mode when existing mode fails to achieve success
New adaptive response modes
  • Uniquely different mode developed as existing and modified fail to achieve success

From Schultz, S., & Schkade, J. (1997). Adaptation. In C. Christiansen & C. Baum (Eds.), *Occupational therapy: Enabling function and well being* (2nd ed.). (p. 476). Thorofare, NJ: Slack.

enced. When the individual is unable to develop anything to meet the challenge, he or she perseverates in using modes that are dysadaptive with respect to the particular challenge. However, adaptive and masterful engagement in occupations that are personally meaningful can lead to development of new modes or modification of existing ones to reach the desired goal.

> **Example 7-12:** *Young adult: Pursuing an active life.* A young woman with arthritis continues to walk but with some difficulty (existing mode). As her disease progresses, she continues to walk but now uses a cane (modified mode). In time, she changes to a motorized cart for mobility (new mode). She continues to use all three of these modes as the occasion demands to respond adaptively and masterfully.

As therapists, our task is to facilitate the client's adaptiveness in either how tasks are done, or changing the task altogether to result in an adaptive and masterful response to occupational challenges.

Adaptive Response Behaviors

Assumption. All three classes of behavior — primitive, transitional, and mature — are always available in the Person's behavioral repertoire. The Person does not "reach" mature behaviors and remain there, but moves around among all three classes of behaviors (Table 7-3).

Assumption. The use of primitive behaviors when the Person feels overwhelmed by the occupational challenge is normative and to be expected. Only when the use becomes protracted is it considered dysfunctional.

Assumption. Transitional behaviors are characterized by variability in the behavior. Therefore, they are more likely to result in a response that is useful because the Person is not stuck in behaviors that preclude adaptive movement as in Primitive behaviors.

Table 7-3   SUMMARY OF ADAPTIVE RESPONSE BEHAVIORS

Adaptive response behaviors are classified as
  Primitive
   • Hyperstabilized in all person systems; "frozen" or stereotypic
   • No adaptive movement (no variety in behavior that can lead to adaptation)
  Transitional
   • Hypermobile in all person systems; high activity level; random; unmodulated; variable
   • Variability can result in behavior more likely to produce response that can lead to adaptation
  Mature
   • Blended mobility and stability in all person systems
   • Goal directed; modulated
   • Most likely to produce adaptive and masterful response to challenge

From Schultz, S., & Schkade, J. (1997). Adaptation. In C. Christiansen & C. Baum (Eds.), *Occupational therapy: Enabling function and well being* (2nd ed.) (p. 476). Thorofare, NJ: Slack.

Assumption. *The sequence of moving from primitive to transitional to mature occurs frequently in adaptive responding.* However, this sequence does not occur invariantly. The Person may move back and forth among these behaviors before successful completion of the task at hand or may move immediately to mature behaviors.

Assumption. *Hyperstability, as a first response to an occupational challenge that overwhelms the Person, is to be expected.* It can function as a beginning to adaptive and masterful occupational functioning. Perseverative hyperstability usually becomes dysfunctional.

Adaptive response behaviors are the third construct within the adaptive response mechanism. These behaviors reside in the Person systems (sensorimotor, cognitive, and psychosocial). As with the energy and mode constructs, adaptive response behaviors also contribute to generating an adaptive response. These behaviors have been labeled as primitive, transitional, and mature. The influence for choosing these labels came from Gilfoyle, Grady, and Moore (1990) in their theory of Spatiotemporal Adaptation. These labels are applied very differently, but it is appropriate to acknowledge the influence of Gilfoyle, Grady, and Moore.

To clarify this distinctive use of these labels, one difference is that Spatiotemporal Adaptation describes the neuromotor development in the child from birth to 5 years. In Occupational Adaptation, these labels are applied to adaptive functioning over the life span. A second difference is that they are applied to three areas of function — sensorimotor, cognitive, and psychosocial. A third difference is that these labels are used as classes of behavior rather than as a hierarchy. In other words, all classes of behavior have a role to play in the adaptive process. The use of mature behavior in one circumstance does not assure that mature behaviors will be the first used in a subsequent circumstance. Also, in some situations, primitive behaviors may be normal.

As each of these classes of behavior are discussed, broken down by Person system (sensorimotor, cognitive, and psychosocial), the Person distinctions are separated to facilitate understanding. Understanding the distinctions can assist in identifying and treating dysfunction in the Occupational Adaptation process. However, when operating in "real time," the distinctions may seem artificial and hard to identify. Nevertheless, the distinctions can be a useful tool in analyzing where the breakdown in an individual's Occupational Adaptation process is occurring.

Primitive Behaviors. *Primitive behaviors* are characterized as *hyperstable*. They represent a kind of "stuckness" that interferes with adaptive movement. Let us consider how these behaviors manifest in each of the Person systems.

Sensorimotor. Primitive sensorimotor behaviors produce excessive stabilization as the individual attempts to gain sensorimotor control of the challenge. Stereotypic or perseverative movement also qualifies as hyperstable, because adaptive movement is prevented.

Cognitive. Piaget's work in cognitive development demonstrates the developmental pattern (e.g. Piaget & Inhelder, 1969; Flavell, 1963). Cognitive hyperstability prevents adaptive movement in the cognitive system. For example, the 3-year-old child employs transductive reasoning. This is a developmental thinking tool that is usual and useful in the developing child. In an adult it may interfere with problem solution. Rigidity of thought also interferes with adaptive movement.

Psychosocial. Primitive psychosocial behaviors such as denial, projection, and avoidance can interfere with adaptive movement. Denial is normative in a 3-year-old but can have limited utility in ordinary life activities of the adult. However, when dealing with traumatic and ego-threatening events, denial as a temporary defense is considered normative (Kubler-Ross, 1969). Persistence of denial beyond the time necessary to regain psychological balance (and this is highly idiosyncratic) is generally considered dysfunctional.

It is important to emphasize that this separating out of system responses is artificial. The person is behaving with a holistic response that involves all three systems. The following example focuses on an employee faced with the occupational challenge of writing a type of report with which he is unfamiliar and with which he has had no experience. This employee will be followed through all classes of adaptive response behaviors.

> **Example 7-13:** *The employee: Preparing a report (1).* An employee must prepare a report for his supervisor. He knows that this report will eventually go to the president of the company. He also knows that he needs a unique premise on which to build his report to receive a favorable response from the president. He has not performed this particular task before and is feeling a bit overwhelmed because he does not know how to begin. His supervisor offers no assistance.
>
> The employee sits at his desk staring out the window. He aimlessly rotates paper clips in his hand. He experiences a sense of cognitive "shutdown" and feels "without a clue" as to a strategy. He believes that if he is nonproductive in this task long enough, his supervisor will rescue him and write the report instead.

As the example above shows, all three Person systems are involved in this hyperstabilized, dysadaptive response.

Transitional Behaviors. Transitional behaviors are characterized as *hypermobile.* This is in contrast to the excessive stability of the primitive behaviors. These behaviors can also be seen in each of the Person systems. Transitional behaviors may follow the use of primitive behaviors; in other words, they often function as a way to break out of the hyperstability. Instead of being excessively stable, the transitional behaviors are excessively mobile. There is much activity that is not goal-directed but almost "action for the sake of action."

Sensorimotor. Transitional sensorimotor behaviors may be excessively active but without apparent goal direction. They may reflect highly energized movement that lacks adaptive modulation. They may appear uncoordinated or random.

Cognitive. Transitional cognitive behaviors may reflect exploratory problem-solving approaches but seem random rather than systematic. Attention may be focused on irrelevant environmental cues rather than relevant ones vis-à-vis the problem at hand.

Psychosocial. Psychosocial transitional behaviors consist of high-energy motivational behaviors without functional boundaries. Behaviors may be psychosocially intrusive if they involve other persons.

> **Example 7-14:** *The employee: Preparing a report (2).* The employee who has to write the report in the example above realizes that he will not be rescued and he will have to write the report if he values his job. He tries several ideas and abandons them, writing them on paper one by one, wadding up each sheet and throwing it in the wastebasket. He walks down the hall to the water cooler several times and goes for two cups of coffee. He goes to the office of a colleague to sit down and talk about something other than his report. The colleague is busy on a task of his own and resents the intrusion into his work.

In the example above, again all three Person systems are involved in this response. The difference is that now his behaviors all reflect hypermobility. He is at least engaging in movement of some sort, but that movement is still not modulated and goal directed.

Mature Behaviors. *Mature behaviors* are characterized by a blend of mobility and stability. In other words, they are modulated behaviors that are an adaptive combination of mobility and stability.

Sensorimotor. With mature behaviors, sensorimotor responses are reasonably coordinated (within idiosyncratic limits) and goal directed. They exhibit the blend of moving and not moving necessary for adaptive movement.

Cognitive. Cognitive behaviors are goal directed, with systematic exploration of problem solution possibilities. They attend to relevant environmental cues. They lead to breaking of perceptual sets that keep the Person from achieving an adaptive response.

Psychosocial. Psychosocial behaviors reflect a directed motivation. They express confidence that the occupational challenge can be responded to adaptively and masterfully.

Example 7-15: *The employee: Preparing a report (3).* Our report-challenged employee suddenly has an "inspiration" for a unique premise on which to build his report. He sits down at the computer and begins to articulate the opening idea. Ideas begin to flow. He identifies a logical sequence for developing his premise. He feels a sense of exuberance because he believes he has hit on a really good idea that will please his supervisor and the president as well.

The employee now exhibits mature behaviors that are characterized by an adaptive blend of mobility and stability. In this example, the Person began as hyperstabilized, then moved into hypermobility, before finally arriving at a blend of mobility and stability with which to respond to this occupational challenge adaptively and masterfully.

Example 7-16. *Independent adult: Reconstructing life after a spinal cord injury.* A young man has recently suffered a C6-C7 spinal cord injury. As his rehabilitation phase begins, he is depressed, unable to articulate any goals, and unwilling to exert any effort to move the muscles with remaining innervation. He expresses a desire to die.

As he recognizes that he is not going to die, he begins to articulate multiple goals, with walking at the top of his list. His family brings in newspaper and magazine articles about cures that are on the horizon and technology that will permit a person with his injury to walk. He wants to try these techniques immediately. Other goals are related to his former social life as a basketball player on the company team. He does not want to learn about things that he can do to feed himself or strengthen muscles that can help him get out of bed independently or groom himself. In his view the wheelchair is only temporary, so he does not want to spend time and energy on becoming competent in its use.

A man with a similar injury visits the rehab unit and shares his experiences. He has resumed his professional life as an attorney. He has modified his adaptive response modes of interacting with his environment using various assistive devices and the help of an aide. He has resumed his amateur athletic life with wheelchair basketball. The attorney helps the patient to see some possibilities short of the "miracle cure" for which the patient is hoping. The patient then begins to collaborate with his therapist and other team members to develop goals that are attainable and that will give him some quality of life despite his injury. He becomes an active member of his rehabilitation team. He still hopes for the miracle cure but realizes that may not be in his near future.

In the example of the man with a spinal cord injury, the sequence also moves from primitive to transitional to mature. It is important for health care professionals to recognize that hyperstability is very common as a first response. To recognize it, acknowledge it as an understandable and frequently occurring response, and accept its legitimacy can be very facilitative to assisting the patient.

Adaptive Response Generation Subprocess (Adaptation Gestalt) (Fig. 7-7)

Assumption

All three Person systems are invariably present to some degree in each occupational response. The particular configuration will vary, based on the perceived expectations for an adaptive and masterful response.

The *adaptation* gestalt is the second major component of the adaptive response generation subprocess. When the adaptive response mechanism has done its work (selected the adaptation energy level, the adaptive response mode, and the adaptive response behavior), the Person must now configure that output into a holistic response to the occupational challenge. Because the Person is viewed as consisting of sensorimotor, cognitive, and psychosocial systems, the holistic response is a configuring of these three systems into a response plan. In general use, the notion of gestalt implies a condition in which the whole is more than the sum of the parts. The adaptation gestalt is a holistic plan in which the contributions of the three Person systems — sensorimotor, cognitive, and psychosocial — come together in a particular integration intended by the Person to produce an adaptive and masterful response.

Visually, the adaptation gestalt is represented as a circle. This representation allows an easy conceptualization of the involvement of the three systems. It is important to note that there is not one best adaptation gestalt. Different occupational challenges require different adaptation gestalts, that is, configuration of the Person systems for a response. Figure 7-8 represents a Person's gestalt in which the sensorimotor system dominates, the cognitive system is less dominant, and the psychosocial system even less dominant.

Adaptation Gestalt

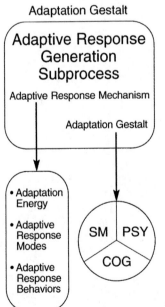

Figure 7-7. Adaptive response generation subprocess — adaptation Gestalt.

Example 7-17: *Ballet dancer: Achieving optimal performance.* The ballet dancer must have a sensorimotor system that is functioning at its peak for a successful performance to occur. The cognitive system is sufficiently involved to permit memory of the steps, cues for entrance onto the stage, and perception of the other dancers around her. The psychosocial system is sufficiently involved to provide motivation to perform at an optimal level and to interact with fellow dancers in a goal-directed manner.

Figure 7-9 represents a gestalt where the cognitive system dominates. In this particular configuration, the sensorimotor system is less dominant and the psychosocial system even less dominant.

Example 7-18: *Student: Taking an examination.* The student taking an important examination has a cognitive system functioning in a dominant role. The sensorimotor system is sufficiently involved to allow the student to remain seated in his chair, turn pages of the examination, and use a pencil to designate his answers. The psychosocial system is sufficiently involved to provide incentive to do well but not so much as to induce a dysfunctional level of anxiety.

Figure 7-10 represents a gestalt in which the psychosocial system dominates. Here the sensorimotor system is involved to a larger extent than the cognitive system, which is minimally involved.

Example 7-19: *Student: Obtaining "justice."* An 8-year-old child at the playground has been angered by a fellow student. The child is picking up objects and throwing them at the offending student; thus, the sensorimotor system has involvement. The cognitive system is minimally involved, sufficient to keep his target in sight; however, the object thrower is not considering potential disciplinary consequences of his actions. Thus, his psychosocial system dominates his response.

The possible variations of the adaptation gestalt are significant in number. The one requirement, from a theoretical perspective, is that all three systems are present in each response.

Adaptation gestalts that are not producing an adaptive and masterful response may need to be modified. One of the most effective adaptations that a Person can make is to change their adaptation gestalt when a change seems indicated.

Example 7-20: *Amateur athlete: Producing a winning performance.* An athlete appears to be "choking" under the pressure of an amateur softball tournament. This athlete has an adaptation gestalt that has too much involvement of the psychosocial system to produce optimal occupational performance. She wants so much to perform well so that her team can win that this desire gets in the way of her best performance. What that athlete would need to do is to reconfigure her adaptation gestalt to reduce involvement of the psy-

Adaptation Gestalt
Ballet Dancer

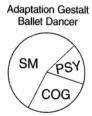

Figure 7-8. Adaptation Gestalt — ballet dancer.

Adaptation Gestalt
Student

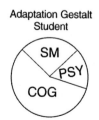

Figure 7-9. Adaptation Gestalt — student.

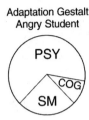

Adaptation Gestalt
Angry Student

Figure 7-10. Adaptation Gestalt — angry student..

chosocial system. The change needs to allow the sensorimotor system to dominate. The cognitive system should be appropriately involved to strategize and perceive response needs for the particular circumstances of the game situation at hand.

One of the potential benefits of this way of visualizing the adaptation gestalt is that it turns a very abstract idea into a simple concrete representation. Its very simplicity is what provides its potential utility as a way of self-monitoring and self-correcting occupational responses that are dysadaptive. If a client is able to depict Person system responses in this visual manner, it points to the potential to also depict a reconfiguration that may lead to a more adaptive and masterful outcome.

Example 7-21: *Occupational therapy student: Achieving successful academic performance.* An occupational therapy student is having significant difficulty mastering the content in a required course on neurophysiology. The student is taking the course for the second time and recognizes the consequences of not succeeding on her second attempt. Failure to pass the course on the second attempt means that she will no longer be a student in the occupational therapy program. This student has had an occupational therapy theory course in which she learned the principles of Occupational Adaptation, including the adaptation gestalt. Her faculty academic advisor meets with her regarding her tenuous state as an occupational therapy student based on her unsatisfactory performance in this particular course at the mid-term mark. The student is very anxious because she realizes the consequences of not succeeding. The faculty advisor draws a picture of what she perceives to be the student's adaptation gestalt with regard to this particular occupational challenge. Because of the student's high level of anxiety, the advisor draws the adaptation gestalt in such a way as to reflect a major involvement of the psychosocial system, with too little involvement of the cognitive system for success with this type of academic material. The student studies the depiction of her adaptation gestalt as the faculty advisor sees it. Her response to the advisor is, "I need to get a tutor." The student then acts to obtain a tutor. At the end of the semester, she not only successfully passes the course but also earns a final letter grade of "A."

What the faculty advisor did was to give the student a simple and rather concrete visual picture of how she was approaching the challenge of passing this particular course. The student then acted to modify her adaptation gestalt to have increased involvement of the cognitive system and much less of the psychosocial system.

The therapist can identify a similar dysfunctional adaptation gestalt manifestation in clients. In recognizing that the client's adaptation gestalt is not adaptively configured for the task at hand, the therapist can facilitate a change in the client's adaptation gestalt so as to produce a response that is more adaptive and masterful. In some cases, the therapist can use this depiction effectively to promote a desired modification in the way the client approaches tasks (i.e., changes in the adaptation gestalt).

The potential for use of the adaptation gestalt in therapeutic intervention has not been adequately explored. One initial attempt to begin this process was in a pilot study conducted by McCament (1996). McCament wanted to know if adolescent clients hospitalized because of mental health issues could use the adaptation gestalt to reflect their way of responding in various situations. She asked four adolescents, two boys and two girls, to depict their adaptation gestalts under certain circumstances. She developed general scenarios that these adolescents might experience at school, at home, and while spending time with friends. She also developed two versions of each scenario, one when things were going well and one when things were going badly.

McCament wanted to know if the adolescents could use this system to literally draw a picture of their responses. In other words, could they discriminate how they responded to these different scenarios and outcomes using a blank "adaptation gestalt" (circle) and color in their Person systems in each case? The adolescents were clearly making some differentiations through their completions of the adaptation gestalts for each scenario.

The hope for this kind of approach depends on the individual's ability to identify and distinguish how the adaptation gestalt appears when things are going well and when things are going badly. If this type of discrimination takes place, the therapist may assist the client to figure out ways in which he or she can change the adaptation gestalt to make it appear more like the positive situation. Individuals in mental health settings have complex lives and circumstances. Much of the therapy by other professionals that involves "talking" therapy is also very abstract and complex. A simple system such as drawing the adaptation gestalt may have the potential to make this complex situation more manageable. In addition, it involves the sensorimotor system through vision and through using the motor activity of filling in the segments of the adaptation gestalt. It also implies that the Person has the capacity to change the adaptation gestalt. This capacity to change can be a potent empowerment tool for the client. The use of the adaptation gestalt in this manner needs to be explored further with various populations and its potential efficacy studied systematically.

Summary

The adaptive response generation subprocess is the subprocess that actually creates or generates the occupational response. Once the Person has a perception of the interacting internal and external expectations, the two major components of the adaptive response generation subprocess come into play. First, the adaptive response mechanism produces a form of adaptation energy for use (primary or secondary), chooses an adaptive response mode for the pattern of interaction (existing, modified, or new), and selects an adaptive response behavior (primitive — hyperstable; transitional — hypermobile; or mature — blended mobility and stability). Second, the Person configures the degree of involvement of each Person system (sensorimotor, cognitive, and psychosocial) into a holistic plan for responding (the adaptation gestalt). The occupational response then becomes manifested as action.

Adaptive Response Evaluation Subprocess (Fig. 7-11)

Assumption

The Person evaluates the response in terms of efficiency (how much were personal time, energy, and available resources used?); effectiveness (to what extent were the performance expectations met?); and satisfaction to self and society (to what extent did the

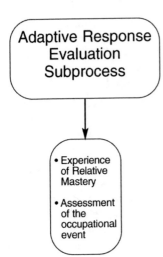

Figure 7-11. Adaptive response evaluation subprocess.

Person experience personal gratification and to what extent did society regard the response as adaptive and masterful?).

Assumption

Relative mastery is not the same as skill mastery that is assessed by an external source. It is a phenomenological assessment, a perception of performance on the part of the Person.

Assumption

Relative mastery can be experienced as positive or negative.

When the occupational response has been created and performed, the Person then evaluates how well the response met the expectations inherent in the occupational challenge. The adaptive response subprocess goes into action. The Person activates this subprocess through raising the question of how masterful was the response. For Occupational Adaptation, the assessment of relative mastery is the primary evaluation avenue.

For an Occupational Adaptation process to be functioning in a healthy manner, the Person must go through the process of self-evaluation. Relative mastery is a way of describing the nature of that self-evaluation. Failure to self-evaluate can result in occupational dysfunction. Failure to self-evaluate can place the Person in a position of not recognizing whether responses are adaptive and masterful.

> **Example 7-22:** *Student: Achieving success in the student role.* An adolescent boy is not succeeding in his role as student. He does not know why nor does he question himself about why. He simply repeats the same dysfunctional responses over and over without assessing how his responses map onto both internal and external expectations for the student role.

Failure to evaluate precludes the possibility of adaptive change that can enhance the likelihood of meeting expectations in life roles. Perseveration in occupational dysfunction occurs instead.

> **Example 7-23:** *Recreational bowlers: Enjoying an evening as friends.* Two friends decide to spend an evening bowling to relax from the stresses of work. One belongs to a bowling

league. She bowls at least twice a week. She is accustomed to averaging in the 195–220 range. The second friend is an infrequent bowler with minimal talent. She is accustomed to bowling in the 80–90 range. On the evening in question, the league bowler performs well below her usual performance, averaging 150. She has fewer strikes and converts fewer spares than usual. She even throws an occasional gutter ball. The infrequent bowler performs well above her usual performance, averaging 110. She throws slightly fewer gutter balls and converts an occasional spare. The league bowler is very unhappy with her score and considers herself to have had a terrible bowling experience at 150. The infrequent bowler is joyous and considers herself to have had a great night at 110. The following week, the league bowler competes with her team and bowls in her usual average range with a score of 210. The league bowler's skill mastery in bowling did not change over this period, but her experience of relative mastery was very different on these two occasions.

Relative mastery can be conceptualized as a simple continuum that ranges from negative to positive with a midpoint that is neither negative nor positive. As the Person evaluates a particular occupational event, she can evaluate each property of relative mastery (efficiency, effectiveness, and satisfaction to self/society) somewhere on the positive to negative continuum.

Example 7-24: *League bowler: Executing a winning performance.* Let's return to the example of the league bowler. On the night she bowled with her friend, she might have assessed her relative mastery in the following way (asterisks are indicators of the Person's self-assessment relative to a positive and negative scale):

Efficiency	− *0 +
Effectiveness	− * 0 +
Satisfaction to self	−* 0 +
Satisfaction to society	−* 0 +

She felt more fatigued after this effort. She certainly felt ineffective. She felt little self-satisfaction with her performance because it was so much below her expectation. When she thought of her bowling league friends, satisfaction to society was low. (Had this been a league performance, her teammates would have been very unhappy with her.) On this occasion she experienced negative relative mastery.

On the following week when she bowled with her league, she might have assessed her relative mastery as follows:

Efficiency	− 0 * +
Effectiveness	− 0 * +
Satisfaction to self	− 0 * +
Satisfaction to society	− 0 *+

She felt more energized after this outing. She felt effective because her score was in the range both she and her teammates expected. She experienced high self-satisfaction and high satisfaction to society because she helped her team win that evening. On this occasion she experienced positive relative mastery.

As the Person considers an occupational event in the aggregate, he or she makes an overall assessment of performance. Since Occupational Adaptation is a process that functions to maximize and increase the Person's adaptive capacity, he or she evaluates whether it was a very adaptive and masterful outcome. The individual may conclude that performance was somewhere between a total disaster and a rousing success. In general, this decision continuum ranges from dysadaptive to adaptive, with homeostasis as a midpoint.

−	0	+
dysadaptive	homeostasis	adaptive

Occupational Adaptation views homeostasis in much the same manner as Frankl (1984). "I consider it a dangerous misconception of mental hygiene to assume that what man needs in the first place is equilibrium or, as it is called in biology, "homeostasis," i.e., a tensionless state. What man needs is not a tensionless state but rather the striving and struggling for a worthwhile goal, a freely chosen task" (p. 110).

Homeostasis is viewed here as a temporary "breath catching" status. It is neither positive nor negative but neutral (i.e., neither adaptive nor dysadaptive). Because it is neutral it does not impact the Person's adaptive capacity. If, however, this neutral point becomes perpetual, there is no adaptive movement that will take place, and this renders the individual unable to perform adaptively and masterfully.

Evaluation by the client of his or her relative mastery in the tasks of the intervention plan is an important empowerment tool for the client. It gives the client a simple framework for evaluating adaptive responses long after active occupational therapy intervention is terminated.

The output of the adaptive response evaluation subprocess is the information. The final subprocess, the adaptive response integration subprocess, uses to reflect on the occupational event. This is the means by which the occupational event becomes integrated and permanently available for the Person to use in subsequent occupational challenges.

After the occupational response occurs, the Person begins to assess how adaptive and masterful was the response. Relative mastery, with properties of efficiency, effectiveness, and satisfaction to self and society, is the primary tool for this assessment activity. The Person reaches a conclusion about the success of the overall occupational event in meeting the occupational challenge with its expectations.

Adaptive Response Integration Subprocess (Fig. 7-12)

Assumption

Integration requires that the Person retain a memory of this event — its genesis from recognition that an occupational challenge exists to its completion as an evaluated experience.

Assumption

Occupational responses that are evaluated as producing either positive or negative outcomes can lead to increase in adaptive capacity.

Assumption

It is the action of the adaptive response integration subprocess transformed into adaptive capacity that leads to generalization of adaptive responses to novel tasks and self-initiation of new adaptive responses.

Now that the Person has generated, performed, and evaluated the response, it is time to integrate the impact of this occupational event into the Person systems. Action of the adaptive response integration subprocess provides the reflective conduit through which the feedback loop to the Person systems moves. This subprocess does the work that culminates in information about the occupational event resulting in long-lasting impact on the Person's adaptive capacity. Its output functions as the terminal point of the feedback loop.

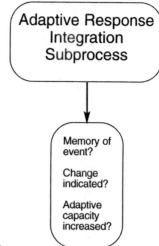

Figure 7-12. Adaptive response integration subprocess.

The minimal form of adaptive response integration is simply a memory of the experience. If the subprocess functions well, this memory becomes the basis for an adaptive reflection. In other words, what has the Person gained in knowledge and understanding of occupational responses that can lead to adaptation and mastery? What went well and what did not go well? Through the action of the adaptive response subprocess, the output of this reflection can be retained for future use.

It seems intuitively obvious that positive relative mastery experiences would enhance adaptive capacity. Memory of occupational responses that result in positive outcomes should enhance adaptive capacity. The potential of negative relative mastery experiences to enhance adaptive capacity is less obvious. Aversive experiences with occupational responses that do not produce adaptive and masterful outcomes can be extremely salient experiences. Therefore, an experience that turns out badly can be highly instructive to the individual. When the Person reflects on the experience and concludes that he or she might have been better served to use an adaptive response that was configured differently, then the adaptive capacity is enhanced according to Occupational Adaptation.

Occupational Adaptation proposes that it is not skill mastery that produces generalization, but rather the adaptive capacity put to use. It is the adaptive capacity to examine an occupational challenge with its role expectations and anticipate how to respond masterfully which produces a successful generalization. Skills unsuccessfully applied to novel tasks do not provide an experience of positive relative mastery. Without the adaptive capacity to anticipate outcomes, the individual is left with an array of specific skills whose applicability is specific rather than general. It is the adaptive capacity that arms the Person with the ability to generalize. It is this same adaptive capacity that the Person uses to produce a new response when a new response is required.

Example 7-25: *Homemaker: Restoring ability to care for self and home (1).* An elderly homemaker with diabetes has returned home from a hospital stay following a severely debilitating period. She is using a wheelchair. Following initial Occupational Adaptation intervention in which the occupational therapist encourages the homemaker to set her own goals, the homemaker integrates for further use each successful goal attainment. Each week she sets new goals for herself and initiates generalizations and new adaptations between therapist visits. The occupational therapist has been successful in facilitating improved adaptive capacity in the client. This enhanced adaptive capacity sets the stage for the client to encounter further occupational challenges in her chosen role of home-maker and respond adaptively and masterfully. This example is based on Ford (1995).

The Person, when confronted with an occupational challenge, creates a response through action of the adaptive response generation subprocess, evaluates the outcome through action of the adaptive response evaluation subprocess, and integrates it into the Person for use through action of the adaptive response integration subprocess. It is impor-tant to remember that progression through these subprocesses may be happening very rap-idly, with the Person responding to multiple challenges simultaneously at different rates.

Assessment and Incorporation by the Occupational Environment (Fig. 7-13)

The occupational environment also assesses the occupational response of the Person. This assessment is based on a comparison with the performance expectations of that environ-ment. Information about the occupational event and its evaluation become incorporated into the occupational environment assessment by those who serve as the evaluation agents of the occupational environment. This information loop provides the possibility that the environment, through action of its agents, can be impacted by the occupational perform-ance of the Person. The environment may use this information to modify the external expectations in some manner or the expectations may remain the same. The expectations may be intensified or they may be lessened.

> **Example 7-26:** *Therapist: Meeting increased work load demands.* A health care facility has reduced its therapy staff. The remaining staff must now treat more clients in the same amount of time. Related documentation must also be included in this time frame. One of the therapists does not meet the expectations for increased productivity because of fail-ure to adapt to this new schedule. The supervisor informs the therapist that she has 2 weeks to demonstrate that she can meet the new productivity standards. Otherwise, she will lose her job.

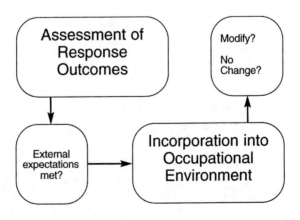

Figure 7-13. Assessment and incorporation by environment.

The above example indicates how external performance expectations may intensify because of feedback to the occupational environment. It may also demonstrate a clash of internal (Person) and external (occupational environment) expectations. When the Person either misperceives the external expectations, ignores their significance, refuses to meet those expectations, or is unable to meet those expectations, the occupational challenge is at its highest difficulty. The need for the Person's internal occupational adaptation process to be at its most functional is apparent. A marginally functioning occupational adaptation process is most likely to result in dysadaptive responses.

The occupational environment, through its agents, assesses the degree to which the Person has met the external expectations. The external expectations for the Person can change (in either a positive or negative direction) based on this assessment. Through this environmental assessment of the Person's occupational response, the Person has the potential to impact the occupational environment and its role expectations.

OCCUPATIONAL ADAPTATION AND INTERVENTION

There are several principles of intervention from an Occupational Adaptation perspective. The practitioner who intervenes from this perspective must understand and commit to these principles.

1. A fundamental treatment assumption in Occupational Adaptation is that adaptiveness leads to enhanced occupational performance. This is in contrast to other approaches which believe that enhancing occupational performance will lead to adaptiveness.
2. The client, through his or her internal adaptive capacity, is the agent of change. The practitioner functions as the agent of the occupational environment (i.e. sets the stage for the client to perform according to both internal and external role expectations).
3. Intervention is focused on enhancing the health and strength of the client's internal adaptive capacity so that the client can maximize participation in desired occupations.
4. The client selects the occupational role for intervention emphasis and is active in the planning of intervention.
5. The client is involved in evaluating the outcomes of intervention.
6. Occupational Adaptation does not tell the therapist what to do. It tells the therapist what questions to ask.
7. Occupational Adaptation is not a collection of techniques nor is it technique specific.

Increased adaptiveness leads to enhanced occupational performance. Figure 7-14 clarifies the distinction between two ways of thinking about intervention. It is important to understand this distinction. Occupational Adaptation is centered on the idea that adaptation is an internal phenomenon. This phenomenon is present in everyday human growth and development. Using Occupational Adaptation to guide treatment, therapists tap into this normal process and orient therapy on the client's internal adaptiveness (adaptive capacity), as opposed to adapting occupations for the client. Each individual has a capacity for personal adaptation. This adaptive capacity can be readily observable in everyday interactions with relatives and friends. Some individuals welcome change and eagerly respond with creative solutions and a high degree of flexibility. At the other extreme, some individuals are reluctant to change. They tend to respond to challenging situations in predictable, long-standing patterns of dysfunction. The therapist who practices from an Occupational Adaptation perspective will focus on the nature and quality of the client's adaptive capacity. For many

	Target	Outcome
Assumption #1	Adaptiveness ⟶	Occupational Performance
Assumption #2	Occupational Performance ⟶	Adaptiveness

Figure 7-14. Comparison of underlying treatment assumptions. (Adapted from Crist, P., Royeen, C., & Schkade, J. K. (2000). Infusing occupation into practice (2nd ed.) p. 99. Bethesda, MD: American Occupational Therapy Association.)

clients with chronic dysfunction it is a deficit in personal adaptiveness that prevents them from becoming functional. Their adaptive capacity may be constitutionally limited, blocked due to developmental issues, or impaired as a result of personal trauma, either physical or emotional. The task of the therapist is to assess the client's capacity to adapt, identify the client's unique process of occupational adaptation (how the person goes about adapting), determine sources of blockage, and intervene to improve the client's process of adaptation.

The Client Is the Agent of Change

The primary target of therapy is to increase and capitalize on the client's adaptive capacity with the client as the primary actor in this effort. Activities that have role relevance and personal meaning are the primary method the therapist uses to affect the adaptive capacity. Such activities are carefully designed to present the client with sufficient but not overwhelming demand for adaptation. The therapist provides only as much direction as absolutely necessary to facilitate a more adaptive response. Determining the type and manner of such direction requires a sophisticated approach in which the therapist is both client-centered and a risk-taker. It is important to clarify what is meant by these descriptors. In Occupational Adaptation, being client-centered means not only focusing treatment on the client's unique needs and interests, but genuinely believing in clients' ability to assume responsibility for self and to become their own source of adaptation. This is in contrast with much of occupational therapy. Many therapists see themselves as the agent of change. It is evidenced by their practice. Their overriding desire to teach the client adaptive techniques, and make modifications in the environment, calls into question their perspective of the client as someone with the ability to be self-reliant. The therapist who is client-centered, as defined in Occupational Adaptation, must by necessity be comfortable with risk-taking. In the highest form of therapy, the therapist provides a very delicate balance of direct action, facilitation, and free-floating presence. Only in this manner can the client become the agent of change.

Focus on Internal Adaptive Capacity

The goal of intervention is that the client can participate in life and societal activities to the extent that health conditions permit. It is important that the client can participate with a quality that is satisfying to the client and significant others in his or her life—family, friends, employers, etc. All human beings who participate in life and societal activities, regardless of any actual or potentially disabling conditions, encounter challenges. Successful participation requires that individuals engage in meeting these challenges adaptively and masterfully. What is meant by successful engagement with these occupational challenges? Successful engagement with occupational challenges means that the individual encounters challenges with which he or she is unfamiliar and has the capacity to consider alternative solutions, generate and perform an adaptive response, and evaluate whether that response met the requirements of a particular challenge. It may require the individual to make more than one try at responding to the challenge. Not every attempt will be successful. The important concern is that the individual possesses a well-functioning internal adaptive capacity that can recognize the efficacy of responses and make adaptations as needed. Occupational Adaptation proposes that those individuals who participate in meeting challenges most successfully are those whose internal adaptive capacity is most functional. This is why intervention from an Occupational Adaptation perspective is focused on the client's internal adaptive capacity.

Client's Role in Intervention Planning

The therapist practicing from an Occupational Adaptation perspective does not make assumptions about appropriate goals for a client based on diagnosis or other group classification systems. It is the client who decides what the focus of intervention will be. A client working toward a goal of engagement in a preferred occupation is much more likely to be an active participant in intervention.

Occupations are always carried out within occupational roles. These roles differ from one individual to another. The occupations that make up those roles will differ from one individual to another, even when the same role is involved. For example, not all homemaker occupations are the same for all homemakers, even though they may be similar. Not all farm worker occupations are identical for all farm workers, although they may bear many similarities. The internal and external role expectations will differ from one individual to another based on the role expectations of a particular occupational environment.

A significant role for the client in intervention planning is to educate the therapist on the expectations for the particular role that he or she has chosen. In this way, the therapist can evaluate the client's ability to carry out the various tasks that are a part of that role. Again, the therapist must not assume what those tasks are, nor the manner in which the client is accustomed to performing those tasks. With knowledge of the specific requirements of a particular role for this particular client, the therapist and client together begin to plan the intervention. The intervention plan focuses on the areas that need to be improved so that the client can carry out his or her role adaptively and masterfully. This plan is directed toward allowing maximal participation in that role despite whatever disabling conditions the client may have.

Client and Therapist Evaluate Outcomes of Intervention

In Occupational Adaptation, it is important that the client engages in his or her own assessment of intervention success. This is where the client assesses his or her experience of relative mastery with regard to progress on occupational goals. Based on the results of this assessment, the client may suggest changes in the plan that he or she believes may increase the desired progress.

The relative mastery assessment by the client does not preclude the therapist from conducting the assessments that facility documentation requires. The therapist will also conduct those required assessments. However, as previously stated, the focus of intervention is to enhance the adaptive capacity of the client. How can the therapist assess whether the client's internal adaptation process has been affected? There are three indicators that this internal process has been affected. One is that the client experiences improved relative mastery. A second indication is that the client engages in spontaneous generalization of previous adaptations without the therapist's suggestion. A third indication is that the client initiates new adaptations in situations not previously encountered.

> **Example 7-27:** *Homemaker: Restoring ability to care for self and home (2).* Let us return to the elder homemaker with diabetes who was discussed in the section on the adaptive response integration subprocess. As the homemaker experienced increasing success in her goals (improved relative mastery), she suggested other goals to meet. When the therapist asked if the client wanted to learn how to transfer from the wheelchair to the commode, the homemaker responded that she had already done that since the therapist's last visit (spontaneous generalization). The therapist had explained and demonstrated other transfers from the wheelchair. The client and therapist had never discussed this type of transfer before. The homemaker also volunteered without prompting that if the coffee maker and coffee-making ingredients were placed lower, she could make coffee herself (self-initiated adaptation). This example is based on Ford (1995).

These are the indicators that the client's internal adaptation process has been enhanced. The homemaker was not learning discrete skills but was learning to think adaptively through the skillful intervention of the therapist, collaborating in pursuit of the client's stated goals.

> **Example 7-28:** *Church member: Shampooing and styling her own hair.* An elderly homemaker sustained a cardiovascular accident (CVA, or stroke). She had been discharged from rehabilitation therapy, as she had reached the highest mobility gains she could obtain. Since her discharge several weeks ago, she has been living at home with her husband of many years. Her primary occupational goal is to be able to shampoo and style her own hair so that she can go out into the community again, to church and to social events with friends. The therapist bases her intervention on achieving this client's goal. The client achieves this goal in a manner that is satisfactory to her. The client believes that she can now return to church (relative mastery). She has generalized her approach to dressing and buttoning her clothes (spontaneous generalization). On one occasion when the therapist arrives, the client greets her with a request to, "Look at me." The client has sewed all the buttons back on her blouse and is expressing great satisfaction to the therapist (self-initiated adaptation). She began to resume numerous activities associated with her primary occupational roles of wife, homemaker, and churchgoer. This therapist had positively impacted the client's internal adaptive capacity through focusing on the client's chosen occupational role. This example is based on Johnson & Schkade (2001).

Occupational Adaptation Intervention Is Based on Questions to Ask

The "Occupational Adaptation Guide to Practice" from Schultz and Schkade (1992) (Table 7-4) consists of a series of questions. There are no statements of what the therapist should "do." The therapist operating from an Occupational Adaptation perspective must always be prepared to ask questions. These are questions that will assist the therapist to collaborate with the client in data gathering, intervention planning, and evaluation of the intervention programming. These questions will also assist in the process of determining which interventions are effective and which need changing to maximize client gains.

> **Example 7-29:** *Student group: Meeting the student role expectations.* A therapist is beginning a group intervention plan in a public school with children who have been

Table 7-4 OCCUPATIONAL ADAPTATION GUIDE TO PRACTICE

Occupational Adaptation Data Gathering/Assessment[a]

What are the patient's *occupational environments* and *roles*?

Which role is of primary concern to patient and family?

What occupational performance is expected in the primary *occupational environment* and *role*?

What are the physical, *social, cultural* features of the primary *occupational environment* and *role*?

What is the patient's *sensorimotor, cognitive,* and *psychosocial* status?

What is the patient's level of *relative mastery* in the primary *occupational environment* and *role*?

What is facilitating or limiting *relative mastery* in the primary *occupational environment* and *role*?

Occupational Adaptation Programming

What combination of occupational readiness and occupational activity is needed to promote the patient's *occupational adaptation process*?

What help will the patient need to assess *occupational responses* and use the results to affect the *occupational adaptation process*?

What is the best method to engage the patient in the occupational adaptation program?

Evaluation of the Occupational Adaptation Process

How is the program affecting the patient's *occupational adaptation process*?
- Which *energy level* is used most often (*primary* or *secondary*)?
- What *adaptive response mode* is used most often (*preexisting, modified,* or *new*)?
- What is the most common *adaptive response behavior* (*primitive, transitional,* or *mature*)?

What outcomes does the patient show that reflect change in the *occupational adaptation process*?
- Self-initiated adaptations?
- Enhanced *relative mastery*?
- Generalization to novel activities?

What program changes are need to provide maximum opportunity for *occupational adaptation* to occur?

[a]Italicized terms are constructs in the Occupational Frame of Reference (Schkade & Schultz, 1992).
From Schultz, S., & Schkade, J. K. (1992). Occupational adaptation: Toward a holistic approach for contemporary practice, part 2. *American Journal of Occupational Therapy, 46,* 925. Copyright 1992 by the American Occupational Therapy Association. Reprinted with permission of the author.

referred as emotionally disturbed or with behavior disorders. She asks the children in the group to take her on a tour of the school. She learns by observation and from asking the children questions what the particular environmental role expectations are for students in this particular school. She knows that her intervention must focus on the role of student in this setting, but she must learn how that role is defined here. She also asks questions of the assistant principal and the teachers. To intervene effectively, she must learn the physical, social, and cultural features of this particular occupational environment. She must learn what are the available opportunities and mechanisms for rewarding successful student role performance here. This questioning approach also allows her to learn what might be obstacles that interfere with successful student role performance. This example was reported by Sally Schultz.

Occupational Adaptation Intervention Is Not About Techniques

Occupational Adaptation intervention is about a way of thinking about your client and your intervention approach. It is not a collection of techniques, nor does it involve specific techniques. The therapist does not throw out everything previously learned about various techniques or methods to enhance occupational performance. The therapist may use many of these in an Occupational Adaptation intervention. What does change is the way the therapist thinks about those methods and the decisions about when or whether certain techniques or methods might come into play. The decision is always based on whether they might enhance the client's adaptive capacity with regard to the client-selected occupational role.

Once the client has determined the occupational role for therapeutic focus, the therapist's assessment identifies what things are facilitating or limiting the client's successful performance in that role. The intervention plan is then developed using two categories of intervention: occupational readiness and occupational activity. The therapist employs these two categories of intervention in achieving intervention goals.

Occupational readiness consists of interventions that are designed to address deficits in the Person systems (sensorimotor, cognitive, or psychosocial) that are interfering with performance in the selected occupational role. These may involve such problem areas as weakness, incoordination, memory or problem-solving loss, and lack of assertiveness. The therapist is the primary actor in occupational readiness intervention. This intervention does not address Person system deficits that are not interfering with the selected occupational role. Only those deficits that inhibit successful performance are addressed.

Occupational activity consists of tasks directly related to the selected occupational role. These tasks must meet the definitional requirements for occupation from an Occupational Adaptation perspective: (1) the client must be actively involved, (2) the activity must have personal meaning for that client, and (3) the activity must involve a process that ends in a product, whether that product is tangible or intangible. If the client wishes to resume his or her previous vocation, the occupational activity must be directly related to that vocation, as the client perceives it. If he or she wishes to resume an avocation as a volunteer in a social service agency, the occupational activity must be directly related to the volunteer role as the agency defines it and the client has experienced it. The importance of the personally meaningfully and occupationally relevant activity cannot be overemphasized. With occupational activity, the client is the primary actor. In this manner, the client becomes his or her own change agent. The therapist simply sets the environmental stage for this to happen.

It is this combination of occupational readiness and occupational activity that comprises the intervention plan. If an intervention plan can be devised that involves only occupational activity, that is the most desirable because the intervention is truly client-centered and the therapist acts as facilitator. If occupational readiness is deemed a necessary part of the intervention, the Occupational Adaptation perspective advocates that it be reduced in importance as quickly as possible with an accompanying increase in occupational activity intervention. Some occupational readiness intervention may be necessary, but we propose that occupational activity produces the fastest gains and engages the client most fully in the intervention. Occupational activity is also more likely to enhance the client's internal adaptive capacity because of his or her active involvement as well as the meaningfulness and the nature of the product-generating process.

It is important that the therapist has a thorough understanding of the comprehensive Occupational Adaptation theory. The therapist must be familiar with the constructs and how they relate to each other. For example, it is important for the therapist to identify when a client is using an existing adaptive response mode that is not resulting in successful occupational performance so that modified or new adaptive response modes can be facilitated. The therapist needs to identify when the client is hyperstabilized so that steps can be taken to facilitate adaptive movement before hyperstability becomes a dominant adaptive response behavior. When the client is working too intensively and expending more energy than is desirable (primary energy), the therapist can change the intervention plan or introduce some other modification that can make the work more smooth, more automatic, and less energy draining (secondary energy). The therapist needs to recognize an adaptation gestalt (a particular involvement of the three Person systems) that is not producing successful occupational performance. Once again, steps can be taken to facilitate the client's reconfiguration or reorganization of the Person systems to produce a more satisfactory adaptive response outcome. If a client is experiencing relative mastery as low, the therapist needs to learn which of the features — efficiency, effectiveness, or satisfaction to self and society — is most responsible for relative mastery that is experienced as negative. In this way, the therapist can undertake intervention that facilitates the changes necessary to bring about a more positive experience of relative mastery.

Population-Based Programmatic Applications

The majority of this chapter uses Occupational Adaptation as a framework for direct interventions. Occupational Adaptation can also be used as a framework on which to base comprehensive treatment programs for specific populations. The following discussion presents such use in three diverse arenas. These are descriptions of actual programs implemented by the second author while serving as a consultant or a therapist/researcher.

> **Example 7-30:** *Consultant in a forensic hospital setting with incarcerated individuals who are mentally ill.* The first program based on Occupational Adaptation was established at a state psychiatric hospital that is a maximum-security facility. It serves individuals who have been either accused or convicted of major crimes and also have severe mental illness. Patients are admitted when they are found "not guilty by reason of insanity" or "mentally incompetent to stand trial." The average age is 29, educational level is 3rd grade, and most common diagnosis is schizophrenia. More than one-third of the patients have committed murder. Although some will be housed in the facility indefinitely, approximately one-third will be discharged to less secure hospitals and community re-entry programs.
>
> The existing rehabilitation program used a variety of modalities to promote skill acquisition. Occupational therapy provided diversion; recreational therapy emphasized group games; music therapy focused on music appreciation; workshops taught elementary horticulture skills, upholstery, and picture-frame–making; and educational classes targeted academic skills consistent with the patient's grade level.
>
> The hospital contracted with the occupational therapy consultant to revamp the psychosocial rehabilitation program. The impetus was a negative accreditation review. Occupational Adaptation was used to assess the program, to design a new program, and to test its effectiveness. A basic assumption of Occupational Adaptation set the stage for the overall process. That is, dysfunction is the result of an impaired ability to adapt. Consequently, the patients were viewed as having blocks in their occupational adaptation process. A program needed to be designed that improved the patient's ability to adapt. For effectiveness, the program also needed consistency across modalities. The consultant developed a curriculum framework that could be universally applied in each of the therapy, work, and educational modalities. It is noteworthy that non-professional staff provided the majority of programming. Regardless of the modality, the staff would use the same generic curriculum framework (i.e., the same structure for content, the same methods to develop each patient's

adaptive capacity, and the same outcome measures). The consultant guided the staff in each modality to develop unique content consistent with the curriculum framework.

The resulting rehabilitation program required a dynamic shift in thinking. It was difficult for the staff to switch from the role of teacher to one of facilitator. It was challenging to recognize that "teaching the right way" was not helping patients become more adaptive. The curricula were different than anything previously used. Role performance was the focus, rather than skill acquisition. Behavioral, social, and internal adaptiveness were organized around practical skill development. Each new curriculum contained three progressive levels of role performance specific to the modality. The design allowed the staff to systematically increase the demand on the patient to adapt. Through each level of role performance new practical skills were acquired, new behaviors incorporated, and new competencies in independent adaptiveness were encouraged.

The outcomes demonstrate the effectiveness of this type of programming. Staff reported an increase in patient attendance, attentiveness, cooperation, and problem solving. Patients reported a higher level of mastery and a desire to learn. As would be expected, skill acquisition also improved. In addition, staff reported that they find the new programming more personally rewarding. In a subsequent accreditation review, the psychosocial program was identified as a "benchmark" service. The effect of this program supports the hypothesis that a program that focuses on improved adaptive capacity may yield a higher level of performance than one which stresses skill acquisition.

Example 7-31: *Therapist/researcher in elementary school setting with children classified as emotionally disturbed or behavior disordered.* The second programmatic use of Occupational Adaptation was a research study conducted in an elementary school of a small town near a large metropolitan area. The objective was to test the viability of Occupational Adaptation to guide group therapy with six special education students having emotional/behavioral disorders. As with the hospital program just described, the concept of role became increasingly significant to the design of the overall treatment program. It is with activities associated with a meaningful role that the demand for mastery interacts with the desire for mastery. The therapist/researcher used an action research design. Changes were made in the program as indicated. Over the 2 years, key premises of Occupational Adaptation were tested in vivo.

The therapist/researcher began by gaining an understanding of the student's occupational environment. Person systems assessments were conducted during practical real-world activities. Meaningful age-related craft activities were the mainstay of the first year. The results verified the assumption that meaningful activity produces a greater desire for mastery, a greater acceptance of challenge, and a correspondingly greater activation of the student's adaptive capacity. The compound effect of role expectation was introduced during the next year. The therapist incorporated an umbrella of positive role opportunities and associated activities with the therapy group. The students began to experience themselves in positive ways through productive school-related events and activities. This approach modified the role experience of the students. As the teachers and other students in the occupational environment began to observe the work of the research-involved students around the school, their expectations regarding those students changed. Involvement in positive meaningful roles changed the students' expectations of themselves. It is important to note that the goal was not to change the environment and its expectations. The goal was to move the student into positive role experiences and improve adaptiveness. The effect on the occupational environment was a naturalistic result of the therapy. The opportunity for intervening in the students' adaptive processes emerged most clearly at the point at which the subjects were involved in activities associated with positive role development. At this juncture, the therapist observed increased determination and openness to exploratory thinking. In other words, their adaptive capacity was being triggered. The students were more receptive to interventions that challenged them to go about activity in a new way. Within this formulation, long-standing patterns of dysfunctional adaptation were observable and could be carefully identified with the student. New approaches could be fostered. Educational skills could be learned. Self-reliance and adaptiveness increased. Teachers reported improved social skills and a decrease in disruptive behavior. At the end of the 2-year study, one of the students was recognized as "citizen of the week" by the principal. In summary, the study demonstrated the powerful effect of therapy focused on the individual's adaptive processes.

Example 7-32: *Consultant in homeless shelter setting with homeless residents.* The third program based on Occupational Adaptation was only recently initiated at a shelter for homeless and disabled in a non-profit organization supported through local foundations and grants. This shelter was established in 1985. The uniqueness of this program is that it has been based on the therapeutic power of "work" since its origin. It provides housing, clothing, education, childcare, and medical services for those who work consistently in the sheltered workshop. Individuals with severe mental illness, cognitive impairment, and physical disability are able to work for the program and obtain services. Work expectations are based on capability. Individuals may move into outreach work programs and continuing education opportunities. All support services continue as long as the individual continues to "work with the program." Some individuals will probably be cared for by the program for the remainder of their lives.

Despite the remarkable opportunities, many individuals drop out of the program and fall into old patterns of dysfunction. The consultant was asked to collaborate with the director to identify the source of this problem and ways to reduce it. Over the past year, the consultant has used Occupational Adaptation to evaluate the program, its staff, and its outcomes.

The severe chronicity of many clients is indicative of their inability to adapt successfully. They are enmeshed in restricted and impermeable patterns of dysfunction. Their characteristic response to challenge is defeat and self-disdain. It is so long-standing that no other perspective is possible without intensive intervention. Despite the comprehensiveness of the facility program, there has been no systematic program to directly target the individual's adaptive capacity. There has been no therapy that is concentrated on interrupting this self-defeating internal pattern of adaptation.

In the past year, the director has hired two full-time and one part-time occupational therapists. They have assumed case manager positions formerly held by social workers. The consultant continues to advise the facility director. She provides training for the medical, psychology, sheltered workshop, and occupational therapy staff. The goal is to improve their ability to identify the client's adaptive capacity, clarify blocks to adaptation, and promote the client's internal process of adaptation. The effects appear promising. Various staff report decreased turmoil with clients, fewer crises, and more self-reliance. They also report that the methods are useful to identify personal dysfunctional patterns and determine adaptation strategies that will yield greater satisfaction in both their personal and work life.

Occupational Adaptation in Intervention

What has been described is an approach to clinical reasoning and therapeutic use of self from an Occupational Adaptation perspective. Whether engaged in one-on-one intervention or dealing with comprehensive programmatic applications, Occupational Adaptation calls on the therapist to be always questioning, evaluating, and modifying intervention in the service of promoting the client's adaptive capacity. In general, the therapist carefully avoids protocol-driven intervention because the client's personal occupational needs will not likely be served well. A therapist using Occupational Adaptation must be creative, reflective, and attuned to client responses. Occupational Adaptation is not for the faint-of-heart therapist but for one who is willing to take therapeutic risks. It requires a therapist who believes in the power of occupation to promote health and well-being. It requires a profound belief that the end goal of intervention is optimal occupational participation in society and that this goal is most likely reached when the client's adaptive capacity (ability to engage adaptively and masterfully) is at its most functional.

STUDY QUESTIONS — BEGINNER

7.1. Occupational Adaptation refers to the integration of occupation and adaptation. In your own words, explain what that means.

7.2. What are the four points guiding the theoretical foundation of Occupational Adaptation as developed at Texas Woman's University?

7.3. How is a CT scan like Figure 7-1?

7.4. Draw a diagram of the process of occupational adaptation. Using an example from your own life, "walk through" an example or two using the diagram you have drawn.

7.5. Compare the definition of occupation put forth by Nelson in Chapter 5 to the one proposed by Schkade and Schultz in this chapter. Which definition is easier for you to understand and why? Which definition could you more easily use in education of the lay public and why?

7.6. List three occupations in which you routinely engage. For each of the three, identify the following regarding the occupation:
   • How the occupation actively engages you.
   • The outcome or product of the occupational process.
   • What meaning the occupation has for you.

7.7. Locate a good dictionary. In it, look up each of the following terms:
   • Adaptive
   • Ability
   • Mastery
   • Efficiency
   • Effectiveness
   • Satisfaction
   For each word, explain how the authors used it in Chapter 7. Further, identify if their use of the word is the same or different from the dictionary definition.

7.8. Think back in your own life over the past week. Identify a single instance of when you were occupationally challenged. Delineate the subsequent adaptive abilities you demonstrated to meet the challenge.

7.9. Right now, rate your own relative mastery of completing the learning activities for Chapter 7. Based on your experience so far, estimate how efficiently, effectively, and satisfactorily you are completing the activities. Compare your rating with a fellow student. Are they similar or different? If different, how are they different and why?

7.10. Identify words that Schkade and Schultz use as synonyms with the word occupation.

7.11. What is an assumption? Schkade and Schultz identify many assumptions which they have about occupation. Do you share their assumptions? Are there any additional assumptions you would like to add?

7.12. In this chapter, the authors refer to the vehicle of occupation. This is a powerful metaphor. Can you explain it?

7.13. Personal mastery is considered to be a constant. Identify an instance of personal mastery that you have displayed.

7.14. The next time you are grocery shopping, think about personal mastery of the environment as a constant. Identify three things that should be changed in the grocery store to enhance the personal mastery of anyone shopping who is older than 60. Speculate as to how these changes would allow for enhanced personal mastery.

7.15. Explain how press facilitates an adaptive response.

7.16. Think about how occupational performance expectations are influenced by the cultural subsystem. Reflect back on your own life and identify at least one example of when you inadvertently violated the "rules of the road" of a cultural subsystem (values, mores, ethics, standards, rules, or communication methods). How did it happen? Why did it happen? How did you cope with it?

7.17. Using the Occupational Adaptation reference, an occupational therapist should have a clear understanding of the demands placed on a client to perform a given occupation in a particular occupational environment. How could an occupational therapist discern these demands? Compare your answer with a classmate's answer.

7.18. What are the adaptive response subprocesses?

7.19. Define adaptive gestalt.

7.20. Do you agree that adaptation energy is a finite supply present at birth? Why or why not?

7.21. Think about your first week of occupational therapy school. What behaviors during that time might be considered as primitive? As you progressed in occupational therapy school, what behaviors might be considered as transitional? As you are now studying in a course and reading this text, what behaviors might be considered as mature? Discuss your answers with a classmate.

7.22. Define and compare the following regarding the adaptive response mode:
- Existing
- Modified
- New

7.23. Speculate as to when you might revert to a primitive behavior if occupationally challenged. Be as specific as possible.

7.24. What is phenomenological about the assessment of relative mastery?

7.25. List 10 questions for a therapist to ask a client that would reflect an Occupational Adaptation perspective.

7.26. Differentiate occupational readiness and occupational activity.

7.27. How can Occupational Adaptation be applied in a population-based approach?

7.28. How do Schkade and Schultz define function and dysfunction?

7.29. Could you employ an approach to therapy using Occupational Adaptation? Why or why not?

STUDY QUESTIONS — ADVANCED

7.30. Compare how culture plays a role in Occupational Therapy Conceptual Foundations by Nelson as contrasted to how it plays a role in Schkade and Schultz's Occupational Adaptation.

7.31. Locate one of the articles on Occupational Adaptation by other authors (such as Spencer & Davidson, 1998; Spencer, Daybell, Eschenfelder, Khalaf, Pike, & Woods-Petitti, 1998; Spencer, Hersch, Eschenfelder, Fournet, & Murray-Gerzik, 1999; or White, 1998). Read their article and compare the complementary but distinct differences in how occupational adaptation is used with what is described in this chapter.

7.32. Discuss the qualitative, grounded theory approach employed by Spencer & Davidson, 1998; Spencer, Daybell, Eschenfelder, Khalaf, Pike, & Woods-Petitti, 1998; Spencer, Hersch, Eschenfelder, Fournet, & Murray-Gerzik, 1999; and White, 1998. Compare the grounded theory approach to the approach used by Schkade and Schultz in this chapter.

7.33. Locate the "Guide to Practice" by Moyers (1999). Explain how occupation is prominent in this publication.

7.34. How does the notion of occupational environment differ from the notion of occupational form?

7.35. Refer to Selye's (1956) seminal work on stress. Identify how his concepts contribute to Occupational Adaptation.

7.36. Where did the term gestalt originate?

References

American Occupational Therapy Association. (1979/1995). The philosophical basis of occupational therapy. *American Journal of Occupational Therapy, 49,* 1026.

Christiansen, C., & Baum, C. (1991). *Occupational therapy: Overcoming human performance deficits.* Thorofare, NJ: Slack.

Clark, F. A., Parham, D., Carlsdon, M. E., Frank, G., Jackson, J., Pierce, D., Wolfe, R. J., & Zemke, R. (1991). Occupational science: Academic innovation in the service of occupational therapy's future. *American Journal of Occupational Therapy, 45,* 300–310.

Flavell, J. H. (1963). *The developmental psychology of Jean Piaget.* Princeton, NJ: Van Nostrand.

Ford, K. (1995). Occupational adaptation in home health: A therapist's viewpoint. *Home Health and Community Special Interest Section Newsletter, 2* (1), 2–4.

Frankl, V. (1984). *Man's search for meaning* (3rd ed.). New York: Simon & Schuster.

Gilfoyle, E., Grady, A., & Moore, J. (1990). *Children adapt.* Thorofare, NJ: Slack.

Johnson, J., & Schkade, J. K. (2001). Effects of occupation-based intervention on mobility in CVA. *Journal of Applied Gerontology, 20,* 91–110.

Kielhofner, G. (Ed.). (1985). *A model of human occupation: Theory and application* (2nd ed.). Baltimore, MD: Williams & Wilkins.

Kielhofner, G. (1992). *Conceptual foundations of occupational therapy.* Philadelphia, PA: F.A. Davis.

Kubler-Ross, E. (1969). *On death and dying.* New York: Macmillan.

Law, M., Cooper, B., Strong, S., Stewart D., Rigby, P., & Letts, L. (1996). The person-environment-occupation model: A transactive approach to occupational performance. *Canadian Journal of Occupational Ther-*

apy, 63, 9–23.

McCament, M. (1996). Application of occupational adaptation in assessing adolescent mental health disorders. Unpublished paper. Texas Woman's University, Denton, Texas.

Meyer, A. (1922). The philosophy of occupational therapy. *Archives of Occupational Therapy, 1,* 1–10.

Moyers, P. A. (1999). Guide to occupational therapy practice. *American Journal of Occupational Therapy, 53,* 247–322.

Nelson, D. (1988). Occupation: Form and performance. *American Journal of Occupational Therapy, 42,* 633–641.

Piaget, J. & Inhelder, B. (1969). *The psychology of the child.* New York: Basic Books.

Reilly, M. (1962). Occupational therapy can be one of the great ideas of 20th century medicine. *American Journal of Occupational Therapy, 16,* 1–9.

Reilly, M. (1969). The educational process. *American Journal of Occupational Therapy, 23,* 299–307.

Schkade, J. K., & Schultz, S. (1992). Occupational adaptation: Toward a holistic approach to contemporary practice, Part 1. *American Journal of Occupational Therapy, 46,* 829–837.

Schultz, S., & Schkade, J. (1997). Adaptation. In C. Christiansen, & C. Baum (Eds.), *Occupational therapy: Enabling function and well being* (2nd ed.) (pp. 458–481). Thorofare, NJ: Slack.

Schultz, S., & Schkade, J. K. (1992). Occupational adaptation: Toward a holistic approach to contemporary practice, part 2. *American Journal of Occupational Therapy, 46,* 917–926.

Selye, H. (1956). *The stress of life.* New York: McGraw-Hill.

Spencer, J., Daybell, P. J., Eschenfelder, V., Khalaf, R., Pike, J. M., & Woods-Petitti, M. (1998). Contrasts in perspectives on work: An exploratory qualitative study based on the concept of adaptation. *American Journal of Occupational Therapy, 52,* 474–484.

Spencer, J., Hersch, G., Eschenfelder, V., Fournet, J., & Murray-Gerzik, M. (1999). Outcomes of protocol-based and adaptation-based occupational therapy interventions for low-income elderly persons on a transitional unit. *American Journal of Occupational Therapy, 53,* 159–170.

Spencer, J. C., & Davidson, H. (1998). Community adap-

tive planning assessment: A clinical tool for documenting future planning with clients. *American Journal of Occupational Therapy, 52,* 19–30.

Trombly, C. A. (1995). Occupation: Purposefulness and meaningfulness as therapeutic mechanisms-1995 Eleanor Clarke Slagle lecture. *American Journal of Occupational Therapy, 49,* 960–972.

White, V. K. (1998). Ethnic differences in the wellness of elderly persons. *Occupational Therapy in Health Care 11,* 1–15.

Suggested Readings

Buddenberg, L. A., & Schkade, J. K. (1998). A comparison of occupational therapy intervention approaches for older patients after hip fracture. *Topics in Geriatric Rehabilitation, 13,* 52–68.

Crist, P., & Royeen, C. (1997). *Infusing occupation into practice.* Bethesda, MD: American Occupational Therapy Association.

Crist, P., Royeen. C., & Schkade, J. K. (2000). *Infusing occupation into practice* (2nd ed.). Bethesda, MD: American Occupational Therapy Association.

Csikszentmihalyi, M. (1990). *Flow.* New York: Harper Collins Publishers.

Dolecheck, J. R., & Schkade, J. K. (1999). Effects on dynamic standing endurance when persons with CVA perform personally meaningful activities rather than non-meaningful tasks. *Occupational Therapy Journal of Research, 19,* 40–53.

Dr. Seuss (1990). *Oh the places you'll go.* New York: Random House.

Garbarini, J., & Pearlman, V. (1998). Fieldwork in home health care: A model for practice. *Education Special Interest Section Quarterly, 8,* 1–4.

Garrett, S., & Schkade, J. K. (1995). The occupational adaptation model of professional development as applied to level II fieldwork in occupational therapy. *American Journal of Occupational Therapy, 49,* 119–126.

Gibson, J., & Schkade, J. K. (1997). Effects of occupational adaptation treatment with CVA. *American Journal of Occupational Therapy, 51,* 523–529.

Jackson, J. P., & Schkade, J. K. (2001). Occupational adaptation model vs. biomechanical/rehabilitation models in the treatment of patients with hip fractures. *American Journal of Occupational Therapy, 55,* 531–537.

Johnson, S. (1998). *Who moved my cheese?* New York: G.P. Putnam's Sons.

Macrae, A., Falk-Kessler, J., Juline, D., Padilla, R., & Schultz, S. (1998). Occupational therapy models. In A. Macrae & E. Cara (Eds.), *Psychosocial occupa-*

tional therapy, a clinical practice (pp. 97–125). Albany, NY: Delmar Publishers.

McGee-Cooper, A. (1992). *You don't have to go home from work exhausted!* New York: Bantam Books.

Pasek, P. B., & Schkade, J. K. (1996). Effects of a skiing experience on adolescents with limb deficiencies: An occupational adaptation perspective. *American Journal of Occupational Therapy, 50,* 24–31.

Ross, M. M. (1994, August 11). Applying theory to practice. *OT Week,* 16–17.

Schkade, J. K. (1999). Student to practitioner: the adaptive transition. *Innovations in Occupational Therapy Education,* 147–156.

Schkade, J. K., & McClung, M. (2001). Occupational adaptation in practice: Concepts and cases. Thorofare, NJ: Slack.

Schkade, J. K., & Schultz, S. (1993). Occupational adaptation: An integrative frame of reference. In H. Hopkins, & H. Smith (Eds.), *Willard & Spackman's occupational therapy* (8th ed.). Philadelphia, PA: J.B. Lippincott.

Schkade, J. K., & Schultz, S. (1998). Occupational adaptation: an integrative frame of reference. In M. E. Neistadt, & E. B. Crepeau. (Eds.), *Willard & Spackman's occupational therapy* (9th ed.). Philadelphia, PA: J.B. Lippincott.

Schroeder-Smith, K., Tischenkel, C., DeLange, L., & Lou, J. Q. (2001). Duchenne muscular dystrophy in females: A rare genetic disorder and occupational therapy perspective. *Occupational Therapy in Health Care, 13 (3),* 79–98.

Schultz, S., & Schkade, J. K. (1994). Home health care: A window of opportunity to synthesize practice. *Home & Community Health, Special Interest Section Newsletter, American Occupational Therapy Association, 1,* 1–4.

Werner, E. (2000). Families, children with autism and everyday occupations. Unpublished dissertation. Nova Southeastern University, Fort Lauderdale, FL.

8

Ecological Model of Occupation

Winnie Dunn, Catana Brown, and Mary Jane Youngstrom

OBJECTIVES

This chapter will help you to:

- Discuss the relationship and interaction of the four constructs of the Ecological Model of Human Performance.
- Differentiate among the five intervention strategies by discussing the focus in terms of single or multiple constructs.
- Explain the assumptions underlying the Ecological Model of Human Performance.
- Apply the Ecological Model of Human Performance to practice situations.
- Discover the suitability of the Ecological Model of Human Performance to research.

⌐ABOUT THE AUTHORS

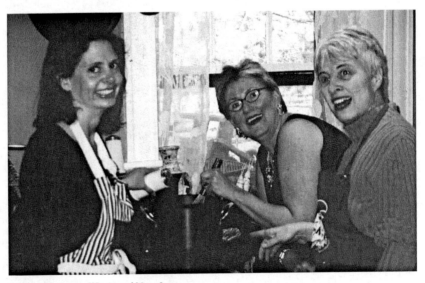

Left to right: Catana, Winnie, and Mary Jane.

"So, what are we going to put into this thing?"

"Oh, I don't know, what do you think will be palatable for our guests?"

"I am tired of serving up the same things over and over again."

"We surely have to provide something familiar at the base of it all, but I would sure like to offer some new ingredients..."

"More things are ripe now than ever before; let's take advantage of that!"

"Yeah, and I think we have some recipes that we can combine to make great new possibilities for people."

You might think this is a conversation among the sous chefs at an interesting new restaurant. In some ways you would not be far from the truth, because we really like to cook, so analogies to cooking always surface in our thinking. Actually, this is how we began our negotiations to construct this chapter. We loved our topic and were happy for it to be on the menu with the other topics, yet we wanted to "kick it up a notch."

This conversation also illustrates our different and complementary styles of approaching tasks like cooking . . . and writing.

Mary Jane is our "stock chef." She keeps the base knowledge simmering and enriching itself with the time that inevitably passes. She cherishes this base ingredient as the necessary starting point for all our tasks. The stock of this chapter resides in the core concepts of the Ecological Model of Human Performance framework, consistency of terminology across old and new sections, and the transitions that hold the material together. Many times the stock is "transparent" to the more recently added ingredients, and yet the maturity of these ideas (the stock) enables the newer thoughts to add interest and texture to this rich base.

Tana is our "ingredient chef." She has cooked (written) long enough to know what goes well together, so she can select and gather knowledge from many other disciplines to inform us about how our core ideas might be expanded, enhanced, and/or reinterpreted. The mix of ingredients for this chapter emerges as the underlying assumptions, background interdisciplinary literature, and the types of examples we selected to represent an inclusive picture. The new ingredients add texture, flavor, and aroma to an already great recipe.

Winnie is our "presentation chef." She has a knack for knowing how an audience can receive the meal so it will be memorable for a long time to come. She sees what will make all the ingredients be noticeable in their own right, while also making sure they complement each other. She adds new ingredients that enrich the meal and connect flavors in a complementary manner. Within this chapter, these skills emerge as the examples of both research and practice, stories illustrating application of concepts, tables, and other embellishments that make the material digestible.

We love to cook.
We love to write.... [arghh]...
We really love LIVING for ourselves and all those we serve...
And, we are confident you will be back for many servings of these great ideas.

INTRODUCTION

The Ecology of Human Performance framework is built around the major constructs of person, context, task, and performance. Although all four constructs are equally important, the model highlights context because it is often neglected in occupational therapy practice as well as many other human service professions and programs. For example, if you consider the assessments commonly used in occupational therapy practice, you will find a number of measures that focus on task performance; even more measuring a person's skills, abilities, interests, and experiences; but few that target the environment or context. A primary purpose of the Ecology of Human Performance is to provide a framework that emphasizes the essential role of context in task performance. This does not mean that the role of the person is de-emphasized, but that the relative importance of person and context factors is considered for each particular task performance.

When all the characteristics of each individual person, context, and task are recognized and appreciated, it underscores the uniqueness of any performance circumstance. No two people can have the exact same task performance because of the sheer complexity of people and environments. Regard for the uniqueness of the individual and the situation is consistent with a client-centered approach. It moves the focus away from the service provider's perspective to that of the service recipient. Consequently, a fundamental value of the Ecology of Human Performance asserts that intervention is directed by what the person wants and/or needs.

Another benefit of greater attention to context is that it expands intervention options. The Ecology of Human Performance outlines five intervention approaches: establish/restore, adapt/modify, alter, prevent, and create. The term intervention rather than therapy is used because therapy tends to imply remediation and illness. Only the establish/restore intervention is aimed exclusively at making changes in the person (remediation). Adapt/modify and alter interventions target the context and task, while prevent and create can address the person, context, or task but take place before a problem occurs or when no problem exists. This expansion of intervention options moves service providers away from a concentration on "fixing" the person to one of considering the totality of the situation. The five intervention options also support an expansion into a wider range of service models, including settings that utilize community-based, consumer-driven, and health promotion values and practices.

Originally conceived by the faculty of the Occupational Therapy Education Department at the University of Kansas Medical Center, the Ecology of Human Performance framework serves as an organizing structure for the department's curriculum, research, and service activities. We are not alone in our zeal for increased attention and thoroughness related to the construct of context; in fact, contemporary conceptual models in occupational therapy have clearly placed a heavier emphasis on context. Occupational Adaptation (Schkade & Schultz, 1992) advocates a holistic approach giving equal importance to the person, the occupational environment, and the interaction of the two. Context is incorporated in Nelson's (1996) view of Therapeutic Occupation through the construct of occupational form, which consists of the physical and sociocultural circumstances outside the person. The Person-Environment Occupational Performance Model of Christiansen & Baum (1997a) and the Person-Environment Occupation Model (Law et al., 1996) are the most similar to the Ecology of Human Performance as all three are built around the constructs of person and environment as related to performance. One difference between the Ecology of Human Performance and the other two models lies in the terminology surrounding occupation and task. Both the Person-Environment Occupational Performance Model and the Person-Environment Occupation Model highlight occupation and indicate that occupations subsume tasks. On the other hand, and perhaps surprising to occupational therapists, the Ecology of Human Performance does not use occupation as a major construct.

Much of the decision around terminology was based on the intended purpose of the Ecology of Human Performance. The Ecology of Human Performance is not designed as a framework exclusively for occupational therapy, but is intended for use by other disciplines as well as a means to facilitate interdisciplinary collaboration. The term "task" is more accessible to individuals outside of occupational therapy because it is familiar and common in everyday language. This decision has resulted in our desired outcome: The Ecology of Human Performance has been used in the work of other disciplines and has served as the basis for several collaborative projects. For example, the Ecology of Human Performance served as the primary framework for special educators to develop funded programs to support individuals with disabilities in adult education and welfare-to-work programs. The Ecology of Human Performance framework provided a structure for designing interventions in these projects. In another example, a center on aging utilized the Ecology of Human Performance to structure the interdisciplinary development of an environmental assessment for stroke research.

Our use of the term "task" does not negate our appreciation for the construct of occupation. In the Ecology of Human Performance, tasks are objective representations of the universe of all possible activities. In the occupational therapy literature, definitions of occupation include the importance of meaningfulness to the person (Christiansen & Baum, 1997b; Clark et al., 1991; Nelson, 1996). Although not explicitly stated previously, in the Ecology of Human Performance framework, occupations exist when the person and context factors come together to give meaning to tasks. The next section will provide definitions and examples for the Ecology of Human Performance constructs and explain the structure of the framework. This is followed by a discussion of the assumptions underlying the framework. The chapter then focuses on applying the Ecology of Human Performance Framework, with a section on application to practice and a section on application to research.

Core Constructs

The Ecology of Human Performance is a framework for considering the relationships among person, task, and context and how the dynamic interactions between these three impact performance. Definitions for each of these four constructs (person, task, context, and performance) are outlined in Table 8-1.

Person

The Ecology of Human Performance is an individually focused, client-centered framework. Individuals are seen as unique and complex. The person brings a unique set of variables including past experiences, personal values/interests, as well as sensorimotor, cognitive, and psychosocial skills. These specific personal values, interests and experiences, and unique ability/skill sets are called person variables. The person variables that an individual brings to tasks influence the tasks that are chosen and the quality of the task performance. The person is also continually surrounded by his or her context and influenced by it. Context may influence the person's interests and choices and may support or inhibit the person's ability to use his or her skills and abilities.

Task

Tasks are objective sets of behaviors that are combined to allow an individual to engage in performance that accomplishes a goal. For example, when a person wants to brush his or her teeth he or she reaches for the toothpaste, unscrews the cap, reaches for the toothbrush, squeezes paste onto brush, etc. These behaviors may be observed, and carrying them out allows the person to reach a goal. The specific behaviors required are determined by the demands of the task. An unlimited number of tasks exists in which a person might engage. However, ability to access tasks will be determined by the person's variables (skills, abilities, interests) and the availability of the tasks within the person's current context.

Table 8-1 **DEFINITIONS OF CORE CONSTRUCTS**

Person: An individual with a unique configuration of abilities, experiences, and sensori-motor, cognitive, and psychosocial skills
  • Persons are unique and complex; therefore, precise predictability about their performance is impossible
  • The meaning a person attaches to task and contextual variables strongly influences performance

Task: An objective set of behaviors necessary to accomplish a goal
  • An infinite variety of tasks exists around every person
  • Constellations of tasks form a person's roles and occupations
  • Tasks are defined differently by different people, and their meaning and performance are influenced by cultural context

Context: A set of interrelated conditions that surrounds a person
  • Temporal contexts (Note: Although temporal aspects of context are determined by the person, they become contextual due to the social and cultural meaning attached to the temporal features):
    1. Chronological: individual's age
    2. Developmental: stage or phase of maturation
    3. Life cycle: place in important life phases, such as career cycle, parenting cycle, educational process
    4. Health status: place in continuum of disability, such as acuteness of injury, chronicity of disability, or terminal nature of illness

Performance: Both the process and the result of the person interacting with context to engage in tasks
  • The performance range is determined by the interaction between the person and the context
  • Performance in natural contexts is different than performance in contrived contexts (ecological validity, Bronfenbrenner, 1979)

Tasks can be categorized at different levels and organized in different ways. On one level, tasks can be conceived of as a large set of behaviors that lead to the accomplishment of an end-goal (i.e., all the behaviors that a person engages in to complete the laundry) or on a smaller level as sets of behaviors that lead to accomplishment of a sub-goal in the larger task (i.e., all the behaviors a person carries out to fold a tee-shirt and put it away). Tasks may also be organized into specific constellations that form a person's roles. Occupational therapists might also understand a specific constellation of tasks as being organized into an occupation — a set of chosen and meaningful tasks in which the person wants and needs to engage.

Context

Context refers to the set of interrelated conditions that surround the person. Two primary types of context are defined. Temporal context includes the aspects of chronological age, developmental stage, life cycle, and health status. Although these conditions reside within the person, they are considered contextual because of the social and cultural meanings attached to them. Environment is the second primary type of context and is composed of physical, social, and cultural dimensions. All these dimensions operate external to the person but at the same time continually influence the person's options and actions. The Ecology of Human Performance framework posits that the interaction between the person and the context (temporal and environment) affects human behavior and performance. Accordingly, in the Ecology of Human Performance model, performance cannot be understood outside of context.

Contexts provide a variety of supports and barriers to performance. These include things such as availability of materials and objects needed to engage in tasks (i.e., a pencil to write with, a car to drive), availability of other people required to perform certain activities or to support a person's performance (i.e., two teams of players needed to play baseball, a teacher to provide feedback to a student), and expectations and norms that guide performance (arriving on time for an appointment, dressing a certain way to go to church). These aspects of the context are called context variables. Context variables are important features that must be considered when understanding performance because they may facilitate or hinder performance.

Performance

Performance occurs when a person acts to engage in tasks within a context. Persons use their skills and abilities to "look through" the context and select the tasks they want and need to do. Performance range, or the number and types of tasks available to the person, is determined by the interaction between the person's variables (their skills, abilities, and motivations) and the context variables (the supports and barriers).

Interactions and Relationship Between the Constructs

The visual depictions that follow are provided to help the learner characterize the constructs of the Ecology of Human Performance framework and to more clearly visualize how the constructs in the framework interact.

Figure 8-1 illustrates how the person is surrounded by and embedded within the context. The person construct includes the individuals' abilities and skills in sensorimotor, cognitive, and psychosocial areas as well as the person's past interests and experiences. The circle surrounding the person is the context. As the picture illustrates, the person and the context are a composite. It has limited meaning to consider one without the other.

Neither the person variables nor the context variables are fixed. The person's variables are continually changing every time the individual has a new experience. He or she may gain skills or potentially lose a skill due to illness or stress. Likewise, persons change their context whenever they go from home to work, develop a new friendship, or change clothes. Context changes with the passage of time as well. For example, morning turns into evening, a stop sign is added at an intersection you cross everyday, or a new boss may be hired at your place of work.

The capital "T"s in the picture signify the many tasks that surround the person and the context. The entire universe of tasks exists for each person. However, it is the person and contextual features *together* that determine which tasks are accessible and feasible for any individual. For example, the task of making homemade noodles exists for everyone. However, whether a person performs this task depends on many factors such as prior experience making noodles; a fair degree of fine motor, visual perceptual and tactile skills; cultural background that values homemade noodles; the availability of certain ingredients and tools; and possibly a special occasion or guests for dinner to promote the motivations or desire to make the noodles.

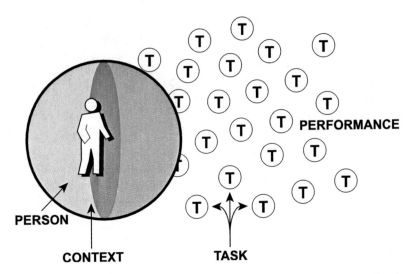

Figure 8-1. Schema for the Ecology of Human Performance framework. Persons are embedded in their contexts. An infinite variety of tasks exists around every person. Performance occurs as a result of the person interacting with context to engage in tasks. (Reprinted with permission from Dunn, W., Brown, C., & McGuigan, A. (1994). The ecology of human performance: A framework for considering the effect of context. *American Journal of Occupational Therapy, 48,* 595–607.)

Figure 8-2 depicts a typical person within the Ecology of Human Performance framework. In this illustration a typical person's performance range is depicted by the megaphone-shaped figure that extends from the person through the context to reach out and encompass a specific constellation of tasks. The tasks within the performance range are those that are available to the person based on his or her skills and abilities and the context supports. The performance range includes those tasks that are meaningful and pur-

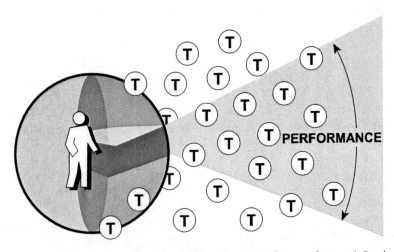

Figure 8-2. Schema of a typical person within the Ecology of Human Performance framework. People use their skills and abilities to "look through" the context at the tasks they need or want to do. People derive meaning from this process. Performance range is the configuration of tasks that people execute. (Reprinted with permission from Dunn, W., Brown, C., & McGuigan, A. (1994). The ecology of human performance: A framework for considering the effect of context. *American Journal of Occupational Therapy, 48,* 595–607.)

poseful to the person. In fact, it is the interaction that occurs between the context and the person that allows the person to derive meaning from the task. For example, baking a cake has a different meaning for a parent making a child's birthday cake than a baker making a cake to sell. The temporal context (in this case the individual's role within the life cycle) influences the meaning that is derived from the task.

Figure 8-3 illustrates how the variety of tasks available in a person's performance range may be organized into a variety of roles. Tasks may overlap into several roles as illustrated in the picture. Just as each person and each context are unique, so are roles. For example, the tasks that comprise the role of parent for a woman who has an infant and a preschooler will be very different from the tasks of a single parent with a teenager or an older woman with five married children. The role is defined for that person within a particular context.

Figures 8-4 and 8-5 depict how performance range may be narrowed when either the person or the context are limited.

Figure 8-4 depicts a narrower performance range because the person's skills and abilities are limited. Although the context is still supportive and varied, the individual is unable to take advantage of the context for as many tasks. The person, due to limitations in his or her capacities, may not be aware of the supports offered by the context or may not have the personal skills and abilities to engage in performance. For example, the person with poor social skills may not recognize opportunities to engage in conversation while in the checkout line at the grocery store. An individual with decreased vision due to macular degeneration may have trouble reading the mail even though the print is large and the lighting is adequate.

Figure 8-5 illustrates how performance range is affected when the context becomes more limited. In this case, the person possesses adequate skills and abilities, but the contextual resources needed to perform are not available. For example, a plumber may be

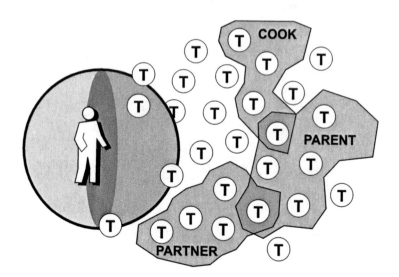

Figure 8-3. Illustration of roles in the Ecology of Human Performance framework. Life roles are a constellation of tasks. People have many roles; some tasks fall into more than one role. These role configurations are unique for each person. (Reprinted with permission from Dunn, W., Brown, C., & McGuigan, A. (1994). The ecology of human performance: A framework for considering the effect of context. *American Journal of Occupational Therapy, 48,* 595–607.)

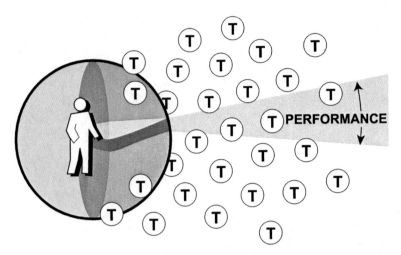

Figure 8-4. Schema of a person with limited skills and abilities within the Ecology of Human Performance framework. Although context is still useful, the person has fewer skills and abilities to "look through" context and derive meaning. This limits the person's performance range. (Reprinted with permission from Dunn, W., Brown, C., & McGuigan, A. (1994). The ecology of human performance: A framework for considering the effect of context. *American Journal of Occupational Therapy, 48,* 595–607.)

unable to fix a leak because he does not have the proper-size wrench. A talented young figure skater may be unable to practice his skill because his parents have moved to Panama.

Individuals with disabilities are faced with a narrower performance range, as illustrated in Figure 8-4. However, their performance is often also impacted by an inadequate context, as illustrated in Figure 8-5. Social attitudes toward disability may place contextual limitations on individuals. They may be ignored in social situations or not invited to

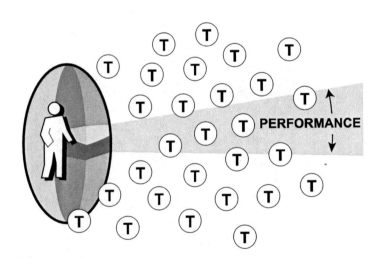

Figure 8-5. Schema of a limited context within the Ecology of Human Performance framework. The person has adequate skills and abilities, but the context does not provide the resources needed to perform. In this situation, performance range is limited. (Reprinted with permission from Dunn, W., Brown, C., & McGuigan, A. (1994). The ecology of human performance: A framework for considering the effect of context. *American Journal of Occupational Therapy, 48,* 595–607.)

participate in community activities. Physical barriers within the environment may also preclude participation (i.e., lack of accessible public transportation for wheelchair users). An appreciation of the interaction between the person and the context is doubly important when planning interventions for those with disabilities. The person variables often cannot be changed, but the context variables can be a prime target for intervention action.

Intervention Strategies

The Ecology of Human Performance framework describes five therapeutic intervention strategies that address the complexity of the person/context/task relationship. Figure 8-6 names the five strategies and points out the variable targets for each intervention. Intervention may be aimed at the person, the context, the task, or in many cases a combination. The ultimate goal of each intervention strategy is to support the performance needs of the individual.

Establish/Restore

In this intervention strategy, the therapist directs intervention efforts at the person's variables and aims to improve the person's skills. The therapist may be facilitating the "establishment" of skills that have not been previously learned, as in the case of a young child who is learning to recognize colors, or the therapist may be intervening to "restore" skills that have been lost due to illness or injury, such as when working with a stroke patient to restore coordination needed to eat.

Although this intervention strategy is targeted at the person's skills, the context in which performance occurs is not ignored. Context features will determine the availability of tasks (i.e., does the young child have other children in his neighborhood with whom he can play), provide supports for performance (i.e., are there grab bars by the toilet), and

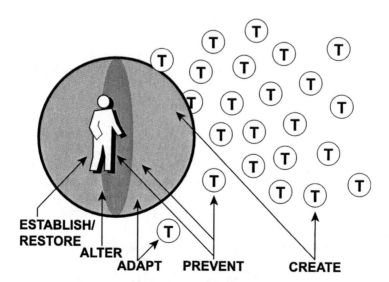

Figure 8-6. Illustration of therapeutic interventions within the Ecology of Human Performance framework. The arrows indicate the variables that are affected by each intervention. (Reprinted with permission from Dunn, W., Brown, C., & McGuigan, A. (1994). The ecology of human performance: A framework for considering the effect of context. *American Journal of Occupational Therapy, 48,* 595–607.)

feedback about performance necessary to learn (i.e., is a caregiver available to provide necessary cues).

Alter

In using this intervention strategy, the therapist focuses on the context in which the person performs. Interventions are aimed at altering the actual context in which tasks occur. An attempt is made to find the best match between the person's current skills and abilities and the context options that are available. For example, persons with substance abuse problems may alter their social contexts (i.e., the friends with whom they socialize) to those that are more supportive of abstinence. An individual with mobility and endurance problems may need to move from a two-story house to a ground floor apartment.

Adapt/Modify

This intervention strategy is applied when modifying the context for performance or the task features of a selected task. The therapist who teaches a one-handed person how to tie shoes by using a one-handed bow-tying method would be adapting or modifying a task feature (i.e., the task method). Modifying the shoe-tying task by providing elastic shoelaces would be another approach (i.e., modification of the objects used in performing the task). This strategy is the one selected when practitioners adapt the environment to support performance. An individual who is experiencing memory loss would benefit by adapting/modifying the environment by placing labels on dresser drawers and cabinets which provided cues about their contents.

Prevent

The aim of this intervention strategy is to preclude the development of performance problems. Therapists using this strategy influence the course of events by changing person, context, or task variables in order to prevent negative outcomes. Examples include providing information to family members about how to manage the symptoms of a family member with mental illness and teaching warehouse workers proper lifting techniques to use in carrying boxes.

Create

This intervention strategy is focused on creating circumstances that support optimal performance for all persons and populations. In contrast to the prevent strategy, the create strategy does not assume that a disability problem exists or is likely to occur. Create strategies maximize performance by targeting person, context, and/or task variables. Providing a stimulating and varied play program in a day care setting for children would be an example of a create strategy. Physical environments that employ principles of universal design promote optimal performance for disabled and non-disabled persons alike.

The five intervention strategies help us to understand more clearly the complex relationship that exists between the person, the context, and the tasks in which people engage. The strategies provide therapists with a comprehensive view of intervention options and help them to recognize that the best intervention occurs when the relationship between context and person is carefully considered.

Tables 8-2 through 8-5 further elaborate the components of context. In the evaluation process, the occupational therapist should identify which aspects of context are most salient for a particular task situation and conduct a thorough assessment of the relevant context features. Likewise, in the intervention planning process, the occupational therapist should consider which context features can be adapted or altered to enhance performance. The tables provide a checklist format to prompt the therapist to think about the contextual features of the temporal, physical, social, and cultural environments.

ASSUMPTIONS UNDERLYING THE ECOLOGY OF HUMAN PERFORMANCE FRAMEWORK

Persons and Their Contexts Are Unique and Dynamic

1. *It is impossible to understand the person without also understanding the person's context.* The complexity and uniqueness of the person's situation is not fully realized without an awareness of context. Knowledge relates to the person's culture, social support system, physical environment, and temporal factors increases the therapist's ability to plan relevant and effective interventions. When occupational therapists focus on the person's physical, social, and psychological limitations, the disability defines the person. However, when professionals include the person's context as a relevant factor, the boundaries between persons with and without disabilities fade.

2. *Persons influence contexts and contexts influence persons.* The person-context transaction is dynamic. The same person acts differently in different contexts, while different persons attribute different meanings to the same context. Furthermore, as a person acts within a context, the context changes. Think about moving into a new house. The physical properties of the house provide certain opportunities and limitations for the person, while the person has the opportunity to act on these physical properties to create a particular living situation. Performance can be enhanced by interventions directed at the person, context, or task.

Table 8-2 **TEMPORAL ENVIRONMENT CHECKLIST**

Temporal Environment

Temporal features of the person (becomes a contextual feature when the environment imposes expectations associated with temporal characteristics)
- Chronological age — consider benchmark ages as they relate to life tasks (e.g., driving, voting, drinking, social security eligibility)
- Developmental stage
- Life cycle — important life phases (e.g., career path, parenting cycle)
- Health status — includes the course of the illness, injury, or disability and where the person is in that course

Temporal features of the task
- Sequential structure — order of the steps of the task
- Duration — how long the task lasts
- Temporal location — when the task takes place (e.g., season, day of the week, time of day)
- Rate of recurrence — how often the task takes place
- Temporal rigidity — how flexible or rigid are the temporal features of the task (e.g., can the steps of the task be rearranged)

Table 8-3 **PHYSICAL ENVIRONMENT CHECKLIST**

Physical Environment

Components of the physical environment
- Objects
- Terrain
- Built environment — home, neighborhood, community
- Natural environment — includes plants and animals
- Weather

Areas to consider in determining physical accessibility of a space — both whether the person can get to the particular environmental feature and, once the person gets there, whether he or she can use it must be considered (e.g., a standard drinking fountain may be too high for a wheelchair user, while a person with limited hand strength may be unable to turn the knob)

- Parking
- Pathways/aisles
- Ground surface
- Curb cuts
- Ramps
- Entrances
- Telephone
- Drinking fountains
- Stairs/elevators
- Alarm systems
- Bathrooms
- Counters
- Kitchens
- Dining areas

Characteristics of the physical environment
- Object use requirements — performance component requirements involved in use of an object (e.g., dexterity, strength, endurance, visual acuity)
- Availability — includes convenience, suitability, and accessibility of objects and settings
- Cultural symbols — inclusion or exclusion of representation of beliefs and values, consistency of symbols with a person's cultural background
- Size features — includes distances between and within settings, use of space, size of objects
- Stimulus/arousal — sensory properties of the physical environment that induce calm or arousal
- Ambiance — use of color, light, objects, etc. to create a mood (e.g., serious, irreverent, homey, rushed)
- Complexity — includes use of cues, orderliness, cognitive demands, efficiency
- Appearance — care and décor of the physical environment that suggest qualities like apathy, opulence, limited resources
- Degree of familiarity — predictability versus novelty

3. *A person's performance range is determined by the transaction between the person and the context.* Experienced therapists recognize that the performance range for persons with similar disabilities can be very different. When two people have a spinal cord injury at the same vertebrae level, one person may get back to work and another may not. The role of worker may be more developmentally salient for one individual, or the social support of the work setting makes the difference. Perhaps the availability of accessible public transportation or financial resources may be a factor. Person factors such as education, work skills, and physical and psychological functioning are also important. Our predictions and consequently our interventions are best when we have a broad knowledge of the person and the context.

4. *It is through engagement in tasks that persons and contexts transact.* The relationship between the person and the context becomes transactional as the person engages in tasks. Sometimes engagement in tasks serves to maintain the person and/or context, when other times the result is a change in the person or context. In

Table 8-4 **CULTURAL ENVIRONMENT CHECKLIST**

Cultural Environment

Cultural associations (groups that contribute to an individual's sense of identity)
- Ethnic
- Social class
- Religious
- Political
- Geographic — e.g., region of the country, rural versus urban
- Age/generation
- Gender
- Sexual orientation
- Schools/clubs/organizations
- Work/career/profession

Ways that culture is expressed
- Beliefs and values — as they relate to a person's world view
- Customs and traditions — include rituals, dress, celebrations, rights of passage, food and eating habits
- Language — verbal and nonverbal communication
- Symbols — physical representations of a cultural group
- Lifestyles — expectations related to gender roles, living arrangements, family, education, work
- Behavior patterns/norms/attitudes — e.g., time orientation, interaction patterns, personal responsibility

one situation a person's participation in a religious service may serve to validate a belief system, while another time a religious service may be a life-changing event. Conversely, the service can be changed by those participating.

Meal preparation is a familiar yet powerful example of the transforming qualities of engagement in tasks. A person puts ingredients together and cooks them so that the food is transformed into a meal. The process of preparing and serving food connects the individuals that share the meal while providing physical sustenance. Meals often have additional purposes as symbols sustaining culture and family. Occupational therapy appreciates the richness of daily activities and uses engagement in tasks as the transforming medium.

Contrived Contexts Are Different from Natural Contexts

1. *When compared to natural environments, contrived contexts may either facilitate or inhibit performance.* Occupational therapy assessments and interventions often occur in contrived contexts, yet performance in contrived contexts may not be the same as performance in natural environments. Performance may be enhanced in the contrived setting because distractions are reduced, positive social support is provided, or the task is simplified. Performance may be inhibited in contrived settings because the environment is unfamiliar or naturally occurring supports are eliminated.

2. *Assessment and intervention best approximate the person's true performance when enacted in natural environments.* The advancement of home-health, school-based, and community-based interventions indicates that occupational therapists are increasingly sensitive to this assumption. Despite the superiority of the natural

Table 8-5 **SOCIAL ENVIRONMENT CHECKLIST**

Social Environment

Microsocietal factors
- Family
- Friends/acquaintances
- Pets
- Neighbors
- Coworkers/colleagues/supervisors
- Caregivers
- Service providers/recipients
- Churches
- Clubs/community organizations

Macrosocietal factors
- Government/political systems — policy and lawmaking groups, political movements
- Economic organizations — includes availability of jobs, social assistance programs, and insurance
- Health services — hospitals, community health centers, private practices, alternative health care agencies/providers
- Social service organizations — governmental and charitable groups
- Educational services — public and private schools and universities, professional and technical education
- Businesses and business group
- Professional organizations

Types of social support
- Practical or instrumental — e.g. transportation, baby sitting, financial
- Informational — sharing knowledge, experience, advice, or guidance
- Emotional — providing support and encouragement

environment for assessment and intervention, there are situations in which this is not realistic. However, when conducting assessments and intervention in a contrived setting, an awareness of the discrepancy with the natural environment is crucial.

Occupational Therapy Practice Involves Promoting Self-determination and Inclusion of Persons with Disabilities in All Aspects of Society.

1. *The occupational therapy process begins when the person served and/or family of the person served identifies what the person wants or needs.* Consistent with consumer-oriented philosophy, this assumption indicates that the person served is the primary decision-maker in the therapeutic process. When the person served sets the priorities by identifying his or her own wants and needs, the person is validated, and involvement in therapy is much more likely to occur. This process includes interventions that promote self-advocacy so that the person served becomes empowered to champion his or her wants and needs in all situations.

2. *Occupational therapy practice includes making changes in systems so that persons with disabilities receive the full rights and privileges they are due.* As a profession that promotes successful and satisfying independent living for persons with disabilities, occupational therapists must be leaders in affecting changes in communities, organizations, businesses, and governments. Occupational therapists can provide information about disabilities to dispel myths or mistaken concerns and play an important role in adapting and altering environments to promote

inclusion. Advocating for individuals with disabilities includes education, confrontation, and involvement at a policy level to eliminate discriminatory practices.

Independence Means Meeting Your Wants and Needs

1. *The use of assistive devices or other persons does not mean a person is dependent.* Everyone uses assistive devices and other persons to meet wants and needs. When persons without disability use written reminders or hire a housekeeper, they are seen as resourceful. There is a tendency to judge persons with disabilities as less competent and sometimes as less of a person when assistive devices or other persons are involved in performing a skill, yet these persons are really asserting independence. Satisfaction with the process is a component of independence.

2. *Intervention strategies that adapt or alter the environment are not reserved for use only when restorative interventions have failed.* Oftentimes the first inclination in intervention approaches is to "fix" the person by practicing memory skills, improving fine motor skills, teaching communication skills, etc. When the desired outcome is not achieved, environmental adaptations are considered. The Ecology of Human Performance indicates all intervention options should be considered as viable options from the beginning. Modify (adapt) and alter interventions can be more expedient and may result in the best outcomes. For example, helping someone with low endurance reschedule daily activities to spread out tasks that are physically taxing (a modify/adapt option) may allow the individual to continue to meet his or her wants and needs right away, whereas increasing endurance (a restorative intervention) may take weeks. It is crucial that the intervention options be presented to the person served and/or the family for evaluation.

APPLYING THE ECOLOGY OF HUMAN PERFORMANCE FRAMEWORK TO PRACTICE

The Ecology of Human Performance model provides a framework for understanding and articulating the important factors that must be evaluated and outlines five strategies that can guide thinking and decisions about the intervention process.

Embedding the Ecology of Human Performance framework into the evaluation and intervention planning process requires consideration of a number of components. For purposes of explanation, these components have been outlined in a linear sequenced fashion. However, evaluation and intervention with the person in context rarely occurs in a set and sequenced manner. In real life the process is fluid and dynamic. Jumping back and forth between steps may occur. For example, you may be assessing a person's temporal context when you discover the person has just been released from a drug rehabilitation program. The knowledge may prompt you to reassess certain psychosocial performance skills that you may not have previously considered significant. Some steps may overlap and/or occur simultaneously (i.e., you may assess the physical environment and analyze the objects and material used in everyday tasks at the same time). Most importantly, the practitioner must attend to all variables that impact performance (person, task, and context) and realize their interdependence.

The basic steps that are used in applying this framework to the evaluation and intervention planning process in practice are outlined below:

1. Prioritize the individual's/population's wants and needs
   - Identify and prioritize tasks that the person(s) considers most important
   - Include task priorities of significant others and organizations or systems that interface with the person(s)
2. Analyze prioritized tasks
   - Analyze a task to understand its skill requirements and demands
3. Evaluate performance
   - Understand how the task is performed differently by this person(s) and what contributes to difficulty of performance
   - Understand how this person(s) views proficiency. What is the acceptable level of performance for this person?
4. Evaluate the contexts
   - Understand the contextual features of the client's situation
   - Identify the contexts in which prioritized tasks occur
5. Evaluate the person/population variables
   - Specifically assess the person variables which hinder and support performance in prioritized areas or tasks
6. Develop goals and choose intervention strategies for identified priorities
7. Evaluate the person/task/context match and select achievable goals and reasonable intervention strategies

The case studies that follow use this process to illustrate how the Ecology of Human Performance framework may be applied in practice. Consider these three examples:

Anthony: **Case Study 8-1**

Anthony is a 10-year-old boy who is in the fourth grade. He attends school in a suburban community that has a large network of special education services. Anthony just moved to this district from another, more rural school. All the children and teachers knew him, understood his idiosyncratic social behaviors, and could make adaptations to support him throughout the day. His parents and Anthony are worried that in this bigger school district, teachers and students will view Anthony negatively and isolate him at a time when he has a strong desire to be part of his peer group. Table 8-6 provides a summary of the priorities that Anthony and his parents have for him as he enters this new school (Step 1 in the application process).

Table 8-7 provides a summary of the data from contextual assessment of his former school, illustrating some of the potentially relevant factors for consideration in planning for Anthony's successful participation in the new classroom. When conducting a contextual assessment, we do not always know which of the contextual factors will support or create barriers for a child; however, by taking note of the factors, the team and Anthony can consider them in planning (Steps 3 and 4).

When applying the Ecology of Human Performance model, the therapist would discuss Anthony's abilities and needs with teachers, parents, and would observe Anthony in several settings (Steps 3 and 5). Table 8-8 summarizes the impressions about Anthony's performance demands. The therapist might also conduct a task analysis on key activities; we provide an example in Table 8-9 for riding the bus (Step 2). The therapist would use all this information and other data from evaluations to generate a number of possible intervention strategies to offer at the team meeting. An example of a list a therapist might generate is provided in Table 8-10 (Step 6).

(continued on page 241)

Table 8-6 **ANTHONY AND HIS PARENTS' PRIORITIES (STEP 1)**

Areas of Occupational Performance	Occupational Performance Issues	Priorities Rated in Order of Importance
Activities of daily living	Being accepted for his idiosyncrasies during the routines of the day/ receiving support and not criticism	1
Work/productivity	Finding where his skills fit in with other children so he can partici- pate and learn	2
Play/leisure	Having friends in his new school	3

Table 8-7 **CONTEXT DATA WORKSHEET FROM FORMER SCHOOL/ COMMUNITY (I.E., BEFORE MOVING)**

	Code[a]
Name: Anthony	
Physical	
• Anthony lived in a small, rural community	c
• His home was located on 4 acres with a pond	?
• He attended the only elementary school in his community, a school with 12 classrooms from kindergarten through fifth grade	c
Social	
• Everyone at school, from the maintenance person to the cooks, knew Anthony	c
• Anthony's mother has part-time employment to regulate Anthony's after school activities	?
• Anthony wants to function in a regular fourth grade classroom	c
• Anthony has one sibling, a 16-year-old brother, who vacillates on living with a brother who is "weird"	?
Cultural	
• Anthony's small rural community had little diversity	?
• The community where Anthony lived values athletic and leadership skills and family involvement in children's activities	b
• Anthony's grandparents live out of state and keep in touch by e-mail	?
Temporal	
• Anthony is 10 years old	?
• Anthony has a chronic condition that interferes with communication and behavior	b
• He is a fourth grade student who succeeded in his familiar school and classroom	?

[a]c, contributing factor; b, barrier to performance; ?, could be either.

Table 8-8 **DATA SUMMARY WORKSHEET**

Name: Anthony

Tasks: daily routines

Person Variables	Activities of Daily Living	Work/Productive Activity	Play/Leisure
Sensorimotor	Anthony gets dressed more efficiently when there is familiar music playing in the background	Anthony completes an after school schedule that includes homework, feeding the animals, walking the dogs, taking out the trash, and taking out recycled products	Auditory defensiveness interferes with peer interactions in large-group, free-play situations
Cognitive	Anthony is full of precise and accurate information about how daily routines must go; making adjustments can be disruptive	Anthony's interests and need for order both help and interfere with his ability to complete tasks in the classroom; he has difficulty terminating activities and tends to perseverate on most tasks	Anthony has difficulty initiating and terminating activities; this can interfere with peer activities such as joke telling and club activities
Psychosocial	Anthony is very focused on wearing "cool" clothes and sometimes perseverates on particular items as critical	Anthony does not have age-appropriate social engagement skills, which interferes with his interacting with peers	Anthony does not use or interpret facial expressions and therefore misses many nonverbal cues, making him an outsider in peer conversations

Table 8-9 **SUMMARY OF TASK ANALYSIS WORKSHEET**

Name: Anthony	Task: riding the bus
Typical Performance of Task	*Anthony's Performance*
• Get on the bus • Find a seat efficiently • Negotiate seating with peers • Greet peers • Engage with others during the ride • Take turns getting into aisles and off the bus • Screen out sounds of traffic, other children, bus noises • Stay balanced in seat during ride	• Gets on and off bus efficiently • Can greet others but does not know what to do next • Becomes overwhelmed with the noises on and around the bus and gets agitated • Need to observe his reaction to the movement of the bus

The school-based team includes the teachers, principal, occupational therapist, Anthony's parents, and the special educator from Anthony's last school. The fourth grade classroom teacher speaks first and reports that her class is very structured, with the same sequence of subjects daily. The parents have observed in this classroom and comment on strategies that this teacher uses that they believe will be useful for Anthony. For example, the teacher has a visual schedule posted in the room, and she walks over to it to let children know when it will soon be time to transition to the next activity (*this teacher is providing adaptive strategies to support the children in her class to participate; she is not waiting for a child to get lost before redirecting*). The parents tell the team that this will be helpful to Anthony, who otherwise is continuously asking what is coming next. The special educator from Anthony's last school cautions that these methods can also be debilitating for Anthony in that if anything changes in the schedule, he becomes agitated and perseverates on "what is supposed to be happening", unable to move on or be flexible. He suggests that giving Anthony a "heads up" when the schedule will be different, with Post-its on the visual schedule, can mediate this interfering behavior (additional *adaptive* strategies). The parents agree that these are potential difficulties that can be addressed with a prior warning.

The teacher also reports that her classroom is crowded and that Anthony's desk will be placed in a group with three other children. The occupational therapist had reviewed a videotape of Anthony from his last classroom (which the last school team provided) and reported that Anthony was fidgety in his desk and distracted by movement and noise. The team decides to place Anthony's desk next to the back wall facing away from the door and classroom and to move three other students to make a group of four in that space (*altering* the context by using spaces and configurations already available). This position restricts the traffic that would be visible to Anthony, thereby controlling distractibility related to the activity of others in the class while allowing Anthony to turn his desk to face the teacher when there is direct instruction.

The teacher reports that her class is using an accelerated math program. The parents are delighted to hear this because Anthony loves math; they tell the team that he frequently uses math concepts to explain all types of relationships around him. The principal suggests that perhaps Anthony can have a role as a peer or younger student tutor for math, as a way for students to view him positively right away (*prevention* intervention). The special educator and teacher decide they will explore this option when he arrives.

Anthony's parents and familiar neighbors have always provided transportation because Anthony always has had difficulty with noise and motion, making the bus a more challeng-

(continued on page 243)

Table 8-10 **WORKSHEET FOR OUTLINING THERAPEUTIC INTERVENTIONS — SAMPLE INTERVENTION SUGGESTIONS FOR SELECTED PERFORMANCE AREAS FOR ANTHONY**

Performance	Establish/Restore	Alter	Adapt	Prevent	Create
Anthony wants to ride the bus with the neighborhood children	Anthony and his parents will ride the bus route together to familiarize themselves with the process	Parents will bring Anthony to school on days when he has extra materials to carry	Anthony will wear concert ear plugs or his Walkman with music on the bus ride; Anthony will sit in the front of the bus	Anthony will meet the bus driver on several occasions so that this person is familiar to him The family will make sure Anthony gets to know some neighbor children who ride the bus	Not applicable
Anthony needs to complete work without being distracted by movement and noise in the classroom	Expose Anthony to sounds[a] using a Walkman; increase volume slowly over time	Anthony completes seat work in the school library during busy classroom times	The teachers place Anthony's desk next to the back wall to minimize his opportunity to notice moving students	Provide auditory and visual cues regarding class-room schedule to prevent Anthony from becoming agitated and then unable to participate with peers	Not applicable

[a]Try fan noise or soft music.

ing option. However, Anthony has expressed the desire to ride the bus in his new neighborhood; the parents want to honor his request but are nervous. The occupational therapist suggests that she could provide support to make bus transportation a positive experience for Anthony. The parents had said that Anthony rocks in a rocking chair at home to calm himself; the therapist points out that the vibration and starting/stopping of the bus could have a similar effect on Anthony, especially if they could minimize the effects of the noise (e.g., using concert earplugs, sitting at the front, using a walkman on the bus; *adaptive* and alternative strategies). The parents agree to a trial period of sending him to school on the bus. The principal agrees to make arrangements for the bus driver to take Anthony and his parents on the bus to introduce him to the experience of the bus (*prevention*) and to monitor his responses. Because the family's new home is toward the end of the bus route, Anthony will not have to be on the bus very long each day.

Anthony has a priority to develop friendships with peers. The team discusses Anthony's interests and discovers that he is an avid baseball card collector and trader. One of the Scout groups at the school has three other boys who collect cards too, so the teacher agrees to contact the Scout leader about Anthony's participation. With Anthony's propensity for math, his memory for sports statistics is large, and the team feels this will be an asset to developing focused relationships (*prevention*).

Because Anthony is coming to a new school, many suggestions are prevention interventions; he has not demonstrated the maladaptive behaviors at this school. The personnel are working to identify ways to keep Anthony's participation positive and are not waiting for him to struggle to design supports for him. Many of these ideas were adaptive or restorative in the last school, since that was Anthony's first school experience.

What If

What if Anthony was 18 years old rather than 10? The team would have to consider community options, including community college, work, and living possibilities. They might implement an *establish* intervention to support Anthony to develop worker roles. They might *adapt* his study environment so he could complete homework for a college course. The family and other team members might use *alter* interventions to identify an optimal living environment. Finally, Anthony might prevent social isolation from peers through internet interest groups and by joining a social group at his church.

Case Study 8-2: *Ella*

Ella is a 78-year-old African American woman who has developed osteoarthritis that is primarily affecting her right knee and her back. She lives alone in a small two-bedroom house and takes great pride in cultivating the flowers in her backyard. She was recently hospitalized for cardiac arrhythmias and hypertension. She has returned home now but has decreased endurance. Her family and doctor are both concerned about her ability to continue to live alone safely. The instability of her knee joints makes her unsteady at times and she is at risk for falling. The occupational therapist has been consulted to assess Ella's safety and functional ability to carry out her daily routine in her home environment.

The occupational therapist began the evaluation process by interviewing Ella in her home. Ella provided a tour of her house, including the basement laundry area and her beautiful flower garden. Table 8-11 lists the occupational performance issues that were identified and notes which ones Ella considered to be most important to her (Step 1).

(continued)

Table 8-11 **ELLA'S PRIORITIES (STEP 1)**

Areas of Occupational Performance	Occupational Performance Issues	Priorities Rated in Order of Importance
Activities of daily living	Has difficulty in the morning in bending her knees to be able to get her pants on easily	3
Work/productivity	Doing laundry on a regular basis is a problem because both the washer and dryer are in the basement; stair-climbing is painful for her knees and unsafe due to joint dysfunction	1
Play/leisure	Although she refuses to give it up, Ella is finding that working in her garden is presenting problems; she has trouble bending over and getting down on her knees and up again	2

Because doing her laundry was the No. 1 priority for Ella, evaluation and intervention planning focused on this task first. The other priorities were addressed later. Tables 8-12 to 8-15 present the evaluation and intervention process. Table 8-12 outlines a brief comparison of the typical task performance and Ella's current task performance (Steps 2 and 3). Tables 8-13 and 8-14 outline the specific context feature and assessment of person variables that support and/or hinder performance. While performing the task analysis, the practitioner will be analyzing the performance components required by the task and noting which components present problems for Ella and which ones may need to be assessed in more depth. The task's context and process will be observed with an eye toward understanding how the tools, materials, processes, and contexts involved in the task performance support or hinder performance. The information presented in Tables 8-12 to 8-14 was collected by interviewing Ella and by asking her to actually demonstrate how she did her laundry.

Ella's specific ability in various performance components required while doing laundry was assessed by watching her go down the stairs to the basement and go through the motions of doing the laundry. Ella talked about how she typically performed this task and what parts were easier and more difficult for her. Based on this observation of performance, the therapist selected specific performance components that appeared to affect performance. Specifically, range of motion and strength of the major joints and muscle groups involved in this activity were assessed (Step 5).

Based on observations of Ella's performance and discussion with her, the therapist next devised several possible intervention plans (Step 6). The range of possibilities that could improve her performance was discussed with Ella. Three types of intervention strategies were developed. Each strategy could improve Ella's performance in this area (Table 8-15).

In considering all the possibilities, Ella decided to initially install a handrail and add a table to the laundry area. She decided to have her granddaughter come over to help with heavier laundry (sheets and towels) only once a month. She decided to take the other suggestions of moving the washer and dryer or using a Laundromat under advisement and perhaps to consider at some future point.

(continues on page 247)

Table 8-12 **SUMMARY OF TASK ANALYSIS WORKSHEET**

Name: Ella

Task: doing laundry

Typical Performance of Task	Ella's Performance
Requires going up and down stairs while carrying laundry Carrying laundry while using stairs increases risk	Able to do, but balance is challenged during stair descent, and Ella complains of pain Using stairs presents a risk of falling
Requires bending over to pick items off the floor	Ella complains of pain when bending over and also supports herself against the washer as she bends

Table 8-13 **CONTEXT DATA WORKSHEET**

Performance Contexts	Personal Contextual Features
Physical	• Ella lives in a small two-bedroom house with a basement • The laundry area (washer and dryer) is located in the basement • Laundry area consists of washer, dryer, and hanging rod as well as one shelf next to the dryer • A flight of 14 steps leads to the basement; a hand rail is on the right side when descending; no rail exists on the left side
Social	• Ella is widowed • Ella has two grown children; her son lives out of town, and her daughter and two granddaughters live in town; in-town family members visit Ella regularly and are interested in helping her • Ella has close groups of friends from her church whom she sees at least twice a week • She has lived in her neighborhood for more than 40 years and sees her neighbors regularly when she is outside gardening
Cultural	• Ella was raised on a farm and values her connection with the land • Ella is a careful housekeeper and prides herself on her cleanliness • She has lived in the same community for many years and feels attached to it and the people in it
Temporal	• Ella has been independent all her life and as she ages her desire to remain independent remains strong • The changes in her physical condition due to her heart and arthritic problems are causing her to slow down in some of her activities; Ella has learned on her own to pace her major activities thoughout the week

Table 8-14 PERSON VARIABLES WORKSHEET

Name: Ella

Prioritized task: doing laundry

Person Variable	Activities of Daily Living	Work/Productive	Play/Leisure Performance
Sensorimotor		• Complains of pain in back when bending over to pick clothes off the floor • She is unable to squat due to instability in her knees • Goes down stairs slowly, holding onto handrail on right • Somewhat less steady as she ascends stairs, because the rail is on the side of her stronger leg and she has no support for her right side	
Cognitive		• Able to remember all steps of doing laundry and organizes task with no difficulty	
Psychosocial		• Talks about how important it is for her to be able to care of herself	

What If

What if Ella's family lived out of town and she did not have a strong social support network available to provide help? Different intervention options under the adapt/modify strategy would need to be selected. For example, Ella might have to choose a more expensive option of moving the washer and dryer to the garage area. The alter strategy of using the Laundromat might also become a more appealing choice.

What if Ella's sensorimotor performance continues to deteriorate? Ella and her family might have to face a decision about whether she could continue to live independently in her own home. Consideration of moving to a more supported living environment, such as a retirement apartment or assisted living where help was more readily available, might be necessary. In either case the importance of both physical and social context in supporting performance is evident.

Case Study 8-3: *EPLAY*

A world wide web company, EPLAY, has contacted Rhonda Mocher, an occupational therapist in EPLAY's home community. The senior executives in the company want their company to be socially responsible; one of the executives has a nephew who has a developmental disability and so the executives have been made aware of the issues that such families face when planning gifts and other purchases. The executives want to market themselves as "family friendly" for all types of family configurations, including families who have a member with a disability. They want to market "playing" as important for everyone to have a satisfying life. They knew that an occupational therapist would be able to help them, since the one executive's family had been exposed to occupational therapy through their early intervention services. In fact, they got this idea when Rhonda had made the family a Christmas shopping list for the child's second Christmas.

In this population-based example, six steps for providing services within the Ecology of Human Performance framework can be applied.

1. Prioritize EPLAY's wants and needs

  Rhonda first met with the executive whose nephew has a developmental disability to identify her perspective on the situation. They decided it would be good for Rhonda to come to one of their senior executive meetings to listen to everyone's "take" on the "Everybody Needs to EPLAY" initiative. They wanted to find a way to emphasize that playing is important during every phase of life.

  During the meeting, the group made a list of whom they wanted to target with their campaign (see Table 8-16 for summary of priorities). They decided that they wanted to target four groups initially:

  a. Preschool children

  b. Midcareer adults who are parents

  c. Midcareer adults who have a parent to care for

  d. Older adults who are retired

  During the discussion, the group decided that they would prioritize preschoolers and parents first, since their company's offerings were more expansive for these audiences. Their strategic plan included expanding offerings for the other groups.

2. Analyze prioritized tasks

  Rhonda suggested that she and some of the staff members collect some data related to the target groups; the executives agreed. Rhonda and one of the staff members conducted

(continued)

Table 8-15 **WORKSHEET FOR OUTLINING THERAPEUTIC INTERVENTIONS**

Name: Ella   Task: doing laundry

Establish/Restore	Alter	Adapt	Prevent	Create
Provide exercise program designed to increase right knee range of motion and strength and to maintain/increase back range of motion	Do laundry at a Laundromat	Move washer and dryer to garage area to eliminate need for using steps Provide table in laundry area so clothes may be placed there and not have to be on the floor; this would eliminate bending Install a handrail on left side of stairs to provide support for going up stairs Have granddaughter visit once a week and do laundry		

focus groups with parents to find out their perspectives about their roles as midcareer professionals and as parents. They discussed the nature of their schedules, pressures that keep them from playing, what they like to do when they can, and what would help them to do what they want to do for play.

3. Evaluate EPLAY's current performance

They also collected information from the EPLAY website, analyzing the demographic profile of those who had used their services. With this information, Rhonda and the staff could see where gaps might exist in the EPLAY services. One of the EPLAY staff members tracked one potential customer through an EPLAY session; the analysis of this transaction is summarized in Table 8-17.

Table 8-16 **EPLAY PRIORITIES (STEPS 1 AND 2)**

Areas of Occupational Performance	Occupational Performance Issues	Priorities Rated in Order of Importance
Activities of daily living		
Work/ productivity		
Play/leisure	Playing for these groups: • Preschool children • Midcareer adults who are parents • Midcareer adults who have a parent to care for • Older adults who are retired	1 2 3 4

Table 8-17 **SUMMARY OF TASK ANALYSIS WORKSHEET — FOLLOWING A PARENT CUSTOMER THROUGH THE WEB SEARCH AND PURCHASE**

Typical Performance of Task	EPLAY's Customer Performance
Log on to network and search engine	Log on to network and search engine
Search for service/website of interest	Select EPLAY
Select proper website	Enter website
Enter website	Select age/interest parameters for search
"Cruise" around in the website	Narrow search based on queries
Make queries	Reroute self when "dead end" occurs
Locate items of interest	(i.e., no items of interest to user show
Select items	up on list, requiring further explana-
Complete payment sequence	tion for search)
Exit website	Select items to study further
	Select items for purchase
	Complete payment sequence
	Enter shipping information
	Read guarantees and safeguards regard-
	ing product
	Exit website

4. Evaluate the contexts of EPLAY

   In this example, the context is the EPLAY website. The EPLAY staff already completed some follow-up work with EPLAY customers, finding out what made the website easy or hard to use, what other connections/windows would be helpful, and what other offerings they would like to see. Table 8-18 contains information about the website itself as a context in this transaction.

5. Evaluate the "person" variables

   For this population-focused intervention service, the person variables would be the characteristics of the preschoolers and the parents/professionals who are likely to use the EPLAY services. It is important to remember that person variables come into play even when systems are the focus. Rhonda recognized that the company wanted to be responsive to this potentially broadened market and therefore wished to understand the characteristics of the target groups. Rhonda offered her knowledge about developmental milestones and other relevant characteristics of preschoolers and adults in their 30s and 40s. She also looked at the person variables that would be required/matched to some of their key products and services on EPLAY, to create a template for an EPLAY PROFILE for each offering. Table 8-19 contains some of this information for the adult parents.

6. Develop goals and choose intervention strategies for identified priorities

   Rhonda and the EPLAY staff collaborated to design several components that the company could use to launch their "Everybody needs to EPLAY" initiative (Table 8-20).

   a. Create an EPLAY PROFILE for each offering that is part of the database so that users can search by any of the variables and enter their profile into the website, enabling the program to prompt them with items that are a good match; include issues that are likely to come up for families with children who have disabilities

   b. Design a database of quick examples of how to play in small bits of time that will come up on the screen during EPLAY transactions

   c. Include, in pop-up screens, pictures of young children and adults with disabilities using EPLAY products

(continued)

Table 8-18 **CONTEXT DATA WORKSHEET (STEP 4) FOR THE EPLAY WEBSITE AS A MEDIUM TO INTERACT WITH CUSTOMERS**

	Code[a]
Physical	
• The website is windows driven, with questions to prompt each decision	C
• The website is very colorful	?
Social	
• The website prompts the users to provide information about the user's play choices	?
• The website has a feedback "room" where users can see what others have said about products	?
Cultural	
• The website attracts savvy computer users	B?
• The website has interest buttons to direct users to categories of products	C
Temporal	
• The website downloads some pictures slowly, illustrating products	B
• The website has age categories in addition to interest categories	C
• The website has trendy headings, logos, and animations	?

[a]c, contributing factor; b, barrier to performance; ?, could be either.

---

    d. Create ads and public service announcements for selected professional society publications and disability groups to let them know the services available on EPLAY

    e. Contract for trials to test some EPLAY products with target disability groups, so EPLAY can use the data in marketing

    f. Identify jobs that are good matches for people with disabilities in the EPLAY organization and hire such individuals

Rhonda became a regular contractor for EPLAY. She worked with a local university to involve occupational therapy students in testing products with various groups, providing a service and research experience for the students as well as data for EPLAY.

APPLYING ECOLOGY OF HUMAN PERFORMANCE TO RESEARCH

Although the Ecology of Human Performance is well suited to practice, providing a structure for assessment and intervention planning, it is also well suited to applied science research endeavors. Because the constructs are presented using generic language, the ideas in Ecology of Human Performance are easily accessible to colleagues from other disciplines; this provides a mechanism for dialogue about each discipline's perspective on the same constructs while simultaneously enabling researchers to draw all their ideas together into a cohesive whole.

    There are several interdisciplinary examples that illustrate these interactions and outcomes. A group of researchers interested in the outcomes of stroke rehabilitation designed a measure of rehabilitation context based on the Ecology of Human Performance. A team of educators and therapists designed and tested an application of Ecology of Human Performance to support both adult education programs and college teaching. Another team

Table 8-19 **DATA SUMMARY WORKSHEET — INFORMATION ABOUT ADULTS IN THE ROLE OF PARENTS OF PRESCHOOLERS**

Name: EPLAY   Tasks: playing for adults who are parents

Person Variables	Activities of Daily Living	Work/ Productive Activity	Play/Leisure
Sensorimotor			Knows what sensory experiences are pleasurable and which need to be reduced/avoided; can provide this information with appropriate prompting
Cognitive	Has a routine to make activities of daily living efficient	Career development is typically the focus, with attention to problem solving and moving to levels of increasing responsibility	Typically enjoys challenges; brain is mature and capable of handling more complex problems to solve
Psychosocial	May be hurried regarding self, with attention focused on preschooler's activities of daily living support needs	Work colleagues serve as a primary socialization outlet, with work meetings as well as lunch and break conversations providing adult interactions	Is likely to seek combination of: • Solitary experiences (contrasting to intensity of child-focused life) • Experiences that enable parent to participate with child • Adult interaction experiences to meet the need for adult companionship

Table 8-20 **WORKSHEET FOR OUTLINING THERAPEUTIC INTERVENTIONS — SAMPLE INTERVENTION SUGGESTIONS FOR SELECTED PERFORMANCE AREAS FOR EPLAY**

Performance	Establish/Restore	Alter	Adapt	Prevent	Create
Provide universal access to EPLAY products/services	Test some of EPLAY products with target disability groups so they can use data in marketing	Design a database of quick examples of how to play in small bits of time which will come up on the screen during EPLAY transactions	Create an EPLAY PROFILE for each offering that is part of the database, enabling the program to prompt users with items that are a good match; include issues that are likely to come up for families with children who have disabilities		Create ads and public service announcements for selected professional society publications and disability groups to let them know the services available on EPLAY
Create a socially responsible company		Identify jobs that are good matches for people with disabilities in the EPLAY organization and hire such individuals			Include, in pop-up screens, pictures of young children and adults with disabilities using products

used Ecology of Human Performance to design a test of grocery shopping and an effective intervention to teach grocery shopping to persons with severe and persistent mental illness who live in the community. Finally, the Ecology of Human Performance constructs underlie the design and validation of the Sensory Profile measures for infants, toddlers, children, and adults. Each example is discussed separately in the following section.

A Measure of the Impact of Context on Stroke Rehabilitation

In this set of studies, a team consisting of a nurse, occupational therapist, physical therapist, and speech language pathologist used the Ecology of Human Performance model to design and then evaluate the integrity of a measure of contextual variables related to the rehabilitation experience, the *Environmental Independence Interaction Scale* (EIIS). Although rehabilitation literature has long acknowledged the importance of person-environment interactions to positive outcomes (e.g., Gentile, 1972), professionals have continued to emphasize improving a person's skills as a means for improving rehabilitation outcomes. These researchers sought to provide an easy and effective method for capturing contextual factors to facilitate consideration of all factors that might contribute to positive rehabilitation outcomes. Beginning with 85 items, they found that 20 items characterize the context and provide adequate stability as a measure. Table 8-21 provides a list of these items.

In initial studies, families and professionals completed the EIIS about their context and in relation to a particular person in their care. The research team has conducted analyses to identify the integrity of the measure itself, with plans for comparing various settings and the relationships between specific rehabilitation outcomes and the EIIS findings in the future (Teel, Dunn, Jackson, & Duncan, 1997).

Some of the items not included on the final version of the EIIS inquired about the frequency of use of alternate forms of communication (e.g., using gestures, a communication board, picture drawing). Only persons with communication difficulty responded to these items, making them less powerful to the overall picture of context. Other excluded items reflect the general social milieu, describing staff as positive, warm, caring, calm, and polite; it is possible that these are necessary and that families do not consider them part of the rehabilitation outcomes per se. Items about the general physical environment were also omitted from the aggregate scale, including inquiries about temperature, smell, lighting, noise, and cleanliness. Items related to home-like environments were also omitted (Teel, Dunn, Jackson, & Duncan, in preparation).

The most striking feature of the items included in the aggregate scale is that they all reflect an active process of implementing the belief that participation is critical to positive rehabilitation outcomes and active participation (Teel et al., in preparation). Factor analysis did not reveal distinct features of context as Ecology of Human Performance describes (i.e., physical, social, cultural, temporal); items from each group loaded together across the four-factor solution. The authors hypothesize that it may be important to consider the context as a collective construct when studying person-context effects in future studies; the EIIS provides a tool for such studies.

Supports for Adult Education

Another team of researchers (educators, special educators, occupational therapists) used Ecology of Human Performance as the theoretical model in a series of research and demonstration projects aimed at designing effective supports for adult basic education,

Table 8-21 **ENVIRONMENT-INDEPENDENCE INTERACTION SCALE (EIIS)**

How well do each of the following statements describe the attitudes, care practices, or features of the rehabilitation program that provides treatment to the individual?
The term "the individual" refers to the person who is receiving rehabilitation services.

Please use the following response categories when you answer these questions.

Not at all	= 1
A Little	= 2
Somewhat	= 3
Quite a Bit	= 4
A Great Deal	= 5

	Not at all (1)	A Little (2)	Somewhat (3)	Quite a Bit (4)	A Great Deal (5)
1. The environment motivates and reinforces the individual to function by himself/herself					
2. A schedule of daily therapies and activities is given to the individual					
3. Staff members are willing to allow the individual to take risks in being more independent					
4. Arrangements can be made to visit places in the community (e.g., grocery store, shopping mall, church)					
5. Care routines support the individual in caring for himself/herself					
6. In a conversation, other people and the individual take turns communicating					
7. There are physical aides (e.g., grab bars in the bathroom, wide doorways) that make it easier for the individual to get around and do things independently					
8. There are plenty of opportunities for the individual to improve in self-care abilities					
9. The individual is encouraged to sit or walk outdoors					

Table 8-21 ENVIRONMENT-INDEPENDENCE INTERACTION SCALE (EIIS) *(continued)*

	Not at all (1)	A Little (2)	Somewhat (3)	Quite a Bit (4)	A Great Deal (5)
10. Rooms are located close enough to each other to make it easy for the individual to get around					
11. Overall, the social environment supports the individual's independence					
12. The individual is expected to improve					
13. The individual has enough time to practice skills needed to become independent					
14. The individual participates in planned activities					
15. Areas to sit or walk outside (e.g., patio, benches, garden path) are available					
16. Caregiving routines (e.g., bathing, grooming) provide an opportunity for the individual to learn to be independent					
17. Overall, the cultural environment of the setting encourages the individual to move toward independence					
18. The individual participates in care and treatment decisions					
19. In general, the physical environment supports independence of the individual					
20. The individual is encouraged to participate in leisure activities (e.g., playing cards, listening to music)					

Subscale	Item #
Physical	4, 7, 10, 15, 19
Social	1, 6, 11, 14, 18
Cultural	3, 5, 9, 12, 17, 20
Temporal	2, 8, 13, 16

welfare-to-work, and community college programs (Bulgren, Gilbert, Hall, Horton, Mellard, & Parker, 1997). These researchers hypothesized that the person-context interaction was critical to understand before designing effective interventions for persons with learning challenges in these settings.

The research team designed an interview process to uncover successful and unsuccessful methods persons had used in the past, to obtain more details about situations that were particularly difficult, and to solicit persons' desires about what they wanted to accomplish. They also used teachers, participants, and the literature to identify the most common complaints about what interferes with success and what adaptations people used most often. Their searches revealed little linkages among ideas; teachers used whatever adaptations they knew about to help someone, without regard to the specific challenges the person described. The researchers used the Ecology of Human Performance intervention format to organize this information into categories, making ideas more accessible and linking ideas for accommodations to appropriate interventions. This process enabled teachers and participants to see the relationships among the accommodations so that they could identify the success of strategies for future situations the participants might face. Figures 8-7 to 8-9 illustrate the use of the Ecology of Human Performance intervention structure to organize ideas for specific learning problems (see Bulgren et al., 1997, for entire notebook of ideas).

In the latest project, the researchers have developed ideas for universal design for classroom and laboratory teaching. The materials include a self-assessment for the teacher, a feedback method for students, and ideas for expanding the teaching/ learning context and repertoire so that a wider range of students can participate successfully without having to have specialized accommodations to support their learning.

Applying Ecology of Human Performance to Grocery Shopping

Researchers (occupational therapist, clinical psychologist, and nurse) used Ecology of Human Performance to develop a skills training program for persons living in the community with severe mental illness. They used grocery shopping as the identified task for the project because it is an important independent living activity and it is an excellent illustration of the complexity of person-environment interaction in daily life. The process of finding the desired items in a grocery store is a cognitively complex task that takes place in a physical environment designed to capture attention and prompt impulsive purchases. Grocery shopping presents workable opportunities to design an intervention that takes advantage of environmental supports to reduce environmental barriers.

Although all aspects of context influence grocery shopping performance, the physical environment is the most conspicuous. The physical environment of the grocery store includes the building, the aisles, the carts, the checkout stations, and the numerous grocery items. This environment brimming with physical information presents a challenge when it comes to finding a particular item. Additionally, the physical environment of the grocery store is organized to encourage the purchase of items the store wants to sell, sometimes obscuring the items for which the customer is looking. At the same time, there are naturally occurring cues in the grocery store's physical environment that support grocery-shopping performance. These cues include the overhead signs, the somewhat consistent layout among stores, item placement, and item labels.

Other contextual factors also play a part. The social environment of the grocery store includes the persons (i.e., other shoppers and grocery store personnel). People can facili-

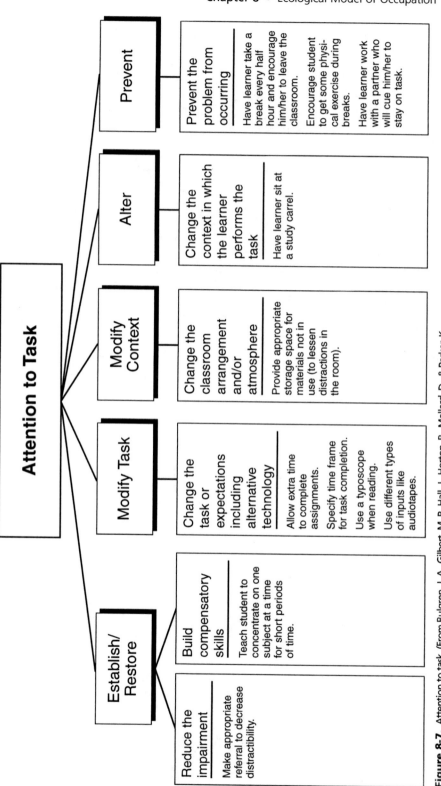

Figure 8-7. Attention to task. (From Bulgren, J. A., Gilbert, M. P., Hall, J., Horton, B, Mellard, D., & Parker, K. (1997). *Accommodating adults with disabilities in adult education programs: National field test.* University of Kansas Institute for Adult Studies.)

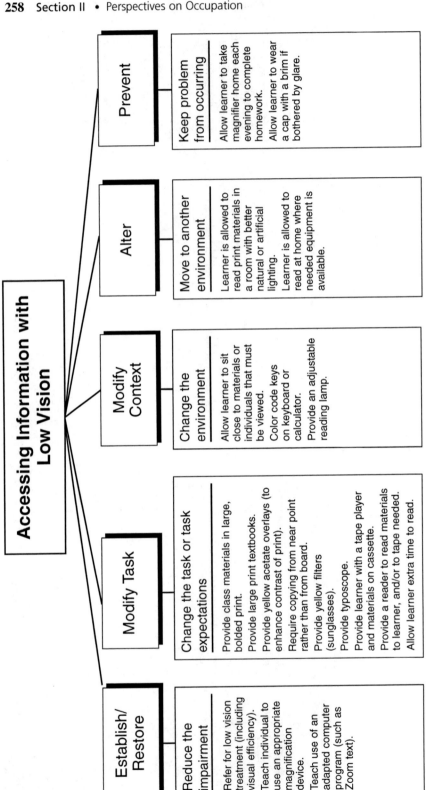

Figure 8-8. Accessing information with low vision. (From Bulgren, J. A., Gilbert, M. P., Hall, J., Horton, B., Mellard, D., & Parker, K. (1997). *Accommodating adults with disabilities in adult education programs: National field test,* University of Kansas Institute for Adult Studies.)

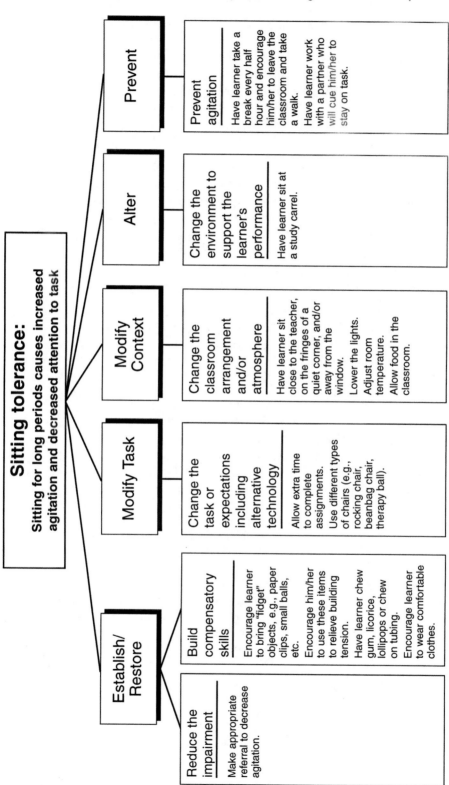

Figure 8-9. Sitting tolerance. (From Bulgren, J. A., Gilbert, M. P., Hall, J., Horton, B., Mellard, D., & Parker, K. (1997). *Accommodating adults with disabilities in adult education programs: National field test,* University of Kansas Institute for Adult Studies.)

tate grocery shopping performance (e.g., when a grocery store clerk helps someone locate an item). They can also create a barrier to performance (e.g., when the store is crowded). Cultural factors include expectations about choices and efficiency while shopping (e.g., shoppers can make progress without interference from others). Finally, the temporal environment includes when and how frequently one shops.

The researchers also used Ecology of Human Performance to organize their intervention plan. According to the framework, understanding the person-environment transaction is the basis for designing interventions that support engagement in chosen tasks. In this case, the person-environment interaction involves the task of grocery shopping for individuals with executive dysfunction in an information-rich environment, the grocery store. The intervention employed *adaptive* methods that increased the accessibility of the grocery store by teaching individuals how to make sense of the process of grocery shopping and the environment of the grocery store. Specifically, they used scripts, environmental cues, and went to the grocery stores to learn in the natural environment to simplify the steps of grocery shopping and provide repeated practice with those steps.

Measuring Sensory Processing in Daily Life

The studies to design and test the Infant Toddler Sensory Profile, the Sensory Profile, and the Adult Sensory Profile also reflect the Ecology of Human Performance principles of person-context interaction. The Sensory Profiles measure the actual person-context interaction. They each contain statements about how persons respond to sensory events in daily life, and persons report on the frequency of those particular responses (Brown, Tollefson, Dunn, Cromwell, & Filion, 2001; Dunn, 1999; Dunn & Daniels, 2002). Studies using the Sensory Profiles indicate that persons with and without disabilities display distinct patterns of performance in relation to each other, suggesting that — when considering the impact of sensory processing — lived experiences are unique for each person and group.

Studying person context interactions through sensory processing points out the importance of person factors as long as we see person factors in relation to contexts and tasks. Sensation is a very personal experience, not only because we interpret sensation within our own nervous systems, but also because those interpretations involve the context and the tasks that contribute to those sensory experiences. Sometimes it is difficult to sort out the person part from the context part of these experiences. Sensation and sensory processing represent by their very nature the "taking in" of the context for the brain's use in constructing adaptive responses.

The Sensory Profile studies illustrate the fact that person factors are still important for us to consider as long as we view person factors within tasks and contexts. Dunn's model of sensory processing provides a method for applying our knowledge about person variables to the daily demands of a person's life (Dunn, 1997a&b), thus applying the Ecology of Human Performance framework in practice. In Dunn's model, we consider both the person's neurologic thresholds and their behavioral schemas for responding to those thresholds. With the neurologic thresholds and behavioral responses intersecting, this creates four general patterns of sensory processing (Dunn, 1997a, 2000). These four patterns incorporate the person variables related to sensory processing and the contextual variables related to the way the person responds within life events. These patterns have emerged in factor analytic studies across the life span, suggesting there is some stability in these features in the human experience (Dunn, 2000; Dunn & Brown, 1997; Brown et al., 2001).

The first pattern represents *diminished registration*; these persons may miss stimuli around them and may seem oblivious to external events that others notice readily. We hypothesize that these persons have high neurologic thresholds and that they are passive in relation to their thresholds, which accounts for them missing many sensory stimuli that others would notice. The second pattern represents *sensation seeking*; these persons enjoy sensory experiences, notice many stimuli around them, and even create more sensation for themselves during activities. We hypothesize that these persons have variable neurologic thresholds, and that their pleasure for sensation generates behaviors that are active to intensify the sensory opportunities available. The third pattern represents *sensitivity*; these persons notice everything and quickly become overloaded or irritated by stimuli around them. We hypothesize that these persons have low neurologic thresholds and are active in relation to their thresholds, accounting for their high vigilance regarding environmental stimuli.. The fourth pattern represents *sensation avoiding*; these persons isolate themselves to reduce stimuli that are too difficult to manage. We hypothesize that these persons also have low neurologic thresholds, but that they have a greater need to keep unfamiliar stimuli away, accounting for their active responses to control their activities and environments.

We can apply the Ecology of Human Performance intervention process using these patterns of sensory processing. Studies on adults suggest that people with and without performance challenges have all these patterns of sensory processing; this leads to the hypothesis that a person's patterns are not functional or dysfunctional by nature, but rather it may be the interaction between the person's sensory processing patterns and the task and context variables in their lives that determine whether they are doing well or poorly. Therefore, the "establish/restore" intervention might address teaching the person/family about the person's sensory processing patterns so they might gain insights about particular behaviors. The "adapt" and "alter" interventions would be directed toward designing and identifying the best matches for a person's sensory processing patterns. For example, we might suggest different home décor or restaurant options for persons who have sensitivity compared with persons who are sensation seekers. In each case, our focus would be on honoring the sensory processing pattern of the person, rather than trying to "fix" it.

Summary Related to Research

There are many ways to approach the application of Ecology of Human Performance to research. The above examples provide illustrations of the ways that our interdisciplinary colleagues have used the concepts to advance our thinking about theory and practice.

SUMMARY

Using Ecology of Human Performance terminology, the practice of occupational therapy focuses on increasing the performance range of people and populations. In other words, occupational therapy practitioners provide interventions that make tasks more available to the person. This may mean that the person can perform a task that he or she was unable to perform or it may mean the person is more satisfied or competent in his or her task performance.

Person, context, and task features must receive equal consideration to make good decisions about intervention approaches that increase the performance range. Although the Ecology of Human Performance was designed to increase attention to context, it is essential that occupational therapists not lose sight of the importance of person and task features. For example, it is ineffective to assess the barriers and facilitators of a particular physical setting with no knowledge of the skills and abilities of the people that use that particular setting. The barriers will certainly vary for different person factors, such as hearing impairments, low vision, limited endurance, or memory loss. Likewise, it is important to know what tasks are performed in the environment and the tools, materials, and processes they employ. Once the person, context, and task factors are identified, the Ecology of Human Performance interventions (establish/restore, adapt, alter, prevent, and create) can then be considered.

A comprehensive analysis of person/context interaction as it relates to task performance has many benefits. First, it facilitates the full participation of all people in their communities. The broadening of intervention options and an expanded appreciation for context means that intervention does not stop at person factors, self-care, and the home environment, but includes all tasks and environments.

A second benefit of the Ecology of Human Performance perspective is a reduction in the disability/non-disability distinction. Daily life for all people involves a complex negotiation of skills and abilities within existing environments. An emphasis on limitations of the person keeps occupational therapists from becoming involved in systems and community change. When context becomes more important, activities such as advocacy and population-based services become central to occupational therapy's role as a human service profession. The belief that all people should be included in all aspects of society compels occupational therapists to become involved at the system, community, and policy levels.

Furthermore, the Ecology of Human Performance promotes consumer empowerment. The tasks that the person wants or needs are determined first before deciding which person and context features need to be assessed. Based on this knowledge, intervention planning involves the consideration of all the possible options, with the assumption that these interventions are discussed with the consumer or caregiver and it is the consumer/caregiver that makes the decision about which approach to take.

Finally, the Ecology of Human Performance supports interdisciplinary collaboration. The constructs of person, context, task, and performance can be applied across human service professions and provide a common, non-discipline-specific language and framework from which providers with varying backgrounds can work together.

STUDY QUESTIONS

8-1. Why does the Ecology of Human Performance emphasize context?

8-2. What doesn't the Ecology of Human Performance emphasize?

8-3. Analyze use of the term task in this chapter. How does, or does it not, relate to occupation.

8-4. Differentiate context from environment.

8-5. Compare the following intervention strategies and generate an example for each:
- Establish/restore
- Alter
- Adopt/modify
- Prevent
- Create

8-6. Generate a "create" intervention strategy for each of the following populations:
- Adolescent males
- Middle-aged females
- Elder males and females

8-7. With whom would you need to collaborate to implement or create intervention strategies presented in 8-6?

References

Bronfenbrenner, U. (1979). *The ecology of human development: Experiments by nature and design.* Cambridge, MA: Howard University Press.

Brown, C., Tollefson, N., Dunn, W., Cromwell, R., & Filion, D. (2001). The Adult Sensory Profile: Measuring patterns of sensory processing. *American Journal of Occupational Therapy, 55,* 75–82.

Bulgren, J. A., Gilbert, M. P., Hall, J., Horton, B., Mellard, D., & Parker, K. (1997). *Accommodating adults with disabilities in adult education programs: National field test,* University of Kansas Institute for Adult Studies.

Christiansen, C., & Baum, C. (1997a). Person-environment occupational performance: A conceptual model for practice. In C. Christiansen & C. Baum (Eds.), *Occupational therapy: Enabling function and well-being* (pp. 46–71). Thorofare, NJ: Slack.

Christiansen, C., & Baum, C. (1997b). Understanding occupation: Definitions and concepts. In C. Christiansen & C. Baum (Eds.), *Occupational therapy: Enabling function and well being* (pp. 2–25). Thorofare, NJ: Slack.

Clark, R., Parham, D., Carlson, M., Frank, G., Jackson, J., Pierce, D., Wolfe, R. J., & Zemke, R. (1991). Occupational science: Academic innovation in the service of occupational therapy's future. *American Journal of Occupational Therapy, 45,* 300–310.

Dunn, W. (1997a). A conceptual model for considering the impact of sensory processing abilities on the daily lives of young children and their families. *Infants and Young Children, April, 10,* 23–25.

Dunn, W. (1997b). The sensory profile: A discriminating measure of sensory processing in daily life. *Sensory Integration Special Interest Section Quarterly, 20.* Bethesda, MD: American Occupational Therapy Association.

Dunn, W. (1999). *The Sensory Profile manual.* San Antonio: The Psychological Corp.

Dunn, W. (2000). Habits: What's the brain got to do with it? *Occupational Therapy Journal of Research, 20* (suppl. 1), 6s-20s.

Dunn, W., & Brown, C. (1997). Factor analysis on the sensory profile from a national sample of children without disabilities. *American Journal of Occupational Therapy, 51,* 490–495.

Dunn, W., Brown, C., & McGuigan, A. (1994). The ecology of human performance: A framework for considering the effect of context. *American Journal of Occupational Therapy, 48,* 595–607.

Dunn, W., & Daniels, D. (2002). *Infant Toddler Sensory Profile.* San Antonio, TX: Psychological Corporation.

Gentile, A. M. (1972). A working model of skill acquisition with applications to teaching. *Quest, 17,* 3–23.

Law, M., Cooper, B., Strong, S., Stewart, D., Rigby, P., & Letts, L. (1996). The person-environment-occupation model: A transactive approach to occupational performance. *Canadian Journal of Occupational Therapy, 63,* 9–23.

Nelson, D. L. (1996). Therapeutic occupation: A definition. *American Journal of Occupational Therapy, 50,* 775–782.

Schkade, J. K., & Schultz, S. (1992). Occupational adaptation: Toward a holistic approach for contemporary practice, part 1. *American Journal of Occupational Therapy, 46,* 829–837.

Teel, C., Dunn, W., Jackson, S., & Duncan, P., (1997). The role of the environment in fostering independence: Conceptual and methodological issues in developing an instrument. *Topics in Stroke Rehabilitation, 4,* 28–40.

Teel, C., Dunn, W., Jackson, S., & Duncan, P. (in preparation). Development of the Environmental Independence Interaction Scale (EIIS).

9

Client-Centered Practice: Implications for Our Professional Approach, Behaviors, and Lexicon

Sue E. Baptiste

OBJECTIVES

This chapter will help you to:

- Differentiate between the traditional and client-centered approaches to practice.
- Discover the historical roots of client-centered practice.
- Describe constructs that reflect the central precepts of client-centered practice.
- Discuss the importance of language in client-centered practice.
- Classify your own therapeutic style on the traditional approach/client-centered continuum and develop strategies to become more client-centered.

SETTING THE CONTEXT

Over the past several years, the occupational therapy profession has undergone widespread change in many key aspects of theory, philosophy, and practice. There has been a return to earlier understanding, to the roots of the profession, and to a reinvestment in the value of occupation as the central construct of practice. There is now nothing for which to apologize

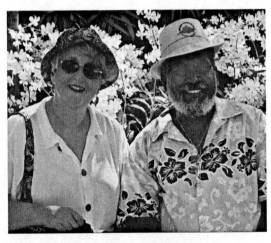

Sue and her husband Doug in Singapore.

in the notion that occupational therapy as a profession gravitates to the community, to the natural place where people meet their environments and are actively engaged within them. We have weathered the storm of reductionism and subscription to a medical model of practice that was essentially a poor fit, both philosophically and practically. Hand in hand with this reawakening of the essence of our practice came the recognition that occupational therapists are enablers, facilitators, and coaches. Consequently, a process was undertaken, within the Canadian occupational therapy context, of determining a set of underlying practice principles, focused on mutual regard and shared objectives, which would best provide a backdrop to developing collaborative partnerships with patients. This search proved rich and rewarding, entailing a new look at professional approaches, behaviors, and language.

Throughout the 1980s and most of the 1990s, Canadian occupational therapists were led through a process of profound reflection regarding their practice by a task force involving membership from the Canadian Association of Occupational Therapists and from the Department of National Health and Welfare, resulting in the development of a model and guidelines for practice in occupational therapy (Department of National Health and Welfare and Canadian Association of Occupational Therapists, 1983; Canadian Association of Occupational Therapists, 1991). These documents served as the underpinnings for the emergence of a new approach to practice, which was reinforced and revisited through constant and consistent application of the principles and model as well as the development of a client-centered outcome measure (Law et al., 1994). The process culminated in the development of *Enabling Occupation: An Occupational Therapy Perspective* (Canadian Association of Occupational Therapists, 1997).

Historical Roots

Thus in a decade, we have seen client-centered therapy develop from a method of counseling to an approach to human relationships . . . it has as much application to the problem of employing a new staff member, or the decision as to who is to get a raise, as it does to the client who is troubled by an inability to handle social relationships. (Rogers, 1951, p. 12)

Carl Rogers, well known for his impact on the field of psychotherapy and his innovative thinking, introduced the concept of client-centeredness. His search focused on developing an approach in psychotherapy that would provide a framework through which individuals could attain greater peace of mind despite the growing complexities of everyday life.

"Each man must resolve within himself issues for which his society previously took full responsibility" (Rogers, 1965, p. 4). The term client-centered practice appeared first in Rogers' book entitled *The Clinical Treatment of the Problem Child* (Rogers, 1939). Within this work, and his work that followed over the next three decades, Rogers identified several core components of what he called client-centeredness. Emphasis was placed on committing to an open and honest clinical relationship, providing the client with the opportunity of playing an active role in the therapeutic experience, and recognizing the critical importance of cultural values (of the client and the therapist) in a successful therapy outcome (Rogers, 1951). Rogers conceptualizes the essence of the move toward client-centeredness as one responsive to constant flux and change:

The picture is one of fluid changes in a general approach to problems of human relationships, rather than a situation in which some relatively rigid technique is more or less mechanically applied. (Rogers, 1965, p. 6)

If we look closely at the details of the application of client-centered principles in a Rogerian context, it would bear little direct resemblance to the emerging paradigm of occupational therapy practice in the second millennium. Regardless, it is of immense relevance and value to spend time in understanding the roots of the concept to more readily understand its more modern derivative.

It was not until the late 1980s that occupational therapists in Canada began to recognize the value and relevance of these ideas to their own practice and search for a congruent framework for an emerging professional persona. A series of working groups were formed during the 1980s to explore and define underlying principles and guidelines for Canadian occupational therapy practice. Clear parameters from which Canadian occupational therapists could derive a comfort and confidence to move forward in defining contemporary practice based on discipline-relevant constructs resulted (Canadian Association of Occupational Therapists, 1991). In the following decades, a strong focus on understanding these principles evolved, resulting in a rich and growing literature base (Canadian Association of Occupational Therapists, 1997; Corring & Cook, 1999; Law Baptiste & Mills et al., 1995; Sumsion & Smythe, 2000; Wilkins, Pollock, Rochon, & Law, 2001). Law (1998) and Sumsion (1999) wrote entire books on the subject of client-centered practice, both offering valuable views of the overall context and underlying principles and being well worthy of readers' attention in their search for further understanding the intricacies of occupation-based, client-centered practice. Law (1998) offers a particularly useful table that provides a synopsis of the concepts common to all models of client-centered practice and encapsulates information, which could be used as a checklist for practitioners wishing to examine their own practices with a view to ensuring a client-centered approach. Others (Clemens, Weltens, Feltes, Crabtree, & Dubitsky, 1994; Gerteis, Edgman-Levitan, Daley, & Delbonco, 1993; Hostler, 1994; King, 1994; Wilkins, Pollock, Rochon, & Law, 2001) explored these ideas from a practice base, identifying and defining the pleasures, successes, difficulties, and barriers associated with trying to practice in a client-centered manner. In 1991, a team of Canadian occupational therapy researchers developed the *Canadian Occupational Performance Measure* (Law et al., 1994), which has become for many occupational therapists around the world a useful starting point for launching, evaluating, and teaching about a client-centered approach to working with clients. This tool has been translated into many other languages and is being used in approximately 30 countries. This in itself introduces fascinating opportunities for evidence-based research to explore the commonalities and differences inherent within the application of client-centered principles across differing cultural contexts.

This chapter explores the underlying notions of client-centeredness, focusing particularly on language, relationships, and applying this new understanding to personal practice. It is hoped that the reader will gain clarity of thought and understanding as well as a clearer notion of how to look at practice through a client-centered lens.

CONCEPTS OF CLIENT-CENTERED PRACTICE

The client, as the term has acquired its meaning, is one who comes actively and voluntarily to gain help on a problem, but without any notion of surrendering his own responsibility for the situation. It is because the term has these connotations that we have chosen it, since it avoids the connotation that he is sick . . . (Rogers, 1965, p. 7)

To think clearly about the impact of client-centered principles on our professional language, the relationships we develop, and the practice styles we adopt, it is essential to become familiar with the essence of the underlying principles associated with being client-centered. These following constructs are considered to reflect the central precepts of client-centered practice:

- *Choice and autonomy*
  Who determines the directions for therapy?
  Who decides what are the important issues to address?
- *Responsibility and partnership; enablement*
  Who is central to the therapy process?
  Who understands the problems and concerns best?
- *Congruence of context*
  How is intervention planned?
  Where does it happen?
  Does it fit with the client's world?
- *Accessibility and flexibility*
  When and where are appointments/meetings held?
- *Respect for difference and diversity*
  Is there respect for and acceptance of cultural/ life style choices?

As we explore the key themes of language, relationships, and practice, these core constructs will provide the threads from which we will weave our own fabric for professional practice.

Language

The application of client-centered practice requires the adoption of new language. Few new words are required but the pattern of word usage must be changed. (Sumsion, 1999, p. 32)

Why is language so important? Language sets the scene for how we see and describe our world, providing a context for our expectations and a sense of the unknown or the familiar. One of the most compelling examples of the graphic importance of language can be elicited from the meaning of the word *lecture*. When hearing that someone attended a *lecture*, one can muster images of a large hall; many rows of chairs ranging upward, all with small desk pallets attached; a teacher speaking from a podium; overheads being projected; and students with expressions varying from somnolence to rapt attention. Now, what if one heard of someone attending a *large group session*? What kinds of images are conjured up now? Chances are that these images are indeed very different. The room is probably conceived to be flat, perhaps with a circle of chairs, or at the very least less rigidly defined rows; many students are interacting with the facilitator/teacher; and the atmosphere is one of less formality.

Learning Activity 9-1

Reflect for a moment on your own day-to-day experience and identify words that provide you with particularly vivid images.

This notion is of particular importance when reflecting on transitioning into a practice style that consciously embraces client-centered principles. There are several words that are employed naturally in such a shift, *client* being, of course, the one of most visibility and the greatest centrality. *Client* is replacing *patient* in this lexicon. Whereas the use of *client* has received much bad press, particularly from individuals who do not readily accept the corporate assumptions inherent with the word, the initial rationale was focused much more on the need to move away from that semantic picture of someone being "done to" instead of being "involved with." *Patient* connotes that picture of passivity, dependence, and waiting for change, cure, or worse.

> *The term client does have certain legal connotations which are unfortunate, and if a better term emerges we shall be happy to use it. For the present, however, this seems the term most appropriately related to our concept of the person coming for help.* (Rogers, 1951, p. 7).

It would appear that, even 50 years later, a better term has yet to be coined.

Undoubtedly, there are many situations within the delivery of health care in which the term *patient* is both relevant and desirable; when being admitted to an emergency room, for example, one would hope to be taken care of, nurtured, and helped. However, as any rehabilitation professional knows, when facing the knowledge of long-term disability and/or illness, the central need for the individual to engage with the process and become invested in the outcome is of paramount importance. It can be professed, therefore, that the image of that involved, invested person is well-captured in a term such as *client*. In this circumstance, the patient/client becomes central to the healing, rehabilitative process, allowing for the desirable degree of autonomy and choice; developing a context within which the individual may feel empowered and enabled; creating the opportunity to assist in the development of an accessible and flexible treatment process and plan; and ensuring respect for the uniqueness of the individual.

Other words and phrases emerge from notions of client-centered practice, not the least of which are those inherent in the underlying principles. Few would argue about the positive influence of ideas related to enabling individuals with occupational performance deficits to access flexible health care services. Few would oppose health care providers responding to these individuals with an understanding of differing cultural expectations. No one would question the meaning of these terms.

To illustrate this element of changing language and understanding, what are the ideas and images we find popping into our minds when we think of autonomy and choice? Undoubtedly, there are concerns around our comfort level with whether our clients have enough information and/or skills to make reasoned and safe choices. If our clients are autonomous, does that not mean that they have the right to do whatever they decide, regardless of what we believe?

LEARNING ACTIVITY 9-2

How comfortable am I with the idea of giving more control to the people who come to me for help with their occupational performance needs?

Can I think of situations in which I have been impressed with my clients' abilities to make difficult choices and decisions?

How did I respond?

Can I think of situations in which I have been concerned about my clients' choices and their inherent risks or dangers?

How did I respond?

Following the direction indicated by the quote from Sumsion (1999) at the beginning of this section on language, we can begin to consider how our interviews would look and how our questions could be framed. In the traditional context, the occupational therapist would likely enter the interview room or sit by the patient's bedside and inform the patient that "Dr. So-and-So has asked me to see you." Then the therapist would continue with a brief but clear litany of who he or she was, what he or she could do for the patient, and what would be the next steps. Client-centered principles turn the whole process around. Instead, the first step would be to ask the client, "Why are you here in this hospital/clinic/agency?" This allows for an immediate appreciation and support of the idea that the client is one, if not indeed the key, decision-maker in this relationship. As the process continues, the more traditional approach would demand that the therapist advise that the assessment indicates a need to do this and this, and then declare the goals for intervention and the schedule for visits and so forth. Once again, client-centeredness offers a very different approach to intervention planning. The client is advised of the results of the assessment and asked if there are any questions or need for further information. "Following receipt of all the necessary information, provided in a way the client can understand, the client then determines the goals for the intervention" (Sumsion, 1999, p. 32).

LEARNING ACTIVITY 9-3

What is my current interview style like?

Where does it lie on the continuum from traditional to client-centered?
Traditional_____Client-centered

Where, along this continuum, would I be comfortable moving toward?
Traditional_____Client-centered

How could I make this shift? What could be my strategies?

Any discussion about language will undoubtedly end up with an exploration of the intricacies of relationships and the manner in which information is imparted. It is here then that the critical elements of partnership and relationship emerge as a primary focus for consideration and analysis.

Case Study 9-1: About Language — Part A

Mrs. Kerr is 80 years old and almost ready to leave the hospital after undergoing surgery for a fractured hip. She had fallen down some stairs at home and was found by her neighbor when she called in to bring her some freshly made cookies. As the occupational therapist, I saw her before her discharge to make sure that she will be okay to return home independently. Upon entering her room, I noted a little lady, sitting up in bed, and wearing a frilly robe and a wide smile. After introducing myself and briefly explaining what occupational therapists do, I asked Mrs. Kerr, now Florence, what were the issues that were concerning her the most about going home and what could I do to help. She replied "Well, dear, you are the expert; you went to school a long time to learn all about this sort of thing; you tell me what would be best."

(continues)

> ### As a Client-Centered Therapist, What Should I Do?
>
> I thanked Florence for recognizing the work I had put in to becoming an occupational therapist, and then suggested that she was the one who understood her life best; that it would be very helpful to me for her to tell me about her house, what her life was like before she fell, and then I could use my knowledge and information to help her get home and stay there safely.
>
> ### Do You Have Some Other Ideas?

Relationships

> *. . . the counselor who is effective in client-centered therapy holds a coherent and developing set of attitudes deeply embedded in his personal organization, a system of attitudes which is implemented by techniques and methods consistent with it . . . the counselor who tries to use a "method" is doomed to be unsuccessful unless this method is genuinely in line with his own attitudes.* (Rogers, 1951, p. 19)

In more traditional approaches to the delivery of health care services, everyone has learned to expect that health care professionals are the experts; that these individuals possess knowledge and skills that are not a part of patients' repertoires. Their expertise is the reason the patient is coming to see them in the first place. Expert/clinical practitioners in turn have been inculcated with the belief and expectation that their patients will be willing to listen, comply with the treatment regimen, and to attend appointments, alert to the moment when the next piece of expert advice will be offered. This is obviously still a good thing in more critical health care situations. However, with the growth of the consumer movement and the emergence of a sense of increased right to information and decision-making, this tenuous balance of dependence and power is being disturbed.

The central notion of power requires some attention, whether we like the term or not. For many reasons, the idea of talking about power or admitting to being powerful or powerless are not easy concepts about which to spend time in discussion. Regardless, within the context of client-centeredness, the power base shifts from the traditional expectations of the roles of expert and patient to become one of sharing, of interdependence, with the client and the practitioner assuming a collaborative stance (Kaplan, 1991; Sumsion, 1993). The client gains power through initially defining his or her own occupational performance issues. Traditionally, as explored earlier, it has been the therapist who, through expert interviewing, assessment, and testing, has developed the intervention plan. The patient's role within that model of care delivery was one of input at the interview and compliance with the plan from then until reassessment. Again, this was not a negative thing for the time in which the model emerged; however, it is incongruent with the principles of both consumerism and client-centered systems. The therapeutic relationship within a client-centered context allows for a reflection of the client's own values, priorities, and goals, being concerned concomitantly with the roles they fulfill within the environments in which they live. In essence, power within this type of relationship is best defined as the process through which the therapist and client achieve what could not be achieved by either in isolation (Crabtree & Caron-Parker, 1991; Law, 1991, 1998). As with any therapeutic encounter in occupational therapy, a key role for the therapist is that of providing input and education as required to the client regarding skills for living, from practical, physical skills to more conceptual skills of problem-solving, self-assertion, and advocacy.

- How comfortable am I with my ability to listen to my clients? What example can I use to illustrate my degree of comfort?
- How comfortable am I with sharing what I know and believe, and then providing my clients space to make their own choices based on that new knowledge? Again, do I have an example to provide me with a cue?
- How comfortable am I in accepting the choices my clients make?

Many clinicians will speak of their concerns about dealing with clients who live totally different lifestyles in comparison with themselves, sometimes on the wrong side of the law and often incorporating habits (such as overuse of drug and alcohol, abusive behaviors) that are anathema to the health professionals. This example was once used to clarify this issue for me: "Well, if your client wants to relearn to drive, you can help him with that. You don't have to teach him to drive the getaway car."

Relationships outside individual therapeutic partnerships will also tend to change in character when a client-centered approach to professional practice is adopted. For example, if we begin acting in a client-centered manner while working within a traditional environment, we can expect to be confronted with many situations in which challenges and the need for negotiation will arise. How we have related to colleagues of long standing from other disciplines may change radically. We take risks by adopting a new professional model for practice. We invite criticism and potentially ostracization or sabotage if we attempt to challenge the status quo. This may seem to be hard language to use in this context; however, we can all reflect on experiences in which we have observed how coworkers who do not fit the mold or the expectations of those around them are treated. The confidence of the therapist in asserting the principles of client-centered practice is critical to the success of assuming this approach to practice. Advocating for a client's decision with others on the health care team can be a daunting proposition. Feeling sure that clients have all the information they need to move forward with their goals takes a good dose of confidence and self-assurance. Knowing that what you know is the most current information available, or at least being confident that you know how to find out what you do not know, is the very basis of evidence-based practice. It is also a core skill in being the strong partner that your client deserves (Sumsion, 1999, p. 33).

- Am I ready to take a fresh look at how I relate to my clients? How will I approach this?
- How will I approach a work place, even if it is far different from the overall culture of my work place? What key words could I use to illustrate my workplace culture?
- Am I prepared to advocate for my clients even in the face of disagreement from my colleagues? What problems could I envision and what strategies could I use to overcome them?

Hand in hand with partnership come responsibilities and accountabilities to one another, as well as to others external to the immediate alliance. Each client must accept the responsibility of honest communication, commitment to the task(s), and engagement in monitoring, evaluating, and redefining progress and goals. More important to this immediate discussion is the responsibility of the practitioner to the client and to the client's support system including agencies with which the client is involved. Often power for the practitioner will translate into advocacy for that client with individuals and agencies with which or with whom there are incomplete matters or difficult issues to resolve. The central importance of developing a respectful and collaborative relationship with clients has been shown to enhance overall client participation and compliance (another word to analyze — but on another day!) as well as improved client satisfaction and enhanced self-efficacy (Dunst, Trivette, Boyd, & Brookfield, 1994; Rebeiro, 2000).

Case Study 9-1: About Relationships — Part B

Florence (Mrs. Kerr) and I went on a home visit to her tri-level detached home in the suburbs. It is a quiet, pleasant neighborhood close to a small street of stores, a church, a few restaurants, a bank, and the local library. She managed to get around her home with relative ease, given her recent surgery. However, I was concerned about the number of stairs and the amount of memorabilia, furniture, and so on that filled the house.

As a Client-Centered Therapist, What Should I Do?

I elected to talk with Florence about the potential hazards that I felt were a problem and could be a hindrance to her smooth return to her own home. She listened and then stated that she totally understood my concerns, however she could not possibly get rid of anything. She suggested that she tidy up a bit and could get her neighbor and her daughter to help her do that. I agreed that this was a good strategy as a first step and that I would be prepared to recommend her discharge given that she did follow through with this idea. Also, I asked her if she felt it would be acceptable for me to come and see her a couple of times after she came home. She agreed.

LEARNING ACTIVITY 9-4

What else would you suggest that I could have done? What would you have done?

APPLICATION TO PRACTICE

Over the past decades of the emergence of the occupational therapy profession, we have undergone many phases of growth and role iteration. What has remained relatively constant are the links to health care systems that were shaped by a medical model of care delivery. Implicit within this notion is the assumption that impairment is the base from which clinical reasoning arises. For many years, occupational therapists tended to modify their vision of ideal practice to fit into the requirements of such a care model, thus ensuring their acceptance into the health care team by communicating through a similar language and visible skill set. This influenced the manner in which care was delivered to the patients referred to occupational therapy, focusing more effort on the cellular, biological issues, thus creating a struggle for occupational therapy to assert its uniqueness through consideration of individual occupational performance issues within the relevant environments. However, this practice approach has been challenged by the changing directions and location of occupational therapy practice environments, and by the move toward client-centered, occupation-centered practice. This has opened the door even further to a conscious declaration of the key nature of occupation to practice and the close alliance with notions of activity and participation, which have become highly visible within the new iteration of the World Health Organization's (WHO) taxonomy, the *International Classification of Functioning, Disability and Health* (ICF) (WHO, 2001).

Thus, given that major changes have been happening already to occupational therapy practice, what are the elements that are specific to assuming a client-centered approach? Perhaps it is most logical to begin with the impact on the system at large. For any health care delivery system, institution, or agency to become truly client-centered, there has to be a shift in how programs are designed, delivered, and funded as well as how clients and families are included in both the planning and the delivery of the required services. (Although some people may use the excuse that payment and reimbursement are different in the United States, the occupational therapist is challenged to be creative in using this approach with clients.) In recent years, it has become much more common that clients and family members or significant others can be found as members of visioning groups, planning committees, boards of treatment centers, and representatives on research and ethics committees. This strategy demands that the processes, which are handled by these groups, are undertaken with more transparency and visibility. It also demands that issues which have been disregarded or hidden for the sake of comfort or an unwillingness to "face the music," can no longer be invisible or ignored. Once an institutional environment embraces a commitment to client-centeredness, the job of front-line practitioners becomes much easier if they too wish to embrace these same tenets. It would appear logical that the chance of the highest level of success with institutional shifts of this nature would necessitate the application of client-centered principles to include employees of the institution (support staff and professional colleagues) as well as community partners, clients, and families. Consequently, the development of a sensitive and responsive working environment would both support and ensure the successful launch of a client-centered initiative. Unfortunately, there have been frequent examples of institutions attempting to make the move to client-centeredness, but neither allocating the necessary resources to make it happen nor recognizing the need for staff to be supported through the transition.

Attempting to move to the client-centered approach without supporting the staff in this move is shortsighted. This approach introduces many potential problems for clinicians who already are feeling pressured to meet clinical expectations and deadlines, and who perceive changes of this nature as "add-ons" to their already overextended schedules. Time, or not having enough of it, however, tends to become a rather convenient excuse. Perhaps it is healthy to take the approach that whenever something new is introduced, there exists an ideal opportunity to review habits and routines as well as to determine priorities and the optimal use of the elusive commodity of time.

LEARNING ACTIVITY 9-5

What would be (or has been) the approach of the place(s) where I work in assuming a client-centered approach to service delivery?

What kinds of strategies would I use to facilitate such a transition?
For the workplace?
For myself?
For my clients?

This brings the discussion to an exploration of the issues for the individual practitioner relative to shifting to a more client-centered approach to practice. Perhaps the most important piece of understanding for adopting such an approach to practice is appreciating the difference between partnering with the client and giving clients free rein to make decisions as they please. True client-centeredness incorporates a strong commitment by the occupational therapist to giving the client the information needed to make reasoned decisions and providing educational input, skill training, and development as required. For example, clients who have always been in relationships in which decisions were made for them will find it very difficult to change that habit, even if they wish to do so. The role of the occupational therapist would focus on ensuring that clients are provided with educational materials and opportunities to practice newfound skills and recognize newfound knowledge in order to assume a more central role in making their own decisions. On the other hand, if the client is offered the chance to assume more responsibility but chooses not to, as is often the case with older clients and clients from differing cultural backgrounds, the responsibility of the therapist becomes one of negotiation: to create a positive climate for clients to meet their needs while taking advantage of any opportunities to educate and inform. This type of relationship is a natural reinforcement for the principles and purpose of evidence-based practice. No longer is it adequate to do what has been done before just because it is so. Also, as clients become more conscious of what they do not know and what they need to know, the therapist in return must become comfortable with the notion of being challenged and questioned and having to produce the evidence and/or rationale for why a certain assessment or intervention approach is suggested.

LEARNING ACTIVITY 9-6

What examples can I think of from my practice (or my experiences as a student) in which my clients have challenged what I have suggested for a treatment plan?

What did I do about it? How did I feel?

Undoubtedly, the core skill sets that occupational therapists must possess to practice in a client-centered manner have been enhanced or changed. Much of what we have done in the past is still required to some degree or another, but when considering client-centeredness in partnership with an evidence-based, occupation-centered practice, then there are some key differences. Initially there is the need to adopt an occupation-centered, client-centered assessment process, such as that exemplified in the *Canadian Occupational Performance Measure* (Law et al., 1994). If this instrument is not used, then the initial interview should be focused on listening to the client and steering away from rote assessment profiles, in which clients are asked standardized questions upon which are based the goals and expected outcomes of treatment. If nothing else, a client-centered practice approach must begin with the client and finding out what is important to him or her and, in the case of a client with cognitive impairment, what is important to his or her family or caregivers.

Very often the goals of the rehabilitation team or the attending therapist may not initially be those of the client. We may believe that a certain client needs to get back home and then back to work. This may be true, but from the client's perspective, we may be very surprised that the immediate, real key issue is for the client to attend his son's university graduation. Intervention approaches geared to this objective will lead naturally into longer-term skill development for accomplishing longer-term goals such as returning to work. If we truly want to know what is important to the clients we see, then we should ask them and not assume we know and understand their life circumstances. They are the experts of their own existence.

Another key question that client-centered practitioners should ask themselves is who is the client in any particular situation. Many times the diagnosed patient within the medical system is not the key client or the total client. Many times the client's family, support system, or caregivers are the true client at the onset of involvement with a certain client system. Similarly, the client is often not an individual but an agency, government department, corporation, or business. It is critical that the identity of the client be clarified early in the relationship to facilitate appropriate assessment and negotiation of interventions and outcomes (Wilkins, Pollock, Rochon, & Law, et al., 2001).

LEARNING ACTIVITY 9-7

Who are the true clients in my practice?

Do I have a range of different kinds of clients? What examples can I draw to identify the different clients with whom I work?

If so, do I deal with them in the same manner when applying client-centered principles?

Case Study 9-2: About Practice — Part C

After Florence went home, I talked with her on the telephone on a few occasions. She talked about how she was happy to be home, how she was tidying up as she had promised, and how much she enjoyed her own place. We made a plan to for me to visit one afternoon, approximately 1 month after her discharge. When I arrived at her house, Florence came to the door looking rather untidy and using a cane. Her gait was slow and uneven as she wended her way through the obstacle course from the front door to the kitchen table. Obviously, nothing much had been done to clear up since her return home. When I approached the subject and told her how uncomfortable I was knowing she was living in a place that could be hazardous for her, she became very introspective. Eventually, after a lengthy pause, she stated very firmly that she had no intention of going anywhere else. She feared that I was there to persuade her to go into a nursing home, and she was not even going to think about that.

As a Client-Centered Therapist, What Should I Do?

I listened carefully and gave reinforcement to Florence as she spoke. I then asked if I could give her some ideas of my own about the situation. She agreed and I outlined how I felt things could be changed around, how some help could be obtained to ensure she did not have go up and down too many stairs, and that she could consider being linked to the emergency call button service in the area. Florence agreed that I could bring my colleague who worked in the community on my last visit to introduce her (since I could not keep coming to see her due to funding and service priorities). I assured her that my goal was not to have her go to a nursing home, but I was concerned and could not ethically leave her in her current situation without some plan in place for improving matters.

Do You Have Some Other Ideas?

FINAL REFLECTIONS

Central to this whole discussion of being or becoming client-centered in our approach to practice is our comfort with relinquishing the role for which we were prepared in our professional education and the perceived and/or real status that we have attained. The practice of occupational therapy is becoming more and more autonomous. More jurisdictions around the world are adopting a view of occupational therapy practice which embraces assumptions of protection of the public and accountability through conscious, responsible practice. As client-centered principles become more commonplace and more accepted, it will be imperative that we recognize their congruence with this emerging vision of professional accountability. If we are to be accountable to the consumers of our service, the public, then we must listen to what they need, heed their perceptions of the services they receive, and adapt our practice in response to their feedback.

STUDY QUESTIONS — BEGINNER

9-1. Explain the historical shift of occupational therapy returning to its roots regarding the focus on occupation. Place your explanation in historical context.

9-2. Discuss the pros and cons of considering occupational therapists to be enablers, facilitators, and coaches.

9-3. Could the manner in which the Canadian Association of Occupational Therapists developed a model and guidelines for practice of occupational therapy be replicated in your country? Explain and justify your answer.

9-4. Describe the essence of the client-centered approach to practice.

9-5. Compare the words patient and client.

9-6. Look up the definitions of the following words:
- Power
- Collaboration
- Consultation
- Rapport
- Compliance
- Value
- Priority
- Goal

9-7. As the author suggests, the role of an occupational therapist is to provide input to a client "regarding skills for living, from practical, physical skills to more conceptual skills of problem-solving, self-assertion, and advocacy." How is that professional role different from that of a psychologist or special educator?

9-8. Explain how power for a practitioner can translate into advocacy for a client.

9-9. Focus on the author's message that increased collaboration with client results in improved client satisfaction. How can you use this information to promote or market occupational therapy within your setting?

9-10. Can occupation-based practice ever be not client-centered? Explain your answer.

9-11. Generate a list of competencies or the skill set an occupational therapist would need to practice client-centered care.

9-12. In your own words, rephrase or paraphrase the following statement: "More jurisdictions around the world are adopting a view of occupational therapy practice which embraces assumptions of protection of the public and accountability through conscious, responsible practice."

STUDY QUESTIONS — ADVANCED

9-13. Look up three of the original publications of Carl Rogers.

9-14. The author alludes to occupational therapy being one of the rehabilitation professions. Speculate as to why Wilcock (Chapter 6) might suggest such a connotation is limiting.

9-15. Speculate potential sources of conflict that would occur if a client-centered approach is implemented in a payment infrastructure using third-party payers.

9-16. Discuss the balance of power and dependence between a client and an occupational therapist.

9-17. Look at your habits and routines as an occupational therapist. How do these habits and routines support or mitigate client-centered therapy? What might you change to foster a more client-centered care approach?

References

Canadian Association of Occupational Therapists. (1991). *Occupational therapy guidelines for client-centred practice*. Toronto, Canada: Author.

Canadian Association of Occupational Therapists. (1997). *Enabling occupation: A Canadian perspective*. Toronto, Canada: Author.

Clemens, E., Weltens, T., Feltes, M., Crabtree, B., & Dubitsky, D. (1994). Contraindications in case management: Client-centered theory and directive practice with frail elderly. *Journal of Aging and Health, 6,* 70–88.

Corring, D., & Cook, J. (1999). The missing perspective on client-centered care. *Occupational Therapy Now, 1* (1), 8–10.

Crabtree, J. L., & Caron-Parker, L. M. (1991). Long-term care of the aged: Ethical dilemmas and solutions. *American Journal of Occupational Therapy, 45,* 607–612.

Department of National Health and Welfare and Canadian Association of Occupational Therapists. (1983). *Guidelines for the client-centred practice of occupational therapy*. Ottawa, Canada: Department of National Health and Welfare.

Dunst, C. J., Trivette, C. M., Boyd, K., & Brookfield, J. (1994). Help-giving practices and the self-efficacy appraisals of parents. In C. J. Dunst, C. M. Trivette, & A. G. Deal (Eds.), *Supporting and strengthening families: Methods, strategies and practices*. Cambridge, MA: Brookline Books.

Gerteis, M., Edgman-Levitan, S., Daley, J., & Delbonco, T. (1993). *Through the patient's eyes*. San Francisco: Jossey-Bass.

Hostler, S. L. (1994). *Family-centered care: An approach to implementation*. Charlottesville, VA: University of Virginia.

Kaplan, (1991). Health-related quality of life and patient decision-making. *Journal of Social Issues, 47,* 69–90.

King, G. P. (1994). *A framework for family-centred service*. Hamilton, ON: McMaster University, Neurodevelopmental Clinical Research Unit.

Law, M. (1998). *Client-centered occupational therapy*. Thorofare, NJ: Slack.

Law, M., Baptiste, S., Carswell, A., McCall, M. A., Polatajko, H., & Pollock, N. (1994). *The Canadian Occupational Performance Measure* (2nd ed.). Toronto, Canada: Canadian Association of Occupational Therapists, ACE.

Law, M., Baptiste, S., & Mills, J. (1995). Client centred practice: What does it mean and does it make a difference? *Canadian Journal of Occupational Therapy, 62,* 250–257.

Rebeiro, K. (2000). Client perspectives on occupational therapy practice: Are we truly client-centred? *Canadian Journal of Occupational Therapy, 67,* 7–14.

Rogers, C. R. (1939). *The clinical treatment of the problem child*. Boston: Houghton Mifflin.

Rogers, C. R. (1951). *Client-centered therapy*. Boston, MA: Houghton-Mifflin.

Rogers, C. R. (1965). *Client-centered therapy: Its current practice, implications and theory*. Boston, MA: Houghton-Mifflin.

Sumsion, T. (1993). Reflections on . . . client-centred practice: The true impact. *Canadian Journal of Occupational Therapy, 60,* 6–8.

Sumsion, T. (1999). *Client-centred practice in occupational therapy: A guide to implementation*. Edinburgh: Churchill Livingstone.

Sumsion, T., & Smyth, G. (2000). Barriers to client-centredness and their resolution. *Canadian Journal of Occupational Therapy, 67,* 15–21.

Wilkins, S., Pollock, N., Rochon, S., & Law, M. (2001). Implementing client-centred practice: Why is it so difficult? *Canadian Journal of Occupational Therapy 68,* 70–79.

World Health Organization. (2001). *ICF: International classification of functioning, disability and health* [Online]. Retrieved December 13, 2001, from the world wide web: http://www3.who.int/icf/icftemplate.cfm

10

Influence of Occupation on Assessment and Treatment

Roger I. Ideishi

OBJECTIVES

This chapter will help you to:
- Differentiate among three ways occupation is used in occupational therapy.
- Discuss the role of occupation used in a top-down approach during evaluation and intervention.
- Describe the role of occupation used in a bottom-up approach during evaluation and intervention.
- Explain the role of occupation used in a contextual approach during evaluation and intervention.
- Apply occupation used in a top-down approach, a bottom-up approach, and in a contextual approach to practice situations.

INTRODUCTION

The practice of a profession has to be viewed as unique and valuable to society. For occupational therapists, the value and uniqueness emerge from what we know, what we do, and how our knowledge contributes to the health and well-being of individuals and society. Occupational therapy intervention is based on an in-depth understanding of the use of occupation and purposeful and meaningful activities as therapeutic agents.

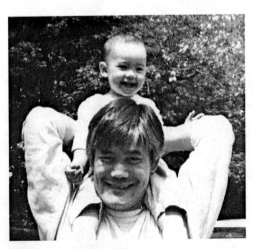

Roger and his daughter Kelia.

Occupation can be used as the therapeutic agent that results in a transformation of the person (Trombly, 1995). Occupational therapists also use occupation as the end-product. The therapeutic tools and the way the occupational therapist organizes his or her interventions may differ depending on whether the therapist is using occupation as a therapeutic agent or an end-product. The relative importance of occupation often varies during the course of an intervention, depending on the status and needs of the client and the perspective of the occupational therapist. For example, independence in dressing might be a goal for an individual, or dressing may be used as a task during the course of an intervention to assist the client in becoming more independent. In the end, effective occupational therapy services allows an individual to have an improved ability to participate in chosen activities and occupations, regardless of the perspective.

There are three ways that occupation is used in occupational therapy that influence the way in which the practitioner organizes practice. These perspectives are the top-down, bottom-up, and contextual approaches. The occupational therapist's individual perspective determines how he or she will develop his or her intervention plan. In the *bottom-up approach*, the occupational therapist focuses on specific skill deficits that create a barrier for an individual's successful engagement in occupations he or she values. In this perspective, the occupational therapist's evaluation begins at the component level. In the *top-down approach*, the occupational therapist focuses on the client's ability to participate in occupations and/or purposeful activities. Evaluation in this approach begins with examining the motivations, routines, habits, and roles of the individual. In the *contextual approach*, the occupational therapist focuses on the person's ability in a specific environment. Evaluation begins by exploration of the person's perceptions of the environment, and the environmental demands influence the individual's performance.

Whichever approach the occupational therapist uses to organize his or her practice, the ultimate goal of occupational therapy is to engage the individual in meaningful and valued occupations as a means to participate in life (see Chapter 1). Our profession has had a long-standing challenge to demonstrate (through education, research, and practice) that occupation is a vital aspect of the human experience and contributes to the health and well-being of a person (Meyer, 1922; Reilly, 1962; Yerxa, 1967, 1994, 1998). Occupational therapy practice includes various perspectives and organizations of practice. Within the various perspectives and organizations of practice, occupation is the thread that keeps the practice of occupational therapy intact. Practitioners realize the full value and scope of occupational therapy when occupation is used either as a means or an end.

INFLUENCE OF OCCUPATION ON ASSESSMENT AND INTERVENTION

Top-down Approach (Fig. 10-1)

In her Eleanor Clarke Slagle Lecture, Trombly (1995) described a hierarchical model of occupational functioning. In this model, the goal of occupational therapy is the achievement of competency and self-esteem in those life roles that a person chooses. The identification of life roles is self-determined depending on what meaning the person ascribes to the role, rather than the role being socially determined. For example, the meaning a person attaches to cooking may determine whether the life role is identified as a work-related role, such as a master chef, or as an exploratory leisure role, such as making cookies.

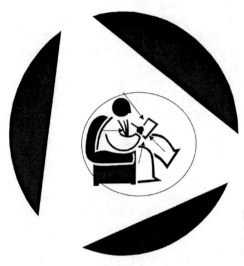

Figure 10-1. Top-down approach. In this approach, everything emanates from the individual's involvement in the occupation. The arrows indicate the focus primarily on the person, down toward the act of writing.

Satisfaction with life roles is determined by a person's ability to perform those tasks inherent in the role (Trombly, 1995). Using the previous example, the life role of a master chef involves the task of cooking. Tasks can be further divided into smaller units of behavior or activities within the task. Hence, for the master chef, stirring a pot is an activity within the task of cooking. To stir the pot, the master chef will require certain abilities such as motor planning and visual motor integration to complete the activity. In addition, more basic capacities, such as grasping the stirring utensil, are required to fulfill the motor plan required for the act of stirring. Keep in mind, the master chef's capacities, abilities, activities, and tasks are hierarchically nested in the chef's desire to be competent and fulfilled in this life role. The top-down approach, as described in Trombly's model of occupational functioning, is based on the top level of the hierarchy or life roles being the primary factor determining how the lower levels or performance components are expressed (Trombly, 1995).

As stated earlier, the top-down approach analyzes a situation beginning from the top of the hierarchy moving downward. The approach first examines the occupations and roles associated with what the person wants or needs to do. Context might be considered as a secondary perspective. The person identifies important roles and the value of each of these roles. Based on the identified valued roles, the occupational therapist analyzes and focuses on the inherent tasks and activities. With this in mind, the occupational therapist assesses the particular abilities or components skills that may limit satisfying participation in the desired occupations (Coster, 1998; Trombly, 1995).

Occupations also have a temporal dimension in that occupations occur over time. This temporal dimension can span from moments to years (Trombly, 1995). Therefore, occupations, valued roles, and abilities change over a person's life just as they may change within the treatment process. The top-down approach also emphasizes the role of purposefulness and meaningfulness in the selection of interventions. In other words, the activities selected for treatment are influenced by the type of participation required of the individual or the tasks involved in the valued roles and occupations of the individual. Specific skill achievement or component remediation may occur through participation in meaningful tasks and activities that the person identifies but, overall, the treatment tasks or activities are determined by the person's life role.

Evaluation in the Top-down Approach

Before the occupational therapist and client begin this process, the occupational therapist establishes therapeutic rapport with the client, the client's family, and significant persons in the client's life. After therapeutic rapport has been established, the occupational therapist and client explore and identify significant roles in the client's life. Some major areas are primary motivators in the client's life, aspirations or goals, self-concept, and efficacy in his or her life role performance.

Following the exploration of life roles, the occupational therapist examines the tasks, routines, and habits relative to the person's life role. Activity and time configurations are often useful and revealing. Recognizing and prioritizing the activities and tasks that are accomplished on a daily basis could form a starting point for intervention. For example, if dressing (which once took only 15 minutes to accomplish) now takes 45 minutes, then dressing tasks, if this is of concern to the individual, may be an important area to address in relation to the person's balance and efficiency of activity and time use. When the priority tasks and activities are identified, the occupational therapist examines why the client is having difficulties in the performance of these tasks and activities. The occupational therapist then identifies which component skills are or are not supporting the task and activity performance.

After a thorough examination and analysis of the client's life role and in collaboration with the client, the occupational therapist formulates or directs the development of therapeutic goals that address the role dysfunction or disruption. When using the top-down approach, the goals and interventions derive from the top of a hierarchy, the client's life roles, motivations, and preferred occupations.

Intervention Using a Top-down Approach

Once the goals for occupational therapy are agreed on, the occupational therapist (in collaboration with the client) selects the appropriate intervention modalities. The information gathered during the evaluation process guides the activity selection and/or contextual modification. In the top-down approach, the higher levels of the hierarchy rule the lower levels. The tasks and activities required for role participation, therefore, are incorporated as the treatment modality for occupational therapy. For example, the evaluation data reveal that one of a client's hobbies and passions in life is gardening. The task and activities of gardening, with its inherent motivating qualities and role identification for the client, are used as treatment. There is familiarity in the role identification and drive to participate in the motivating qualities. These factors have a positive influence on learning and development. The tasks and activities are adapted to meet the immediate lower level constraints, such as limited range of motion, poor attention span, or visual-perceptual dysfunction, so the client experiences success in the familiar role performance.

Case Study 10-1: *Bobby*

Bobby is an 11-year-old boy with cerebral palsy resulting in mild spastic quadriplegia. He lives with his parents and one brother in a one-story ranch home in a suburban neighborhood. He is independent in his self-care activities and participates in home chores such as taking out the garbage. Bobby attends a local public school where he earns average academic grades

(continues)

in the fifth grade. His handwriting is legible but he requires additional time to complete assignments. Bobby wants to learn how to ride a bicycle like the other kids in the neighborhood. A cautious child, he does not readily attempt new activities. Bobby is ambulatory but has mild spasticity in his extensor muscles of his lower limbs and flexor muscles of his upper limbs. At times, he cannot make efficient and appropriate postural adjustments during quick moving activities such as running and jumping. Bobby was referred to occupational therapy to improve his motor and postural efficiency during functional activities.

The first objective for the occupational therapist, regardless of the particular therapeutic approach, is to establish a therapeutic rapport with the client and significant persons in the client's life. In Bobby's case, it is important that the occupational therapist establish a rapport with Bobby, his parents, and his brother. Before meeting with Bobby and his family, the occupational therapist reflects on the child's culture and the developmental needs of 11-year-old children in general. This perspective assists the occupational therapist in understanding Bobby as a young child with typical developmental needs.

When the occupational therapist decides to use a top-down perspective, the occupational therapist begins by identifying what occupations are important for the child in his particular situation. In Bobby's case, two of his primary occupations are going to school and playing in the neighborhood. Each of these occupations has a set of tasks and activities that Bobby must be able to complete. For example, the occupation of going to school may involve the activity of reading from a book, listening while another person reads, completing worksheets, copying from the board, using a keyboard, and using various tools such as a pencil, scissors, or chalk. The tasks involved with these activities may require sitting, standing, reaching, writing, turning a page, or typing. The occupation of playing in the neighborhood may involve the activities of riding a bike, playing ball, or playing a game. The tasks involved with these activities may also require a variety of postures, running, throwing, catching, steering, and pedaling. Using the top-down approach, the assessment and treatment are grounded in Bobby's occupations. One of Bobby's specific interests related to his occupation of play is riding a bicycle. Riding a bicycle would allow him to satisfy his desire and image of himself as a neighborhood kid who plays with his neighborhood friends.

Once the specific occupation has been identified, the occupational therapist completes an activity analysis of the activities and tasks to understand the basic requirements for activity participation. For example, riding a bicycle requires confidence that one can learn a new task, a certain degree of postural control for maintaining balance, and the willingness to risk falling. The occupational therapist analyzes the intersection between Bobby's tasks and activities with his skill set. Bobby has spasticity in his extremities, has difficulty with postural adjustments during quick movements, and is cautious and hesitant to participate in new tasks and activities. The occupational therapist, therefore, needs to assess Bobby's use of his extremities, how he makes postural adjustments with the identified tasks and activities, and how he explores his play and school occupations. In Bobby's case, riding a bicycle may form the basis for a therapeutic goal and intervention since both he and his mother expressed a desire for him to ride a bicycle in the neighborhood.

The treatment activity derives from Bobby's occupation of play and desire to ride a bicycle in his neighborhood. Treatment may involve direct participation in riding the bicycle on the street or driveway. Engaging in the occupational performance of actually riding a bike directly influences the development of Bobby's postural control and confidence. This is an example of how the higher levels of the hierarchy rule the lower levels in this approach.

In Bobby's case, the occupational therapist first had him walk with the bike to gain familiarity and confidence with it. Then, while seated on the bike, Bobby pushed off with his feet along the curbside, which enabled him to gain a sense of balance. When Bobby developed enough confidence and balance on the bike, he cruised down an inclined driveway without peddling. Each of these modifications challenged Bobby's skills and helped him to develop confidence and balance skills. The sessions then progressed to Bobby riding the bike in an enclosed parking lot. First riding in a straight line, then in graded curves, and stopping and restarting. Eventually he progressed to riding on the sidewalk with decreased physical space demands. The occupational therapist requested the mother to bring her bicycle to ride alongside of Bobby. The intervention resulted in Bobby riding his bike around the block in his neighborhood.

Bobby's motivation of wanting to be a "neighborhood kid" and the occupation of riding a bike were used as the treatment interventions. Bicycling remained the focus of the intervention throughout the treatment process while at the same time addressing his skill development of postural control and confidence. His lower level skills, for a time, constrained his ability to ride a bicycle. In the end, however, it was his higher-level motivation and occupation that drove the development of his lower-level skills.

Case Study 10-2: *Malik*

Malik is a 4-year-old boy whose mother contacted early intervention services with concerns that her son is having difficulty with handwriting. The early intervention team evaluated Malik and determined that he is functioning at a 34-month (or 2.8-year-old) level for fine motor skills. He primarily uses a pronated grasp and occasionally a palmar grasp for crayon use. He attends a preschool where he engages in games, reading, circle time, coloring, crafts, and playing with balls. Malik was referred to occupational therapy to improve fine motor dexterity and develop pre-handwriting skills. Initial therapy modalities were tabletop activities (e.g., worksheets, coloring books, drawing). Malik needed coaxing and coercion to participate in the worksheet activities. The occupational therapist became frustrated with Malik's slow progress and his resistance toward therapy. The occupational therapist examined her approach and decided to use a top-down approach.

The top-down perspective begins at the top of the hierarchy, the roles and motivations of the client. In Malik's case, one of his primary roles is as a preschooler who engages in play. His preschool participant role includes his play development. Gathering information about the routines, tasks, and activities at the preschool is important to understand the flow of Malik's day. One possibility for Malik's resistance to participate in tabletop crayon and paper activities is that those activities may already be a part of his typical preschool daily routine. Thus, when the occupational therapist arrives to do more of what he has already completed, a novel interest in therapy may be lacking. When Malik was presented with other novel activities related to writing, he would say, "I can't." In addition, Malik might have been removed from the typical activities and the other children to have "therapy."

The occupational therapist analyzed the time schedule of Malik's preschool routine and noted that playground time and circle time reading are in the morning. Following lunch, tabletop, craft activities, and additional playground time are at the end of the day. Therapy was subsequently rescheduled during playground time, and the playground activities that Malik initiated were done first. This is an example of how the occupational therapist examined Malik's patterns of daily occupations relative to his role participation and motivations.

Moving down the hierarchy, the occupational therapist identified the tasks and activities that Malik initiated on the playground such as racing games and imaginary role-playing. Analyzing the skill requirements of these tasks, the occupational therapist concluded that his fine motor skill development could be capitalized in his typical established play routines. The occupational therapist created a new racing game that involved pre-writing skills

(continues)

while on the playground, chalk races on the wall of the building. The treatment activity derived from Malik's own desire and goal of winning a race. The environmental conditions can be changed to the classroom or to the tabletop using paper and crayons. Despite the variety of environmental changes, the driving force for Malik's participation was his role as a child at play and the task and activities involved with racing. Malik used various tools and tool sizes, and adapted his prehension patterns to meet the object demands. He was persistent in participating in the writing racing games. His imaginary role-play of being a champion provided him with a sense of efficacy in his pre-writing abilities. Due to his persistence, Malik self-initiated his own pre-writing activities and developed age-appropriate prehension skills.

This case demonstrates the power of role identification and motivation as a driving force for activity engagement. The developments of Malik's fine motor dexterity were embedded in the tasks and activities that comprised his role. The higher-level occupational role and motivation of wanting to be a "champion racer" and the task of writing races were used as the treatment. Racing remained the focus of the intervention throughout the treatment process while at the same time addressing his skill development. His lower level skills, for a time, constrained his ability to use tools in a mature manner. In the end, it was his higher-level motivation and role image that drove the development of his lower level skills.

Three months following the initiation of the writing racing games, Malik would comment, "Oh, that's easy. I know I'm good," when the occupational therapist would provide positive feedback about him winning the games.

Bottom-up Approach

The bottom-up approach (Fig. 10-2) has similarities to the top-down approach in that both are hierarchical and analyze a situation using occupation and activities. The difference lies in the focus and implementation of the intervention issues. The bottom-up approach focuses first on the specific performance component deficits or underlying capacities that are creating barriers to successful occupational performance.

The bottom-up approach is historically embedded in the profession's concern for the underlying psychological, physical, and physiologic components and processes of behav-

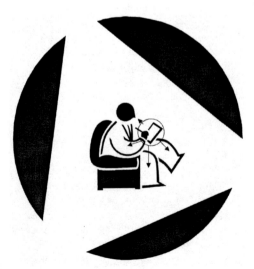

Figure 10-2. Bottom-up approach. In this approach, everything emanates from the performance components involved in the act of writing. The arrows indicate the focus primarily on the act of writing and move up toward the person.

ior and activity engagement (Ayres, 1954, 1958, 1963; Fidler & Fidler, 1963; Llorens, 1970, 1977; Mosey, 1968). Component skills are viewed as the basic units for complex behavior and thinking. Basic actions or skills must be developed before learning another more mature or adaptive action or skill. The bottom-up approach focuses on the development of components or capacities as leading to higher-level skills and role performance. In bottom-up approaches the intended outcome or rationale for the development of component skills is for purposeful function, engagement with objects, interpersonal and social relations, successful participation in expected social roles, and the mastery of particular skills, abilities, and relationships. Bottom-up approaches have been developed to evaluate and treat specific component deficits that affect occupational performance including sensory and perceptual dysfunctions, psychosocial adjustments, neurodevelopmental deficits, biomechanical dysfunctions, and sensorimotor and cognitive impairments.

Evaluation in the Bottom-Up Approach

The bottom-up evaluation is also hierarchically based, with the assessment beginning by identification of the underlying capacities or skills that are creating barriers to occupational performance. The process then continues to examine other areas and levels of the hierarchy including performance areas and contextual concerns. The occupational therapist begins the assessment by establishing therapeutic rapport with the client, client's family, and significant persons in the client's life. After therapeutic rapport has been established, the occupational therapist explores and identifies problems and concerns that the client has with participating in desired roles or occupations. The participation in desired roles may serve as an indicator for the remediation or elimination of the underlying psychological, physical, or physiologic reasons for performance dysfunction.

Following an exploration of the client's life roles, the occupational therapist may examine the particular capacities or skills that are impeding participation in those desired life roles. The occupational therapist examines particular tasks and activities that the client performs on a routine basis or directly assesses the underlying pathologies or impairments that are contributing to the occupational dysfunction. An appropriate assessment tool should be selected depending on the particular pathology or impairment. For example, if a person has muscular weakness that is the primary impairment limiting a person's ability to raise his or her arms overhead to groom or dress, then an assessment addressing muscular strength would be appropriate. The occupational therapist would select assessment tools to examine a child's vestibular sensory system if he or she has difficulty with standing balance and cannot ride a bike. In the bottom-up approach, assessment begins at the component level but therapeutic goals address all areas of dysfunction.

Intervention Using a Bottom-Up Approach

In the bottom-up approach, remediation of the component deficits can facilitate the client's ability to engage in meaningful occupations. For example, a client with increased range of motion for shoulder forward flexion by 20° degrees will have increased independent performance of self-care activities requiring overhead limb use, such as grooming and dressing. When using the bottom-up approach, the treatment focus and methods may derive from the bottom of the hierarchy but the ultimate performance outcomes are generated from the top of the hierarchy.

Once the occupational therapist determines appropriate goals, the occupational therapist, in collaboration with the client, selects tasks and activities or adaptive devices to use as the treatment modalities. The information gathered during the evaluation guides the activity selection. In the bottom-up approach, a focal point of treatment is the remediation of the lower level skills and capacities that constrain the higher level task engagement and role performance. Therefore, the underlying physical, psychological, or physiologic impairment is addressed directly. Using a previous example, an evaluation revealed that one of the client's hobbies and passions in life is gardening. After an analysis of the client's gardening routine and tasks, it is discovered that overhead reaching is a required activity for the client to pick apples from a backyard tree. The treatment may emphasize stretching and strengthening activities of the upper limb for overhead reaching. Activities that require overhead reaching that have some interest and motivating qualities for the client are then selected. These activities may include picking apples from a tree but may also involve participation in simulated yet purposeful reaching range of motion activities such as making a vertical upright macramé plant holder. One of the beauties and skills of an occupational therapist is to embed the underlying physiologic, physical, or psychological components in meaningful and purposeful activities. Meaningful and purposeful activities have the greatest potential for learning and adaptive responses.

Case Study 10-3: *Leon*

Leon is a 58-year-old man who was a history teacher in a public high school. He had a left cerebrovascular accident 4 years ago and received acute and outpatient rehabilitation. He lives with his wife in a ranch-style home that includes a pool and well-kept landscaping in a suburban neighborhood. He has two children who attend college out of the state. Following his initial rehabilitation, Leon was ambulatory without an assistive device; independent in self-care; participated in household tasks such as meal preparation, laundry, and yard maintenance; and needed extra time and effort for bilateral activities. He decided not to return to work after his rehabilitation.

Before the cerebrovascular accident, Leon and his wife, a successful businesswoman, enjoyed traveling and socializing with friends. Four years after the accident, he is again referred to occupational therapy for spasticity management due to increasing spasticity and shoulder pain as well as decreased range of motion of his right upper extremity. His wife's concern is that he is no longer active in household tasks. A physical therapist recently issued Leon a cane because of increasing incidences of loss of balance due to decreasing postural trunk control.

The evaluation based on a bottom-up perspective might not differ greatly from the top-down approach. All the hierarchical levels need to be assessed. Thus, in Leon's case, it is important to understand Leon's role as a husband and social partner to his wife. In addition, he also had a role as a household manager. Leon was particularly proud of the landscaping of his home. After identifying Leon's roles, the occupational therapist must identify and then analyze the tasks and activities involved in his life roles.

The tasks involved with his role of household maintainer include instrumental activities of daily living such as laundry, cooking, and yard maintenance. Since Leon expressed an interest in his landscaping, the therapist used his yard maintenance role as one of the focal points and goals of intervention. After interviewing and observing Leon participating in yard activities, the following tasks were identified as part of his yard maintenance role: weeding, watering, mowing, and raking. After identifying the tasks in which Leon participates, it is important that the occupational therapist examine the demands of the activities. These tasks require activities such as standing to water the plants, squatting and bending to weed, pushing the lawnmower, and grasping the water hose and yard tools.

Following the activity analysis, the occupational therapist must determine whether Leon's abilities match with a satisfying and effective engagement in those activities. Leon's upper extremity spasticity limits his ability to grasp, hold, and release yard maintenance tools. In addition, his difficulty with rotating his trunk to make postural adjustments, his increased shoulder pain, and his decreased range of motion limit his ability to make sweeping motions for watering the yard, pushing the lawnmower, raking leaves and weeds, squatting and bending to weed the garden beds and grass, and performing other large motion activities. His wife expressed concern that Leon did not participate in these activities at the same frequency as he used to and believes this is a contributing factor toward the increased spasticity and muscle tightness of his upper extremity. His wife reported, and Leon concurred, that he used to engage in yard tasks on a daily basis. Now, he tends to the yard once a week and some weeks not at all. He reports most of his time is spent watching television. He stated that the increasing muscle tightness made it more and more difficult to participate in the yard activities. Leon expressed that he valued a nice landscaped yard but did not have the same energy to do all the work. Following the evaluation and analysis of his yard maintenance role, it became clear that Leon highly valued his home landscaping. The occupational therapist inquired about whether hiring a landscaper would help the situation. Leon said, "They never do it right," and expressed that he would like to continue performing these tasks.

After exploring and assessing Leon's occupations and his performance deficits, the occupational therapist in the bottom-up approach needs to select appropriate frames of reference to address the specific component deficits and to guide the intervention. In Leon's case, the occupational therapist selected the proprioceptive neuromuscular facilitation frame of reference (Voss, Ionta & Myers, 1985) to remediate the underlying motor deficits that were limiting his participation in desired occupations. The treatment activities are derived from Leon's own desire and goal of resuming his participation in yard maintenance at the same frequency and effectiveness as before the increase in spasticity of his upper extremity. Using the bottom-up perspective, adjunctive treatments and therapeutic activities were selected to remediate or manage his upper extremity spasticity and trunk control so he could resume the tasks of watering, weeding, raking, and lawn mowing. The evaluation revealed that his upper extremity spasticity and trunk control directly impact the efficiency with which he participates in yard activities. This is an example of how the lower levels (performance components) of the hierarchy constrain the higher levels (role participation). Leon, with the occupational therapist's guidance, developed a goal to resume his yard maintenance tasks three days per week without losing his balance or expending excessive amounts of energy during the task.

Beginning at the bottom of the hierarchy, treatment focused on Leon's ability to move his upper limb in a bilateral and smooth manner. Neuromusculoskeletal support, stretching, and resistive techniques were used so Leon could experience efficient movement sensations. Leon received tactile and proprioceptive input according to the proprioceptive neuromuscular facilitation frame of reference to guide rotational and reaching movement patterns. Graded movement and activities were introduced when Leon demonstrated efficient movement patterns in small graded ranges. For example, watering activities in standing emphasize midline trunk alignment and postural adjustments.

Moving up the hierarchy, the activities and tasks of the role were introduced when Leon was able to move his upper extremity and trunk with ease and greater range of motion. Turning on the water hose provided a natural resistive force for Leon to maintain his trunk alignment. At first, the force of the water pressure was low but was gradually increased as Leon

(continues)

experienced greater success with maintaining midline trunk alignment. The lawn provided a natural feedback mechanism for Leon's trunk rotation and shoulder range of motion. Natural feedback for Leon's trunk and shoulder rotation and range of motion was provided through his ability to water the lawn. Initially, only small patches of the lawn received water due to his limited shoulder range of motion and motor control. In time, greater areas of the lawn received water as his shoulder range of motion and motor control improved.

Continuing up the hierarchy, watering the lawn three times per week was incorporated into Leon's daily routine. Leon used time management sheets to monitor the frequency of his participation. Eventually, Leon did not require cuing from the time sheets to initiate watering the lawn.

Using the bottom-up perspective, it may be hypothesized that his decreased activity participation resulted from the increased spasticity and decreased trunk control. For him to resume yard activities, the limiting performance skills needed to be addressed. In the end, the ultimate goal was his engagement in valued occupations and his desire to participate in those occupations that provided a learning environment to address his motor deficits.

Case Study 10-4: *Liam*

Liam is a 26-year-old man who had a left cerebral hemorrhage due to an aneurysm resulting in a right hemiplegia. Liam was admitted to the neurologic intensive care unit with no movement of his right upper and lower extremity. He is left-handed. Initially, his extremity muscle tone was flaccid but gradually developed dominant flexor posturing in both his right upper and lower extremities. He does not appear to have any difficulty with his cognitive abilities, his vision, or his speech. He lives with his partner on the second floor of an apartment building in a large city. The building has an elevator. Before to his illness, Liam commuted to work on the subway. He worked in advertising sales for a major television network company. Liam also pursued another career as an actor and singer outside of his sales career. He attended acting and singing lessons two times a week. Although Liam had a few acting jobs over the past years, his primary source of income was from his sales position. Liam's other recreational interests were working out at the gym and participating in outdoor activities such as hiking and canoeing. Liam was energetic and motivated to begin therapy. After receiving occupational therapy in the neurologic intensive care unit, Liam was referred to an acute inpatient rehabilitation unit.

At the inpatient rehabilitation clinic, the occupational therapy evaluation began with an interview to establish therapeutic rapport. Since Liam had such an effervescent personality and expressed motivation to begin therapy, therapeutic rapport was easily achieved. He readily expressed what he wanted to do and hoped that physical and occupational therapy were going to assist him in achieving his goals. His primary goal was to return to work as a sales representative and to continue pursuing an acting career. Liam expressed great confidence that the "paralysis" was going to "go away" with therapy. The occupational therapist was very deliberate and cautious in expressing any prognostications of the therapy outcome, while at the same time trying to capture Liam's motivation.

A comprehensive evaluation requires that the occupational therapist assesses all areas of Liam's occupational functioning. This ensures that intervention and treatment, while aimed at impacting the hemiplegia, have occupation-centered outcomes. In Liam's case, the occupational therapist began by assessing the status of Liam's sensory and motor functioning due to the hemiplegia. While assessing his sensory and motor functioning, the occupational therapist skillfully explored Liam's daily roles and his typical daily habits and routines. The occupational therapist concludes that remediation of Liam's sensory and motor disabilities must be the focal point for organizing and prioritizing the interventions. This conclusion is consistent with a bottom-up approach that begins at the component level.

During the evaluation, it is noted that Liam has significant limitations in his abilities to move his limbs, manipulate objects, and ambulate. These sensory and motor disabilities directly limited his participation in daily activities including his ability to work and pursue his acting career. The occupational and physical therapists determined that both the neurodevelopmental treatment and biomechanical frames of references should be used given Liam's sensory and motor disabilities. They begin the treatment regimen by stimulating the muscle spindles, proprioceptive, and joint receptors to initiate muscle activity by active movement and handling techniques. Liam was unable to support or move his upper limb, and the upright sitting postures created increased tensile and shearing forces at his glenohumeral joint that could potentially cause abnormal joint separation and subluxation. Therefore, consistent with the biomechanical frame of reference, Liam was provided with education and training in trunk and limb positioning.

As his extremities developed flexor dominant muscle tone, the sensory and motor training techniques were applied so he could easily alternate his movement directions and to counter the dominant flexor pattern. The occupational therapist suggested ways he could incorporate the positioning and movement techniques during grooming and dressing. Since Liam was highly motivated to do anything "therapeutic" for his extremities, he readily incorporated the positioning and weight-bearing postures while he engaged in his daily morning self-care. After several weeks, Liam achieved self-care ambulation independence using compensatory methods and assistive devices and was discharged from the hospital to his apartment. It was recommended that he continue his occupational therapy on an outpatient basis. The goal of outpatient rehabilitation was to improve the efficiency of his motor skills so he could return to work and resume his acting classes. As his motor skills improved, he became able to manipulate large objects in his hand, raise his arm to approximately shoulder height, and ambulate without an assistive device. Although his motor skills improved, he continued to lack controlled forearm rotation and thumb opposition. He believed he could return to work.

Based on Liam's improvements, the occupational therapist changed the focus of intervention from sensory and motor skill development to a focus on his ability to engage in occupations. The occupational therapist analyzed the specific activities and tasks that were required for him to complete his roles as a salesperson. Primary activities were conversing on the phone and writing reports. Conversing on the phone required grasping the phone, holding the phone to the ear and mouth, sitting upright at a desk, and writing notes while on the phone. In addition, the average phone conversation lasted 15 minutes. Because one of Liam's current motor impairments involved the rotary ability of his forearm, the telephone was strategically placed on his desk to maximize his forearm rotation when he reached for the telephone with his right hand. Other motor tasks were analyzed for the rotary motor component and then synthesized into his daily routines to increase the frequency of muscle stimulation and activity. Thus, the motor skills were the driving force behind the task and activity reorganization of one of Liam's valued roles.

Contextual Approach

The contextual approach (Fig. 10-3) has similarities to the top-down and bottom-up approaches in that it is hierarchical and analyzes a situation using occupation and activities. The difference in the contextual approach is the initial focus and implementation of the intervention. The contextual approach first considers the influence of the environment or context on occupational performance. The context is not only defined by the physical elements of the environment but also by the social, cultural, and temporal ele-

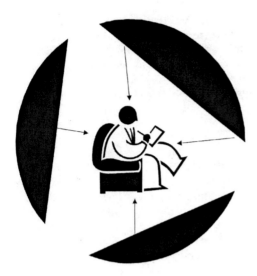

Figure 10-3. Contextual approach. The primary focus is on the context and how it affects the individual's involvement in the occupation of writing.

ments in the surroundings (Dunn, Brown, & McGuigan, 1994). When an occupational therapist decides to begin with a contextual approach, the occupational therapist first examines the dynamic interaction between multiple systems acting on and influencing each other (Dunn, Brown & McGuigan, 1994; Kielhofner, 1995; Law et al., 1996). For example, in their Person-Environment-Occupation Model, occupational performance is viewed as the result of the transaction of the person, the environment, and the occupation. Occupational performance is the result of an interaction between the person, the occupations, and the environment (Law et al., 1996). A contextual approach considers the opportunities and demands in the environment that either support or limit a person's performance. This dynamic interaction changes as the different interacting components change.

In the contextual approach, occupational therapy intervention begins by considering that a person is embedded in a context. The person performs through that context, and the context supports the performance. The person's performance depends on the person's skills and abilities and the cues for action that are derived from the context (Dunn, Brown, & McGuigan, 1994).

Evaluation in the Contextual Approach

A contextual approach evaluation is also hierarchically arranged, with the assessment beginning with a consideration of the interaction between the environment, the person, and the occupation. The importance here is the environment within which the occupation exists. The initial objective of the evaluation is to identify the key environmental factors that create barriers to occupational performance. Factors that are important are temporal features such as chronological age, developmental age, place in the lifecycle, and disability status as well as environmental factors such as physical, social, and cultural factors. An assessment of all the interacting systems is necessary to have a full view of a person's occupational performance. After consideration of these systems, the occupational therapist continues to assess other areas including performance areas and performance components.

As is characteristic of all occupational therapy evaluations, the occupational therapist begins by establishing a therapeutic rapport with the client, client's family, and significant persons in the client's life.

Since contextual approaches have dynamic qualities, the assessment process may begin at any of the interacting systems but must always consider contextual factors. When assessing systems that focus on the person, similarities to the bottom-up approach might exist. In this case, the occupational therapist considers the context's influence on the client's capacities and skills. When assessing the systems, the occupational therapist focuses on occupational and task behaviors, similarities to the top-down approach, but again considers the influence of the context on how the occupational and task behaviors are performed. Contextual approaches consider the environment or context of the performance to be just as important as the person or the occupation.

When a thorough examination and analysis of the interacting systems have taken place, the occupational therapist and client develop therapeutic goals that address the influence of context on role dysfunction or disruption. When using contextual approaches, the goal of the occupational therapist is to create a match between the different systems so the systems are working synchronously for optimal occupational performance.

Intervention Using a Contextual Approach

Once the goals for occupational therapy intervention are established, the occupational therapist must consider the contextual factors and the context in which the person will engage in the activity to determine how it will influence the person's ability to perform. One contextual approach, the Ecological Model of Occupation (see Chapter 8), outlines five intervention approaches: establish/restore, adapt/modify, alter, prevent, and create. Dunn, Brown, and McGuigan (1994) point out that in this approach to therapy goes beyond focusing on "fixing" the person to dealing with the total situation.

As in the top-down and bottom-up approaches, the information gathered during the evaluation guides activity selection. Treatment may focus on the areas in which the systems are not interacting or are minimally interacting. For example, if a noisy and disorganized environment is not supporting the person's capacities to perform the desired occupation or task of cooking, then the treatment may focus on adapting the environment for successful performance. A physical or social environmental mismatch, such as the noisy or disorganized environment, may not be conducive for a person with cognitive impairments. Therefore, arranging the location and organization of frequently used pots and pans or limiting the number of persons in the kitchen to reduce social distractions could create a better match between the person, the task, and the environment. In addition, the type of food might influence performance. For example, preparing a culturally familiar dish would be an example of a sociocultural environmental match and would likely result in a meaningful experience and optimize the occupational performance.

Case Study 10-5: Tanya

Tanya is 7-month-old infant who was born prematurely and exposed to drugs in utero. She is delayed in prone gross motor skills. She does not tolerate being placed on her stomach, is unable to prop or push up in prone, has difficulty with transitional movements, and does not

(continues)

have any rudimentary sitting or righting skills. She has a palmar grasp and only occasionally demonstrates a tendency toward grasping objects with the radial side of her palm. She lives with her parents who both have full-time jobs. The parents alternate their work schedules to care for Tanya. The occupational therapist identified that she spends most of her playtime supine on the bed or in an infant seat.

Approaching this case using a contextual perspective requires the occupational therapist to examine the interaction of the person, the tasks, and the environment for occupational performance. In Tanya's case, an assessment of the person reveals that she lacks specific motor skills and experiences in her daily life. In addition to assessing the client, it is important to gather information from caregivers or other significant persons in the client's life. Gathering information from Tanya's parents is extremely important. In this case, the occupational therapist explored the reasons why the parents only place Tanya in the supine position. The parents expressed that the pediatrician told them not to allow her to sleep on her stomach due to the risk of sudden infant death syndrome (SIDS). The parents were very receptive to additional education and assistance in helping Tanya develop.

Following an assessment of the person, an assessment of the daily tasks in which she and the parents participate was conducted. Due to Tanya's developmental delays, she was only able to engage and interact with the immediate environment at the moment. Overhead mobiles were always in her reach, and her parents provided constant auditory stimulation. Tanya is beginning to hold a bottle independently but cannot maintain the hold for more than 10 seconds. She is able to hold an eating utensil but is inefficient in getting food to her mouth. The parents were attentive to Tanya's needs, feeding and playing with her.

Finally, her skills and the tasks she participated in were examined in context. The parents provide a loving and attentive home. They are motivated to educate themselves on current parenting issues. For example, they followed the recommendations for sleeping position to reduce the risk of SIDS. Tanya has access to toys and objects for play as long as they are within her reach. After gathering the information, the occupational therapist discusses the parents' expectations, goals, and outcomes for Tanya. The parents express that they would like Tanya to sit up so she can have other play experiences.

The occupational therapist then analyzed the match between the person, tasks, and environment. The therapist concluded that Tanya and the parents have many potential skills that have not been expressed or experienced due to the environmental constraint of the SIDS precaution. While the specific tasks of sitting, playing, and eating are limited due to her postural instability, her postural skills are not maximized due to her constant supine positioning and her lack of opportunity to experience weight-bearing through her arms and tummy and simple mobility or transition experiences.

The treatment focused on reorganizing the interaction of the environment, primarily the parents' interpretation of the SIDS precautions and the parental play interactions. The occupational therapist provided the parents with education on the value of diverse play experiences while the infant is alert and interactive, which includes different postures. In addition, it was explained that the SIDS precaution is not inconsistent with this perspective because the recommendation is for sleeping positions or positions when the infant does not have immediate visual adult supervision. This is how the occupational therapist modified the social environment through education to create a greater match for the goal of Tanya being able to sit and play.

The parents were motivated to help Tanya but were concerned about having Tanya play on the floor. The occupational therapist explored this concern and discovered that the parents felt that a floor is not a clean play surface. Because Tanya was typically placed on elevated surfaces such as a sofa, bed, or table (while in an infant seat), she was constantly monitored and limited in her mobility exploration for safety reasons. The occupational therapist and parents explored various environmental settings and surfaces that would be suitable considering the parents' concern for cleanliness and safety. The occupational therapist suggested placing a picnic blanket on the living room floor. The parents liked this suggestion. Providing Tanya with floor time on a blanket served multiple purposes. The parents were no longer concerned that she was playing on the floor or that she might fall. The floor time provided opportunities for Tanya to develop novel play routines in prone postures. This suggestion is an example of how physical environmental adaptations are made to create a better match between the task demands, the person, and the environment.

During treatment, the occupational therapist modeled for the parents many different ways to interact and play with Tanya that included prone positions. Then, the occupational therapist assisted the parents to develop those routines and tasks within theirs and Tanya's daily activities. This is how the occupational therapist modified the tasks or occupations to create a greater match with the sitting and playing goal. Within weeks, Tanya began to develop new skills and postural control that led to upright sitting and new play experiences.

In this case, the occupational therapist identified that the various parts of Tanya's occupational functioning were inhibiting her skill development (e.g., her parents' understanding of SIDS risk, the social and physical environment). The occupational therapist provided information and alternatives that allowed the context to aid in facilitating Tanya's development through play and exploration.

Case Study 10-6: Jonathon

Jonathon is a 34-year-old man who holds two master's degrees, one from an Ivy League business school and one from an Ivy League school of government. His academic career has been punctuated with periods of high achievement and then paralyzing depression. He has held several jobs in the public and private sector, enjoying the public sector jobs more, viewing them as having more meaning and relevance for society and being more consonant with his values.

He also feels he is destined for great things, should not settle for any job, and should be earning a huge salary, despite the stress of these high aspirations. About 2 years ago, he was fired from a management consulting job because, as he says, "I crashed and burned." Jonathon was referred for occupational therapy to assist him in returning to work after 6 months of unemployment.

The contextual approach examines the various systems and the interrelationship of those systems. The assessment looks at the person's specific qualities or abilities, the environment in which the person participates, and the specific task or occupational demands that are needed. There is no particular starting point for assessment using the perspective, because the contextual approach does not have a hierarchical order to constrain the organization of the assessment or treatment.

In Jonathon's case, he described his personal abilities or qualities that influenced what he did each day. He was unable to get out of bed in the morning or to engage in job search activities, especially when he was alone. In fact, he described a pattern of needing to be in the presence of his wife to complete many of the tasks that made up his last job. He also described spending endless hours either watching television or surfing the internet with no specific purpose in mind. Jonathon had limited problem-solving skills, rigid thinking, and demoralization. He struggled to recognize his severe depression as a disability and struggled against the concessions he needed to make to take care of himself well. One of the goals of treatment based on these personal qualities was to identify strategies he could use to counter the inertia he experienced on a daily basis.

After assessing his personal abilities, it is important to assess the task demands and occupations. In Jonathon's case, he and the occupational therapist identified the occupations in

(continues)

which he wanted to participate. They included returning to work and stress management. He seemed to focus on a patient self-image while at the same time an image of himself as a high rolling executive in the private sector. Some of the task demands of an executive that he expressed included managing a large number of people, preparing reports and proposals, reviewing contracts, making deals, and maintaining business networks.

The contextual approach examines the environment as a critical piece for occupational performance. As Jonathon painted a picture of being a "high roller," the environment in which "high rollers" discuss work was examined. The image of the well-known term "power breakfast" emerged. The idea of shifting the locus of intervention from the pathologic association where the occupational therapy office was located to the normalized atmosphere of the local coffeehouse seemed an obvious choice. The emphasis was on the occupational therapy concept of environmental adaptation and the importance of context in the intervention process. A meeting location that capitalized on a setting where people might meet to discuss jobs, hold preliminary interviews and make deals was a logical treatment environment for a meeting with a man who sees himself in a "high roller" position.

Using the contextual approach to treatment, the occupational performance and treatment emerge from the overlapping interrelationship of the person, task, and environment. The "power breakfast" location interlocked with his executive self-image, and occupational task demands created a relevant and meaningful experience for Jonathon to get out of bed, to stimulate his problem-solving skills, and to engage him in activities other than television and the internet. The experience led to more in-depth exploration of an ideal work setting as well as matching his skills and interests with his need to diminish stress in the workplace. This exploration resulted in his decision that although the private sector held the promise of great riches, the public sector offered an environment in which job security and the protection of the government bureaucracy held some safety.

Within weeks of the environmental shift to sessions in the coffee shop, Jonathon had created a job hunt flow sheet, had begun to contact former associates with whom he had past successes, and began to use his pleasant personality as an asset in the quest. Within a few more weeks, he had obtained a job as budget director in a large city agency.

He has successfully held that new job, despite brushes with recurring depression. All these interventions can be framed as additions to his environment, in the form of social supports needed for him to function successfully.

Theory to Practice: An Occupational Therapist's Challenge

From the above examples, it can be seen that occupational therapy practice can be organized in many ways. There is one common link and process, however, that all the approaches and perspectives use. All occupational therapy practices — whether top-down, bottom-up, or contextual — are linked by a common goal of engaging the individual in meaningful and valued occupations. The challenge for the occupational therapist is to transform and articulate our theoretical concepts into daily practice. If we can articulate what we do and why we do it, then our clients, our communities, our colleagues in other disciplines, and the institutions that pay for our services will understand the unique contribution that occupational therapy provides society.

STUDY QUESTIONS —BEGINNER

10-1. Which of the following approaches would you, or could you, use in occupational therapy practice and why?
- Top-down
- Bottom-up
- Contextual

10-2. Apply a top-down occupational perspective to your own life. Identify occupations in which you engage. Delineate the purposeful activity comprising each of your occupations. Choose one of the purposeful activities and conduct an activity analysis on it.

10-3. Explain how and why a top-down and a bottom-up assessment might superficially appear similar.

10-4. Specify the behaviors of an occupational therapist that would promote therapeutic rapport with a client.

10-5. Provide an evidence-based argument supporting the author's assumption that meaningful and purposeful activities have the greatest potential for learning and adaptive responses.

10-6. Explain the concept of theory to practice.

STUDY QUESTIONS — ADVANCED

10-7. Discuss the importance of context in the bottom-up perspective illustrated in the case of Leon.

10-8. If the contextual approach to intervention adapts the environment and looks at the match between the person, task, and the environment, how and why should it be considered occupational therapy?

Acknowledgments

Case stories contributed by Siobhan Kelly-Ideishi, OTR/L, CIMI, and Susan L. Haiman, MPS, OTR/L, RPRP.

References

Ayres, A. J. (1954). Ontogenetic principles in the development of arm and hand functions. *American Journal of Occupational Therapy, 8*, 95–99, 121.

Ayres, A. J. (1958). The visual-motor function. *American Journal of Occupational Therapy, 12*,130–138.

Ayres, A. J. (1963). The Eleanor Clarke Slagle lecture: The development of perceptual motor abilities: A theoretical basis for treatment of dysfunction. *American Journal of Occupational Therapy, 17,* 221–225.

Coster, W. (1998). Occupation-centered assessment of children. *American Journal of Occupational Therapy, 52*, 337–344.

Dunn, W., Brown, C., & McGuigan, A. (1994). The ecology of human performance: A framework for considering the effect of context. *American Journal of Occupational Therapy, 48*, 595–607.

Fidler, G. S., & Fidler, J. W. (1963). *Occupational therapy: A communication process in psychiatry*. New York: Macmillan Co.

Kielhofner, G. (1995). Introduction to the model of human occupation. In G. Kielhofner, (Ed.), *A model of human occupation: Theory and application* (2nd ed.). Baltimore, MD: Williams & Wilkins.

Law, M., Cooper, B., Strong, S., Stewart, D., Rigby, P., & Letts, L. (1996). The person-environment-occupation model: A transactive approach to occupational performance. *Canadian Journal of Occupational Therapy, 63*, 9–22.

Llorens, L. A. (1970). The Eleanor Clarke Slagle lecture: Facilitating growth and development, the promise of occupational therapy. *American Journal of Occupational Therapy, 24*, 93–101.

Llorens, L. A. (1977). A developmental theory revisited.

American Journal of Occupational Therapy, 31, 656–657.

Meyer, A. (1922). The philosophy of occupation therapy. *Archives of Occupational Therapy, 1,* 1–10.

Mosey, A. (1968). Recapitulation of ontogenesis: A theory of practice of occupational therapy. *American Journal of Occupational Therapy, 22,* 426–432.

Reilly, M. (1962). The Eleanor Clarke Slagle lecture: Occupational therapy can be one of the great ideas of 20th century medicine. *American Journal of Occupational Therapy, 16,* 1–9.

Trombly, C. A. (1995). 1995 Eleanor Clarke Slagle lecture: Occupation: Purposefulness and meaningfulness as therapeutic mechanisms. *American Journal of Occupational Therapy, 49,* 960–972.

Voss, D. E., Ionta, M. K., & Myers, B. J. (1985). *Proprioceptive neuromuscular facilitation: Patterns and techniques* (3rd ed.). New York: Harper & Row.

Yerxa, E. J. (1967). The Eleanor Clarke Slagle lecture: Authentic occupational therapy. *American Journal of Occupational Therapy, 21,* 1–9.

Yerxa, E. J. (1994). Dreams, dilemmas, and decisions for occupational therapy practice in a new millennium: An American perspective. *American Journal of Occupational Therapy, 48,* 586–589.

Yerxa, E. J. (1998). Health and the human spirit for occupation. *American Journal of Occupational Therapy, 52,* 412–418.

11

Ethical Concerns: Human Occupation

Aimee J. Luebben

Aimee J. Luebben

OBJECTIVES

This chapter will help you to:

- Differentiate among three traditional ethical frameworks.
- Discuss how professional ethics help structure ethical reasoning in a discipline.
- Compare three AOTA documents related to ethics.
- Apply the DECIDE Process of ethical reasoning to practice situations.
- Consider ethical aspects of human occupation related to four key phrases: occupation-focused, client-centered, evidence-based, and continuing competence.

INTRODUCTION

This chapter begins with an ancient form of teaching, the dialectic method, to introduce ethical concerns of human occupation embodied in the conversation of two occupational therapy patients, Rachel and Midori, and especially in the conversation of two occupational therapists, Miguel and Linda. The considerably different viewpoints these four peo-

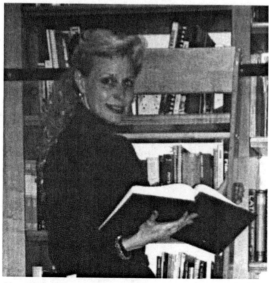

Aimee J. Luebben.

ple have about the practice of occupational therapy provide an ethical slant on *occupation-focused*, *client-centered*, *evidence-based*, and *continuing competence*, four key phrases in the occupational therapy profession.

To start this chapter with the dialectic method, also called *Socratic method*, is only fitting since Socrates was the first person in Western civilization to turn philosophy inward from investigating the external universe (cosmology) to studying the life of man, seeking to establish universal standards of conduct (ethics). That Socrates chose to die rather than repudiate his beliefs — sacrificing his life because of his moral principles — is known only through secondary sources: the writings of two of his many students, Plato and Xenophon. The earliest form of critical reasoning, the dialectic (from the Greek word διαλεκτικός, meaning "discussion") predated both inductive and deductive reasoning. Although Plato's student, Aristotle, developed the more rigidly structured pro and con form — still used in formal debating today — the following ethical dialectic uses the more rambling form of the Socratic method.

ETHICAL DIALECTIC

For the past few weeks Rachel and Midori, outpatients in the Prima Clinic for Upper Extremity Rehabilitation, have seen each other almost daily in occupational therapy. Often following one another on a similar strengthening circuit, they decide to stop for lunch after therapy. Miguel and Linda, two seasoned occupational therapists from a rival clinic, are sitting at the next table and beginning to eavesdrop on the conversation just as the two women get ready to pay the check.

"I can hardly wait for the day to begin — I just love occupational therapy," said Rachel sipping the last of her bottled water as she raked her fingers through her hair, damp from her exertions in therapy.

"You're kidding, right?" Midori exclaimed, ransacking her purse, filled to overflowing with her grocery list, makeup case, latest novel, and finding not her wallet, but her youngest son's homework he needed earlier that morning. "I dread every session — in the Prima building, time seems to slow down to a worm's wiggle — I can hardly wait to leave."

"Speaking of leaving, I'm late for my class," said Rachel scraping the chair legs across the glazed tile floor.

"Oh no, I should have called to say I'd be running late," Midori cried. "Our family owns a specialty grocery store, and I told my father-in-law I'd be right back to help with deliveries."

Watching Rachel and Midori collect their things and move toward the door, the two therapists sat in a stunned silence and then began staring at diners at opposite ends of the restaurant before looking at each other.

When the door slammed shut behind Midori and Rachel, Linda mused, "Why is it that some of our patients love occupational therapy and others hate it?"

"Probably because many patients don't receive authentic occupational therapy," Miguel replied.

"What do you mean *authentic* occupational therapy?"

"To me, authentic occupational therapy is a service provision that's occupation-focused."

"Occupation-focused! Not you too — I thought occupation-focused was just another fad in our profession."

"No," Miguel said emphatically pounding the table. "Occupation-focused service happens to be the core of our profession, our uniqueness. Occupation is not just a passing fad."

"Those women who were just sitting here . . . do you think they're receiving authentic occupational therapy?" Linda questioned while stirring artificial sweetener into her iced tea.

"I don't really know — we'd need more information. But I'm willing to bet you: the woman who dreaded occupational therapy sessions probably wasn't getting authentic occupational therapy."

"So, exactly what kinds of activities do you consider to be occupations, Miguel?"

"I equate occupations with doing. Occupations, to me, are those everyday things people do in their lives," clarified Miguel. "And I believe occupations are described by words ending in the suffix, -ing. As I remember, my high school teacher called those types of words 'present active participles' — something like that. A person must actively participate for an activity to be called an occupation. There's no passivity involved in an occupation."

"But, but, but," Linda interrupted while digging into her coat pocket for lipstick. "Those women talked as if they had identical occupational therapy regimens. They even looked about the same age. So how could the same intervention be authentic occupational therapy for one but not the other woman?"

"For the one woman, weight training — notice the *ing* word, Linda — might be a vital aspect of her life," replied Miguel patiently as he placed his rumpled napkin on the table. "Maybe she loves exercising for leisure, or perhaps she's a person who has chosen to actively participate in a strengthening program because she's high risk for osteoporosis. Linda, that woman could even be into bodybuilding. Strengthening would probably qualify as an occupation-focused, everyday activity for that woman. I would consider that she is receiving authentic occupational therapy services."

"But what about the other woman, the one dreading therapy," asked Linda as they walked out the door.

Using a keyless remote to unlock the car doors, Miguel replied, "If exercising, weight training, strengthening — again, the *ing* words, Linda — are not part of her everyday life, she may not be an active participant so her intervention plan may not include authentic occupational therapy services."

"So give me an example of how you would modify her intervention plan to be occupation-focused," challenged Linda, snapping her seatbelt into the buckle.

"Of course, I'd need to complete a formal evaluation, but we picked up some clues just sitting at the next table," answered Miguel, turning the key in the ignition. "At the end she talked about missing deliveries at the family-owned grocery. I'm betting the woman and I could design an intervention plan that would incorporate that into some of her occupations; for example, unpacking boxes and stocking shelves at various heights." Rolling down the window, Miguel said, "Basing intervention on her occupations would not only constitute authentic occupational therapy, the woman might also begin anticipating and not dreading her therapy."

"You said 'the woman and I could design a plan' earlier, Miguel," said Linda, turning her head to look at him. "What did you mean by that?"

"Haven't you noticed? I work with each of my patients to design a customized intervention plan. It's called 'client-centered.' Where've you been, Linda?"

"You know where I've been, Miguel," scoffed Linda, rummaging through her pockets looking for a mint. "In the clinic, pushing up the productivity units. I haven't been to a workshop for 3 years. Don't you remember when administration decreased our continuing education budget to next to nothing?"

"Actually, I picked up the phrase *client-centered* from my readings," said Miguel, activating the right turn signal while slowing to turn. "I haven't been away from the clinic either, but attending workshops is just one method of keeping up on what our profession now calls *continuing competence*. I prefer independent study. I guess my occupational therapy professors really did some brainwashing . . . all that preaching about the need for lifelong learning must've sunk in. You know, my approach to continuing competence is updating the professional development plan I started in occupational therapy school. I even do journal club."

"Journal club?"

"Yep, journal club, another habit left from occupational therapy school. In classes we read two research papers a week for four semesters — I read over 100 articles before I even graduated!"

"Fascinating, Miguel, tell me more."

"Journal club these days, though, is really small — just me! You know how I always leave work on Wednesdays for lunch," queried Miguel, slowing the car to wait for a child in the crosswalk. "I pick a quiet place for eating and reading. I usually manage to finish at least two research articles. Linda, that's how I know about the hot phrases, occupation-focused and client-centered."

"I've heard of client-centered practice, but dismissed the whole idea. It takes too much time," declared Linda, looking at the brown and white spaniel playing in the side yard of a house. "Besides, I know what's best for my patients."

Flipping down the visor to shield his eyes, Miguel responded, "I disagree on both counts. I used to think I knew what's best for people, but realized that individuals are different. I just can't treat them all the same. As for taking more time, that's not true either. After reading about the *Canadian Occupational Performance Measure* (COPM) (Law et al., 1998) in one of my journal club sessions, I advocated for purchasing the assessment instrument." Swinging the visor to the left to block the sun in the side window, Miguel continued, "The *Canadian Occupational Performance Measure* structures my formerly haphazard intake interview and evaluation. In addition, I never have to worry about my documentation when an accreditation team comes to town. Remember, Linda, how everybody freaked last year when the Joint Commission on Accreditation of Healthcare Organizations visited us? Well, the *Canadian Occupational Performance Measure* provides evidence that patients actively participate in the intervention planning and collects outcomes on performance and satisfaction. If all of us in the department collected *Canadian Occupational Performance Measure* outcomes, just think about the evidence we could provide about our effectiveness!"

"Evidence? As in evidence-based? You certainly know all the professional buzz words, Miguel!"

Glancing toward Linda and lifting his eyebrows, Miguel responded, "Yes, evidence-based. You know, I read Margo Holm's Slagle Lecture in the last *American Journal of Occupational Therapy* issue of 2000 during journal club last week and the beginning really made me think."

"Oh?"

"Lecturing on our mandate to provide evidence-based practice, Dr. Holm began by questioning what would happen if our patients asked about the effectiveness of occupational therapy. She asked audience members whether they would be able to provide research evidence of our profession's effectiveness similar to that contained in the pamphlets of prescription medications." Turning into a parking lot and finding an empty place close to the entrance, Miguel slowed to stop and said, "She ended by challenging everyone to become evidence-based practitioners."

He said, throwing the gearshift into park, "Thanks for taking me out to lunch! Next time we go, you're driving and I'm paying."

Closing the passenger door, making sure the lock was engaged, Linda replied, "How about next Wednesday? And . . . how about telling me what you're reading for the week — we'll double the size of your journal club!"

ETHICS 101

Although a deep philosophical and historical discussion about ethics is beyond the scope of this chapter, the following brief review of ethical basics provides a foundation for the ethical concerns of human occupation. At one time in Western civilization, philosophy encompassed all knowledge. With specialization, content areas (e.g., science, mathematics, political science) separated from philosophy and became individual fields of study. Much of philosophy today can be essentially categorized into three areas dealing with being, knowing, and acting. The formal names for these philosophical fields of study are ontology (being), epistemology (knowing), and ethics (acting). For occupational therapy practitioners, the word *acting*, derived from the participle form *actus* of the verb *ago*, is of particular importance. From this word, which also translates into two significant occupational therapy words, "doing" or "performing," the word *activity* is derived. That the Greeks considered ethics to be the practical philosophy is apparent from the English translation.

Interestingly, the words *ethic* and *ethnic* have a common origin in the Greek word εθω (etho) meaning "to be accustomed to" or "to be in the habit." From *etho* came the derivatives: (a) εθος (ethos), "custom," "habit," and (b) εθνοσ (ethnos), "a number of people accustomed to living together." The word *ethnic* has assumed a more broad definition — associated with culture — whereas the more narrowly defined word *ethic* describes one aspect of culture. In the ancient Greek world, the words *ethical* and *moral* came from the same word, ηθικος and were used synonymously. At that time, to be "ethical" and "moral" were not merely habitual ways of acting; both terms were ways that were approved by a larger group or society. The separate meanings of ethics and morals came when the Romans transliterated the Greek into *ethics* and used *mores*, the plural from of *mos*, which means "character," "behavior," "customs," "laws." From the Roman model, the words *moral* and *ethic* continue to have separate meanings with ethics being a subset of morality.

According to Purtilo (1999), morality "is habitual" (p. 8); "concerns the relations between people and how, ultimately, they can best live in peace and harmony" (p. 7); and consists of "values and duties based on beliefs people take for granted most of the time" (p. 7). Morality, therefore, is what society deems to be right and wrong. Ethics, on the other hand, is the systematic reasoning of and critical reflection on morality.

Table 11-1 delineates three broad categories of theoretical ethics approaches. Although this table summarizes information related to traditional ethical frameworks, please note that some ethicists may argue that this graphic organizer is an oversimplification. For example, deontological ethics is sometimes split into "act" and "rule," resulting

Table 11-1 **THREE TRADITIONAL ETHICAL FRAMEWORKS**

	Deontological	*Teleological*		*Aretaic*
Also known as	Nonconsequentialism	Consequentialism		• Virtue ethics • Values ethics
Greek derivation	Δεον	τελεο		αρετη
English translation	• Things needful/ proper • Advantages • Duties	• Having reached its end • Finished • Complete		• Goodness • Excellence • Virtue
Basis	Act/action	Act/action		Agent
Emphases	• Means • Process • Duty driven	• Ends • Outcomes • Goal driven		• Character
Focus	Doing	Doing		Being
Forms		Act	Rule	
Theorists	Kant	Bentham, Mill: Utilitarianism	Fletcher: Situational ethics	Aristotle
Description	A person should fulfill duties by following rules without regard to consequences	A person should perform that **act** that will bring about the greatest good for all involved	A person should perform the *rule* that will bring about the greatest number of good consequences for all involved	Virtuous character and moral habits allow a person to be good and therefore act right

in confusion with those designations and act and rule teleological ethics. Some ethicists add a fourth category, divine command or exceptional man, but other authors classify divine command as rule deontology. At times a fourth category is a combination of deontological and teleological ethics with situational ethics often classified into this united duty-consequence theoretical framework. For the most part, people practice an integrated ethical approach, retaining faithfulness to their duties while honoring the rights of others, considering the consequences of their actions, and remaining virtuous individuals with principled moral habits.

Professional Codes of Ethics

Professional ethics, according to Edge and Groves (1999), are "applied ethics designed to bring about the ethical conduct of a profession" (p. 40). In fact, adoption of a formal code of ethics is one of many characteristics that distinguish a profession from a field of study. Professional codes of ethics provide structure to help make what Edge and Groves (1999) call "value-laden decisions" or to resolve moral issues and problems. In ethical situations Purtilo (1993) differentiates between an ethical issue, "one in which one or more moral norms or principles are present, but do not create a problem," and an ethical problem, "one in which two or more moral norms or principles create a challenge about what to do" (p. 37).

For professions, codes of ethics systematize basic ethical principles developed to help practitioners determine right and wrong. The principles provide a structure for professional ethical reasoning since there are no easy, cookbook answers to tough issues. Medicine was one of the first professions with a code of ethics. Indeed, many professions modeled their initial codes of ethics on the medical field's *Hippocratic Oath*. One of the shorter works within the *Corpus Hippocraticum* (a library of medical treatises written by many people), the *Hippocratic Oath* is actually attributed by the ancient commentator Erotian to Hippocrates. Although the year the oath was written is not known, the *Hippocratic Oath* has provided a foundation for biomedical ethics for millennia.

OCCUPATIONAL THERAPY DOCUMENTS RELATED TO ETHICS

In 1977, the American Occupational Therapy Association (AOTA) first adopted a code of ethics, which was revised in 1979, 1988, 1994, and 2000. Once Hippocratic in nature, the *Occupational Therapy Code of Ethics* has evolved into a sociological model of ethical conduct. At first glance, the 2000 revision seems to have one additional main principle — seven compared with six main principles in the 1994 version. Although three principles (1.C, 6.D, and 7.D which are subsumed under existing main principles) are original to the *Occupational Therapy Code of Ethics* (AOTA, 2000), the newest main principle (inserted as number 2 and titled "nonmaleficence") was created by moving two principles, which had been under the first main principle (labeled as beneficence) in the previous version. The main change seen in the comparison of the *Occupational Therapy Code of Ethics* (AOTA, 2000) and the *Occupational Therapy Code of Ethics* (AOTA, 1994a) is the significantly different use of the terms *personnel* versus *practitioner* as the agent of the ethical principles, $\chi^2(1, n = 56) = 9.565, p < 0.005$, with a standardized effect size, w = 0.413, which is indicative of a medium value. Results of the changing pattern of these two words indicate the 1994 version of this professional ethical code provided standards of behavior to everyone involved in providing occupational therapy services — from aides and secretaries to therapists — shown by using the word *personnel* 4.2 times more often than *practitioner*. The 2000 version, in contrast, became more focused on practitioners — occupational therapists and occupational therapy assistants and those in the student role — as evidenced by *practitioner* being used 1.5 times more frequently than *personnel* compared with the 1994 version.

The *Occupational Therapy Code of Ethics* (AOTA, 2000) is intended to be used in conjunction with two other documents, *Core Values and Attitudes of Occupational Therapy Practice* (AOTA, 1993) and *Guidelines to the Occupational Therapy Code of Ethics* (Hansen, 2000). According to Hansen (2000), these three documents are "aspirational rather than legal documents . . . designed to be used together in the deliberation of ethical concerns" (p. 14). Table 11-2 provides the seven principles of the *Occupational Therapy Code of Ethics* (AOTA, 2000) with corresponding seven core concepts of the *Core Values and Attitudes of Occupational Therapy Practice* (AOTA, 1993) and 10 topic headings of the *Guidelines to the Occupational Therapy Code of Ethics* (Hansen, 2000).

Ethical Reasoning in Occupational Therapy

To identify and examine ethical dilemmas, occupational therapy practitioners can choose from many ethical decision-making models and processes, which vary in number of steps,

Table 11-2 **COMPARISON OF THREE AOTA DOCUMENTS RELATED TO ETHICS**

Occupational Therapy Code of Ethics (2000) (Principle Number)[a]	Core Values and Attitudes of Occupational Therapy Practice (Core Concept Number)[b]	Guidelines to the Occupational Therapy Code of Ethics (2000) (Topic Heading Number)[c]
Beneficence (1)	Altruism (1)	Ensuring the common good (3)
Nonmaleficence (2)		Conflict of interest (6) Impaired practitioner (7) Sexual relationships (8)
Autonomy, privacy, confidentiality (3)	Equality (2) Freedom (3) Dignity (5)	Confidentiality (5)
Duties (4)	Prudence (7)	Competence (4)
Justice (5)	Justice (4)	
Veracity (6)	Truth (6)	Honesty (1)
Fidelity (7)		Resolving ethical issues (10)
		Communication (2) Payment for services (9)

[a]AOTA, 2000.
[b]AOTA, 1993.
[c]Hansen, 2000.

ease of remembering, and complexity. Purtilo (1999) has a six-step process that includes utilization of theoretical ethical approaches; the short list helps with remembering. Kyler (1998) provides a seven-step factual assessment procedure and also an eight-step analysis model/system. Pfeiffer and Forsberg's (2000) nine-step RESOLVEDD Strategy is fairly easy to memorize because of the acronym. In Kornblau and Starling's (2000) CELIBATE Method for Analyzing Ethical Dilemmas, the acronym stands for clinical ethics and legal issues bait all therapists equally; however, the acronym does not match the ten steps. For students, in particular, the DECIDE Process (Luebben, 2000) offers a shorter process — six steps — and a catchy mnemonic:

- *D*etermine the dilemma and gather information
- *E*stimate the ethical and legal options
- *C*heck out the consequences of options
- *I*dentify all possible solutions
- *D*ecide the best solution
- *E*valuate the outcomes of the selected solution

These six models/processes provide organized methods of resolving ethical issues. Of the ethical decision models and processes reviewed, the CELIBATE Method is the most comprehensive and includes a checklist to confirm legal issues outside regulatory issues.

ETHICAL ASPECTS OF HUMAN OCCUPATION

Although previous sections (the ethical basics, professional codes of ethics, occupational therapy documents related to ethics, and ethical reasoning in occupational therapy) of this chapter are professional building blocks that provide background information, the focal point is the ethical dialectic. Miguel talked about "authentic occupational therapy" when he first spoke, replying to Linda's question, "Why do some patients hate occupational therapy?" Authentic is not a new term to describe occupational therapy. Using "Authentic Occupational Therapy" as the title of her 1966 Slagle Lecture, Yerxa (1967/1985) presented many ideas that foreshadow this chapter's four key phrases: occupation-focused, client-centered, evidence-based, and continuing competence. In the discussion that follows, evidence-based and continuing competence have separate sections; however, occupation-focused and client-centered have been purposefully kept together in the same section to show the interdependence of these two key phrases.

Occupation-focused and Client-centered

In her Slagle Lecture, Yerxa (1966/1985) argued for the profession's purpose and uniqueness, using four key phrases: choice; self-initiated, purposeful activity; reality orientating; and perception. Her key phrases *self-initiated, purposeful activity* and *choice* correspond respectively to *occupation-focused* and *client-centered* today.

Of the *Occupational Therapy Code of Ethics* (AOTA, 2000), Principle 3A deals with recipient or caregiver autonomy: "Occupational therapy practitioners shall collaborate with service recipients or their surrogate(s) in setting goals and priorities throughout the intervention process" (AOTA, 2000, p. 614). Therapists who work with service recipients in teams to establish goals throughout treatment will ensure occupational therapy services that are client-centered. When client-centered services are assured, interventions are very likely to be occupation-focused.

In the ethical dialectic, Miguel feels so passionately about occupation-focused service delivery that he pounds the table when he responds to Linda's question about authentic occupational therapy. Equally emphatic about client-centered practice, Miguel tells Linda, who is focused on productivity units not people, that he uses the *Canadian Occupational Performance Measure* (Law et al., 1998) to provide structure for his evaluation and also to determine customized intervention. To Miguel, authentic occupation therapy is both client-centered and occupation-focused.

The ethical dialectic serves a secondary purpose: to showcase the utility of narrative reasoning in determining the occupations of the four people involved. Remember Miguel saying to Linda that they had picked up some clues just sitting at the next table? Readers of the ethical dialectic probably picked up some clues from the very first reading. Keeping in mind Miguel's thoughts (an occupation is equivalent with *doing,* and a true occupation takes the form of a present active participle), use narrative reasoning to reread the ethical dialectic for occupations — words ending in the suffix, *ing* — for the two patients, Rachel and Midori, and the two occupational therapists, Miguel and Linda. Verify the list of occupations for each person with Table 11-3.

Miguel spoke strongly that no passivity be involved in an occupation — that a person must actively participate for an activity to be called an occupation. Interestingly, WHO (2001) recently adopted a new taxonomy, the *International Classification of Functioning, Disability, and Health* (ICF), with a component called "Activities and Participation." The ICF is structured remarkably similar to Uniform Terminology III (UT III), an AOTA (1994b) taxonomy that is being replaced by the Occupational Therapy Practice Framework (2002). (Tables 11-4 and 11-5 show comparisons of the ICF and UT III.) Authentic occupation correlates with UT III's (AOTA, 1994b) performance areas and with ICF's activities and participation

Table 11-3 **OCCUPATIONS OF RACHEL, MIDORI, MIGUEL, AND LINDA**

Two patients	Rachel	Midori
	1. Following one another on a similar strengthening circuit 2. Sipping the last of her bottled water 3. Scraping the chair back on the glazed tile floor 4. Weight-training 5. Exercising for leisure 6. Body building 7. Strengthening	1. Following one another on a similar strengthening circuit 2. Ransacking her purse 3. Running late 4. Missing deliveries at the family-owned grocery 5. Unpacking boxes and stocking shelves at various heights 6. Anticipating and not dreading her therapy

Two occupational therapists	Miguel	Linda
	1. Sitting at the next table 2. Beginning to eavesdrop 3. Watching Rachel and Midori collect their things 4. Looking at each other 5. Staring at diners at opposite ends of the restaurant 6. Pounding the table 7. "Willing to bet you" 8. Using a keyless remote to unlock the car door 9. Rolling down the window 10. Activating the right turn signal while slowing to turn 11. Eating and reading . . . journal club 12. Flipping down the visor to shield his eyes 13. Swinging the visor to the left to block the sun in the side window 14. Reading about the *Canadian Occupational Performance Measure* 15. Glancing toward Linda 16. Lifting his eyebrows 17. Turning into a parking lot 18. Finding an empty place close to the entrance	1. Sitting at the next table 2. Beginning to eavesdrop 3. Watching Rachel and Midori collect their things 4. Looking at each other 5. Staring at diners at opposite ends of the restaurant 6. Stirring artificial sweetener into her iced tea 7. Digging into her coat pocket for lipstick 8. Snapping her seatbelt into the buckle 9. Turning her head to look at him 10. Rummaging through her pockets looking for a mint 11. Pushing up the productivity units 12. Looking at the brown and white spaniel playing in the side yard of a house 13. Closing the passenger door, making sure the lock was engaged

(WHO, 2001). Within the ICF activities and participation component (WHO, 2001), the majority of items ends in *ing* (e.g., managing daily routine in the general tasks and demands domain, moving around the house in the mobility domain, caring for hair in the self-care domain, and disposing of garbage in the domestic life domain).

Table 11-4 **COMPARISON OF TWO TAXONOMIES: INTERNATIONAL CLASSIFICATION OF FUNCTIONING, DISABILITY, AND HEALTH (ICF) (WHO, 2001) AND UNIFORM TERMINOLOGY III (UT III) (AOTA, 1994B)**

UT III (AOTA, 1994b)		ICF (WHO, 2001)	
Element	Parameters	Components	Parts
Activities of Daily Living	Performance Areas — occupations	Activities and Participation (limitations/ restrictions)	I: Functioning and Disability
Work and Productive Activities			
Play or Leisure Activities			
Sensorimotor	Performance Components	Body Functions and Structures (impairments)	
Cognitive			
Psychosocial			
Environment	Performance Contexts	Environmental Factors (barriers/ facilitators)	II: Contextual Factors
Temporal aspect		Personal Factors	

Evidence-based

Yerxa (1967/1985) began her 1966 Slagle Lecture by discussing research — building and using a scientific body of knowledge — as a step toward professionalism. In the Slagle Lecture 34 years later, Holm (2000) emphasized the need for occupational therapy practitioners to use the profession's body of knowledge as a basis for practice, thus providing *evidence-based* occupational therapy. Evidence-based has become one of the hottest topics in the profession in recent years, starting when Law and Baum (1998) advocated modeling evidence-based practice in occupational therapy after evidence-based practice in medicine. Tickle-Degnen (1999) then launched a new evidence-based forum in the *American Journal of Occupational Therapy*.

Although not explicit, evidence-based practice is implicit within the *Occupational Therapy Code of Ethics* (AOTA, 2000), particularly in Principle 3B: "Occupational therapy practitioners shall fully inform the service recipients of the nature, risks, and potential outcomes of any interventions" (p. 614). Without research evidence of treatment effectiveness, occupational therapy practitioners would be hard pressed to fully inform persons who receive occupational therapy services of the intervention variables listed in this ethical principle.

In the ethical dialectic, Miguel talks to Linda about evidenced-based practice. Accepting Holm's (2000) challenge to become an evidence-based practitioner, Miguel then openly fantasizes about everyone in his facility collecting *Canadian Occupational Performance Measure* outcomes, thereby demonstrating the effectiveness of the department.

Table 11-5 COMPARISON OF TWO TAXONOMIES: INTERNATIONAL CLASSIFICATION OF FUNCTIONING, DISABILITY, AND HEALTH (IFC) (WHO, 2001) AND UNIFORM TERMINOLOGY III (UT III) (AOTA, 1994B)

ICF (WHO, 2001)					
Parts	I: Functioning and Disability			II: Contextual Factors	
Components	Activities and Participation (Limitations/Restrictions)	Body Functions and Structures (Impairments)		Environmental Factors (Barriers/Facilitators)	Personal Factors

UT III (AOTA, 1994b)								
Parameters	Performance Areas—Occupations			Performance Components			Performance Contexts	
Elements	Activities of Daily Living	Work and Productive Activities	Play or Leisure Activities	Sensorimotor	Cognitive	Psychosocial	Environment	Temporal Aspects

Continuing Competence

In occupational therapy, the purpose of professional training and credentialing is to protect the public by assuring practitioner competence. Derived from the Latin *competo* ("to be suitable" or "to be adequate"), competence implies meeting minimum standards but not a particular position along a continuum of excellence. Minimum standards, therefore, protect the public but do not ensure quality. Although initial competence requires occupational therapy practitioners to demonstrate mastery of entry-level concepts on credentialing examinations, continuing competence was considered for years to be an internal aspect of professionalism: individual occupational therapists and occupational therapy assistants were expected to assure they were keeping current in the field. For example, continuing competency has been addressed in earlier versions of the *Occupational Therapy Code of Ethics*. Of the seven principles of the *Occupational Therapy Code of Ethics* (AOTA, 2000), Principle 4 is: "Occupational therapy practitioners shall achieve and continually maintain high standards of competence" (p. 615). Specific duties for occupational therapy practitioners listed under this fourth principle include: (a) holding appropriate credentials,

(b) using procedures that conform to AOTA documents relevant to practice, (c) maintaining and documenting competence by participating in professional development and educational activities, (d) critically examining and keeping current with emerging knowledge, (e) protecting service recipients, (f) providing supervision, and (g) referring to or consulting with other service providers.

More recently, AOTA and the National Board for Certification in Occupational Therapy (NBCOT) became interested in more formal methods of assuring and documenting continuing competence. To structure the internal process of assuring continuing competence, AOTA began by designing a self-appraisal guide (Thomson et al., 1995), which includes a competency self-appraisal tool as well as a listing of 13 methods of achieving competence and 10 methods of documenting competence. The self-appraisal guide was followed by the *Standards for Continuing Competence* (AOTA, 1999). In the ethical dialectic, Miguel talks about preferring independent study (in the form of journal club), one of Thomson et al.'s (1995) 13 methods of achieving competency, but he does not indicate which of the 10 methods of documenting continuing competency he is using.

Continuing competence in occupational therapy has moved from an internalized aspect of professionalism to being explicitly addressed in the profession's code of ethics. In fact, Yerxa's (1967/1985) conclusion on professional authenticity heralded the profession's formalization of planning and documenting achievement of competence beyond entry level. Although inherent in continuing competence, the ethical aspect is further emphasized with the addition of ethical reasoning as one of five continuing competence standards (AOTA, 1999).

CONCLUSION

To predict that ethical concerns will end when occupational therapy practitioners demonstrate continuing competence and provide evidence-based practice consisting of authentic occupational therapy — both occupation-focused and client-centered — is unrealistic. Ethical concerns of occupation will likely never cease, but will change as new ideas, theories, and practices enter the field. This chapter concludes with a few considerations.

Consider first the ethical dialectic and changes that might be seen 3 months from now when Midori transfers to the rival clinic with Linda as her occupational therapist. In the meantime, Linda has used the competency self-appraisal tool in Thomson et al.'s (1995) guide to develop her own professional development plan. No longer relying on her company's largess to pay for continuing education workshops, Linda has chosen independent study and mentoring as her primary methods of achieving competence. She and Miguel have decided they want to supervise students in an alternative fieldwork experience they read about in their much-loved Wednesday journal club lunches. They plan to share two students at a time from a nearby university with an innovative occupational therapy curriculum. Linda has made Midori the center of decision-making in the clinic and has focused intervention around Midori's priorities, so now Midori looks forward to her occupational therapy sessions because she is receiving authentic occupational therapy.

Next, consider continuing competence — which ends in *ing* — to be an occupation for occupational therapy practitioners. For occupational therapists and occupational therapy assistants, the five continuing competence standards encompass five primary occupations of knowing, thinking, interacting, doing, and acting. Formally, these standards are knowledge, critical reasoning, interpersonal abilities, performance skills, and ethical reasoning, respectively (AOTA, 1999). Consider the possibilities if all occupational therapy practitioners demonstrated and documented increasingly more sophisticated competence every year for each of these five standards.

Then, consider a growing cadre of practitioner-scholars working together across the country, systematically studying all aspects of occupational therapy. Partnerships will form between universities and clinics as students and faculty work with practitioners to methodically build the profession's body of knowledge, thereby showing evidence of occupational therapy's effectiveness.

Finally, consider the future, when each person who receives occupational therapy services is offered a pamphlet expounding on the effectiveness of occupational therapy. Instead of declaiming toxicity (which after all is the primary purpose of pharmaceutical literature), site-specific occupational therapy literature will provide a listing of benefits the various interventions have to offer along with the concomitant research findings explained in a language anybody can understand.

STUDY QUESTIONS

11-1. The dialectic method is also called the Socratic method. What is it?

11-2. What is cosmology?

11-3. What is ethics?

11-4. What was a major accomplishment of Socrates?

11-5. What is a synonym for critical reasoning?

11-6. In terms of origin of development, chronologically order the following methods into proper sequence:
- Deductive reasoning
- Inductive reasoning
- Dialectic

11-7. Compare Plato's method of instruction to Aristotle's method of instruction.

11-8. Define authentic occupational therapy. Generate an example to illustrate the concept.

11-9. Explain how "...occupation-focused service is the cornerstone of our profession."

11-10. Define each of the following:
- Client-centered
- Continuing competence
- Evidence
- Evidence-based practice
- Mores
- Morality
- Ethics
- Ethical
- Epistemology
- Ontology

11-11. How could you organize and implement a journal club?

11-12. Differentiate each of the following:
- Ethical issue versus ethical problem
- Field of study versus a profession
- Competence versus excellence

11-13. Explain how the occupational therapy code of ethics has changed from an ethical code based on the Hippocratic Oath to one based on a sociologic model.

11-14. Discuss the concept of autonomy pertaining to client-centered and occupation-focused intervention.

11-15. Explain the role of narrative reasoning related to occupation-focused intervention.

11-16. For a given intervention strategy, what is its nature, potential outcomes, and potential negative side effects?

11-17. How can you participate in a university-clinic partnership?

References

American Occupational Therapy Association. (1993). Core values and attitudes of occupational therapy practice. *American Journal of Occupational Therapy, 78*, 1085–1086.

American Occupational Therapy Association. (1994a). Occupational Therapy Code of Ethics. *American Journal of Occupational Therapy, 48*, 1037–1038.

American Occupational Therapy Association. (1994b). Uniform terminology for occupational therapy — third edition. *American Journal of Occupational Therapy, 48*, 1047–1054.

American Occupational Therapy Association. (1999). Standards for continuing competence. *American Journal of Occupational Therapy, 53*, 599–600.

American Occupational Therapy Association. (2000). Occupational Therapy Code of Ethics (2000). *American Journal of Occupational Therapy, 54*, 614–616.

American Occupational Therapy Association. (2002). *The Occupational Therapy Practice Framework* (final version). AOTA website.

Edge, R. S., & Groves, J. R. (1999). *Ethics of health care: A guide for clinical practice* (2nd. ed.). Albany, NY: Delmar Publishers.

Hansen, R. A. (2000). Guidelines to the Occupational Therapy Code of Ethics (2000). In P. Kyler (Ed.), *Reference guide to the occupational therapy code of ethics* (pp. 14–18). Bethesda, MD: American Occupational Therapy Association.

Holm, M. B. (2000). Our mandate for the new millennium: Evidence-based practice-2000 Eleanor Clarke Slagle lecture. *American Journal of Occupational Therapy, 54*, 575–585.

Kornblau, B. L., & Starling, S. P. (1999). *Ethics in rehabilitation: A clinical perspective*. Thorofare, NJ: Slack.

Kyler, P. (1998). Frameworks for ethical decision making. In AOTA Commission on Practice (Ed.), *1998 reference guide to the Occupational Therapy Code of Ethics* (revised ed., p. 34). Bethesda, MD: American Occupational Therapy Association.

Law, M., Baptiste, S., Carswell, A., McColl, M. A., Polatajko, H., & Pollock, N. (1998). *Canadian Occupational Performance Measure* (3rd ed.). Ottawa, Ontario, Canada: CAOT Publications ACE.

Law, M., & Baum, C. (1998). Evidence-based occupational therapy practice. *Canadian Journal of Occupational Therapy, 65*, 131–135.

Luebben, A. J. (2000) *DECIDE process of ethical reasoning*. Unit of the course: OT 320: Professional Communication, Evansville, IN: University of Southern Indiana, Occupational Therapy Program.

Pfeiffer, R. S., & Forsberg, R. P. (2000). *Ethics on the job: Cases and strategies* (2nd ed.). Belmont, CA: Wadsworth Publishing Company.

Purtilo, R. B. (1993). *Ethical dimensions in the health professions* (2nd ed.). Philadelphia: W. B. Saunders.

Purtilo, R. B. (1999). *Ethical dimensions in the health professions* (3rd ed.). Philadelphia: W. B. Saunders.

Thomson, L. K., Lieberman, D., Murphy, R., Wendt, E., Poole, J., & Hertfelder, S. D. (1995). *Developing, maintaining, and updating competency in occupational therapy: A guide to self-appraisal*. Bethesda, MD: American Occupational Therapy Association.

Tickle-Degnen, L. (1999). Evidence-based practice forum-Organizing, evaluating, and using evidence in occupational therapy practice. *American Journal of Occupational Therapy, 53*, 537–539.

World Health Organization. (2001). *ICF: International classification of functioning, disability, and health: Final draft* (English full version) [Online]. Retrieved June 15, 2001, from the World Wide Web: http://www.who.int/icidh/ICIDH-2%20Final%20Draft%20ENG%20Website%2022_04.pdf

Yerxa, E. J. (1967/1985). 1966 Eleanor Clarke Slagle Lecture: Authentic occupational therapy. In American Occupational Therapy Association (Ed.), *A professional legacy: The Eleanor Clarke Slagle Lectures in occupational therapy 1955–1984* (pp. 155–173). Rockville, MD: American Occupational Therapy Association.

12

Reaffirming the Importance of Occupation

Paula Kramer, Aimee J. Luebben,
Charlotte Brasic Royeen, and Jim Hinojosa

OBJECTIVES

This chapter will help you to:

- Summarize various ways occupation is used in this text.
- Reflect on your own understanding of perspectives of human occupation and ideas of occupational therapy.
- Consider future challenges in occupational therapy.

The previous chapters illustrated the rich and diverse state of our current theoretical perspectives of occupation. For some occupational therapists, the ideas proposed move closer to the perceptions of the beliefs about the roots of the occupational therapy profession. These perspectives, as a group, focus on occupation as a major construct of the profession and a primary means for bringing about change with clients. For other occupational therapists, these perspectives challenge their thinking about the importance of occupation and its relevance to practice. For all occupational therapists and assistants, it is critical that they explore the construct of occupation and what it means to people to arrive at a personal definition of what occupation means to themselves.

OCCUPATION: A KEY CONSTRUCT

Each contributor to this text presents a theoretical perspective in which occupation is a seminal, key construct. We are fascinated by the varying ways the authors use the construct of occupation to explain what we do, why we do it, and how we should be thinking. Around the construct, many authors have developed intervention models. It is interesting to see the varying ways the authors use the concept of occupation to explain what is done in occupational therapy practice, how it is done, and what occupational therapists should focus on during interventions. To be sure, some authors have been more definitive about specific areas than others. Certain contributors stay in a more theoretical realm, whereas others are more explicit about practice and intervention. All authors challenge and attempt to stretch our conception of the construct of occupation.

The various authors' perspectives represent the breadth of current views on human occupation. Whereas the perspectives presented in this text often use the same terms, these words or phrases are frequently used and defined differently, or at least with a slightly different twist. Although the authors agree on the importance of the construct of occupation, they approach and use that concept in different ways. Such diversity represents a healthy growth in our profession as we deepen our understanding of what we do. Although the reader may wish to have all definitions clearly laid out with distinctions regarding the way each perspective defines and uses the word occupation clearly, this is not possible. The authors, at this point, are more concerned with developing their whole theoretical perspectives rather than drawing parallels and focusing solely on definitions. At present, they are still refining their own perspectives and are not at a point of exploring how each perspective relates to the others. Maybe comparing perspectives will occur at some time in the future or perhaps that will always be left up to the reader. A revised clarity in our language may also occur in the future. For now, this compilation demonstrates the current state of our profession's views on occupation. This diversity represents the healthy growth of occupational therapy.

VALUE OF HUMAN OCCUPATION

It is important to learn how each chapter's contributors have conceptualized the term *occupation* and how they have integrated occupation into their individual theoretical perspectives. It is also important to recognize that for some occupational therapists, the term *occupation* is not held in high regard. These occupational therapists, while ultimately concerned with human occupation, continue to examine the importance of activities, modalities, and other legitimate tools of the profession. As discussed in the first chapter, activities and related tasks are the foundations for human occupation. Although these occupational therapists are not putting occupation in the forefront of their thoughts, they do believe in the power of doing and the value of this engagement to the individual. These occupational therapists believe that only the client can ascertain the value of an activity to determine for himself or herself whether that activity can be considered a human occupation. Ultimately, it is the individual occupational therapist in the context of his or her responsibilities and roles that will lead to a personal perspective on human occupation.

VIEWS OF OCCUPATION

The chapters in this book present views of occupation on many levels. Each chapter could be the beginning of a book; certain perspectives already have books written solely on that subject. Some of the chapters are looking at occupation in terms of individual interaction, and others are looking at the construct from a greater societal perspective. These chapters demonstrate the wide variety of thinking as to how occupation influences participation as a building block to lives at all levels. The reader cannot think of each chapter as being equal or equivalent to each other, but must look at the different aspects of the construct and how they might influence the profession.

Furthermore, as a whole, this book explores the breadth of the concept of occupation and the robustness of how this concept can be integrated into a theoretical perspective that explains its influences on individuals' lives. In its own way, each chapter speaks to the breadth of the profession and gives the reader an understanding of one of the many ways to look at this concept when working with people within the context of their lives. There is no one way to look at occupation in our society; instead, there are many ways of exploring the same thing. It is an aspect of the maturity of our profession that we can tolerate these different views, expecting the perspectives to be looking at different aspects of the same concept and not to be saying or doing the same things. This current generation of various theories is powerful, and each increases our knowledge and understanding of the field of occupational therapy without the need for discussion of any as right or wrong. Scholarship requires the continued discussion of topics such as occupation without the need for reaching a consensus. Agreeing and disagreeing can be a springboard for producing more thoughts. The diversity of these perspectives is healthy and relates to the depth of the subject matter. We are not at a point of bringing them together or choosing one over the other but of embracing the diversity.

FUTURE INQUIRY RELATED TO HUMAN OCCUPATION

This book has many foundational points on which future research can be based. It is incumbent on all of us, as professionals, to make the links between occupation and practice in three critical areas: education, research, and treatment. The next step is to move forward, to research each of these theoretical perspectives, and to assess their efficacy and effectiveness in interventions. We need to explore occupation in the context of the various guidelines for intervention used by occupational therapists. Simultaneously, we need to focus on evidence-based research and use various forms of inquiry and a multitude of methodologies, including qualitative, quantitative, and integrated approaches, to refine and apply the concept of occupation systematically into the body of knowledge of the occupational therapy profession. It would be important to consider that an appropriate outcome to demonstrate the effectiveness of an intervention is an individual's ability to engage or participate in human occupation and thereby increase his or her life satisfaction. Consistent with this idea, we should develop research that assesses how well we, as occupational therapists, are able to accomplish this.

PERSONAL AND PROFESSIONAL PERSPECTIVES

Working on this book changed our individual perspectives in many ways. Compiling different, current perspectives on occupation seemed like a simple job, but the sum is greater than each of its parts. More than just a compendium of thoughts on one critical topic, this book is a statement on the vitality of our profession: We have returned to a concept that was key in the development of the profession and have expanded on it. The scholarship of the profession has been enriched by all the theoretical developments related to occupation, and the growth of the profession is evident because we have embraced differing views and have not focused on one to the exclusion of others. The fact that we do not agree is healthy and not negative. If we tried to develop a common framework at this point, we would lose some of the richness that comes from the stimulation of thought by different people.

Interestingly, at a time when multiple thoughts about occupation abound, the American Occupational Therapy Association has organized the profession into a framework for practice. During a routine 5-year review process, *Uniform Terminology, Third Edition* (AOTA, 1994) was not revised into a fourth edition. Instead, the *Occupational Therapy Practice Framework: Domain and Process* (AOTA, 2002) "was developed in response to current practice needs — the need to more clearly affirm and articulate occupational therapy's unique focus on occupation and daily life activities and the application of an intervention process that facilitates engagement in occupation to support participation in life" (p. 1). The fact that the process required 18 drafts and needed 3 years beyond the usual revision deadline indicates the Commission on Practice's valiant effort to synthesize many complex ideas.

The occupational therapy profession just may not be ready for this integration yet. At this time, the *Practice Framework* (AOTA, 2002) may not do justice to the different thoughts about occupation that are discussed here, and some of the richness that comes with the diversity of multiple perspectives may have been lost in this process.

We believe this book is a starting point for a dialog, allowing us to build on the concept of occupation. Currently, it is more productive that there is no consensus, as it allows us to develop our ideas further. We began to see this book not just as the conceptual models of separate groups of authors, but also as different ways to view the profession as a whole. Our profession is alive and well in its ability to support all these perspectives concurrently.

At the same time, it is important to note that this book is basically a Western conceptualization of occupation and occupational therapy. Our authors are predominantly American, with most being from the Western hemisphere, whereas occupational therapy is a worldwide profession. As globalization continues to become more prevalent, it will be a challenge to explore how these conceptualizations are realized in the world at large, and whether these perspectives can be translated successfully.

The profession of occupational therapy has operated on a philosophy that has been relatively consistent for almost 100 years. The current focus on occupation is very much a return to our basic beliefs, as noted in Chapter 2, and yet so far advanced. We still have the same basic beliefs, assumptions, and values that were part of the founding of the profession: changing how people live their lives through doing with meaning. This consistent philosophy regarding what we do is what the founders of our profession did in 1917 and is what occupational therapists will do in 2017. Whether we call it occupation or activity is less important than the fact that our basic beliefs have remained intact for a prolonged period. Our beliefs, assumptions, and values have evolved in many ways, but basically they remain the same — by allowing people to engage in doing with meaning, individuals can participate in life.

STUDY QUESTIONS

12-1. When the occupational therapy profession is studied 300 hundred years from now, what do you want people to find?

12-2. What is the occupational therapy profession's purpose?

12-3. In what way do occupational therapists serve society?

12-4. How will the refinement and development of theoretical perspectives add to the evolution of the profession of occupational therapy?

12-5. Do occupational therapists really change lives?

12-6. How does the occupational therapy profession use occupation to change lives?

References

American Occupational Therapy Association. (1994). Uniform terminology for occupational therapy (3rd ed.). *American Journal of Occupational Therapy, 48,* 1047–1054.

American Occupational Therapy Association. (2002, January). Occupational therapy practice framework: Domain and process (draft XVIII.). Bethesda, MD: Author.

Index

Note: Page numbers followed by f indicate figures; those followed by t indicate tables; and those followed by b indicated boxed material.